Hemodynamic Waveform Analysis

Hemodynamic Waveform Analysis

THOMAS S. AHRENS, DNS, RN, CCRN

Clinical Specialist
Critical Care
Barnes Hospital at the Washington University Medical Center
St. Louis, Missouri

LAURA A. TAYLOR, MSN, RN

Barnes Hospital at the Washington University Medical Center
St. Louis, Missouri

W.B. SAUNDERS COMPANY

Harcourt Brace Jovanovich, Inc.

Philadelphia ○ London ○ Toronto ○ Montreal ○ Sydney ○ Tokyo

W.B. Saunders Company
Harcourt Brace Jovanovich, Inc.

The Curtis Center
Independence Square West
Philadelphia, Pennsylvania 19106

Library of Congress Cataloging-in-Publication Data

Ahrens, Thomas.
    Hemodynamic waveform analysis / Thomas Ahrens, Laura Taylor.
      p. cm.
    Includes bibliographical references (p.   ) and
index.
    ISBN 0-7216-4009-5
    1. Hemodynamic monitoring. I. Taylor, Laura (Laura Ann)
II. Title.
RC670.5.H45A37   1992
616.1'0754—dc20   91-42950

Editor: Michael J. Brown
Developmental Editor: Lee Henderson
Designer: Bill Donnelly
Cover Designer: Charles Smith
Production Manager: Peter Faber
Manuscript Editor: Linda Weinerman
Illustrator: Juan Ortega and David Strong
Illustration Specialist: Peg Shaw
Indexer: Roger Wall

Hemodynamic Waveform Analysis   ISBN 0-7216-4009-5

Last digit is the print number: 9 8 7 6 5 4 3 2 1

To the most special person in my life—my wife, Pat, for all her patience, support, and love during the many hours I spent on this and other endeavors

Thomas S. Ahrens

To Lauren and Carli, who, despite the many interruptions during the writing of this book, provided me with love and endless hours of happiness

Laura A. Taylor

PREFACE

In our critical care nursing experience, perhaps the most commonly seen clinical problem has been the interpretation of hemodynamic waveforms and the application of waveform values. This is a problem experienced by both physicians and nurses. This text has been written in response to the need of all critical care clinicians for an easy to read resource for the interpretation of hemodynamic waveforms. It covers all the key problems seen in the critical care setting.

We are indebted to the many people who have helped make this book possible, especially the nurses and technicians at Barnes Hospital. They are responsible for obtaining many of the waveforms as well as helping to illustrate the problems associated with interpreting and applying hemodynamic waveforms.

Thomas S. Ahrens
Laura A. Taylor

ACKNOWLEDGMENTS

We wish to thank all our friends and colleagues in the critical care units at Barnes Hospital, especially the nurses and technicians in the cardiac care unit. Thanks also are extended to Ed Fry, MD, for his support during this project. Without their help and encouragement, this text would have been much more difficult to complete.

CONTENTS

I INTRODUCTION

1 The Need for Accurate Waveform Analysis

Hemodynamic monitoring is one of the most important components of critical care. Nurses and physicians rely heavily on hemodynamic data and routinely analyze the data to help identify appropriate treatment modalities for critically ill patients. As much as we rely on hemodynamic data, however, clinicians do not routinely analyze the actual hemodynamic waveforms—either alone or in conjunction with electrocardiograms (ECGs).

Some clinicians read hemodynamic values from the pressure monitor, while others use a single-channel strip recorder to obtain these values. This is unfortunate. Use of monitors or single-channel strip recorders alone presents many problems in the identification of waveform values—problems that are explained in detail in the chapters that follow. *The most accurate method of obtaining hemodynamic data is to use a dual-channel strip recorder, which records the hemodynamic waveform and the ECG simultaneously, and to analyze the waveform itself and the ECG together.*[1,2]

Manufacturers of monitors have done an excellent job of developing algorithms to determine hemodynamic values. These algorithms are, however, designed to be used only in situations when waveform analysis is not complex, unlike abnormal waveform, artifacts, marked respiratory distortions. Monitors have been designed as an *aid* to the clinician, not as a replacement for the clinician's interpretation of the waveforms.

Single-channel strip recorders are also very limited. With a single-channel strip recorder, the ECG cannot be used to verify specific waves. If specific waves, such as A and V waves, cannot be identified, correct analysis of central venous pressure (CVP) and pulmonary capillary wedge pressure (PCWP) is difficult. Moreover, abnormal waves (e.g., giant A, C, or V waves) and waveform artifacts cannot easily be identified with a single-channel strip recorder.

In today's critical care environment, nurses and physicians *must* be proficient in the interpretation of hemodynamic data. The most acutely ill patients in a critical care unit are the most likely candidates for invasive hemodynamic monitoring. Proficiency in the interpretation of hemodynamic data will facilitate accurate assessment of these critically ill patients. Because this assessment serves as the basis for treatment, proficiency in interpretation of hemodynamic data can make the difference between appropriate and inappropriate therapeutic interventions.

For example, one of the key components of hemodynamic information is cardiovascular pressure. Cardiovascular pressure measurements are employed to infer function of the left and right ventricles. Cardiovascular pressure is generated in arteries and veins through atrial and ventricular contractions that move blood throughout the circulatory system. Because atrial and ventricular contractions are not constant but episodic, the cardiovascular pressure rises and falls. These pressure changes are detected on a hemodynamic monitor as waves. To interpret the hemodynamic pressures correctly and to intervene appropriately based on this interpretation, a clinician must understand the waveforms created by these cardiac actions.

Unfortunately, in many undergraduate nursing programs, hospital education programs, and graduate medical programs, in-depth waveform analysis is not taught. This may be because of the limited amount of information on waveform analysis available in the literature, or because of the assumed accuracy of monitors. Whatever its cause, inconsistent clinical education in waveform analysis increases the potential for misinterpretation of the hemodynamic data used to guide therapy in an acutely ill population. It may be interesting to check your ability to read a few common waveforms. The following section provides some waveforms for your review.

CLINICAL SCENARIOS

The following scenarios include Practice Waveforms typical of those that occur routinely in any critical care unit. After reading a scenario and interpreting the Practice Waveform, turn the page to check your interpretation.

CLINICAL SCENARIO 1–1. The following waveform is obtained on a 67-year-old man with a diagnosis of acute congestive heart failure during an attempt to ''wedge'' the catheter. The physician cannot get the catheter to wedge and tells you not to try to do so. What is your analysis of the waveform?

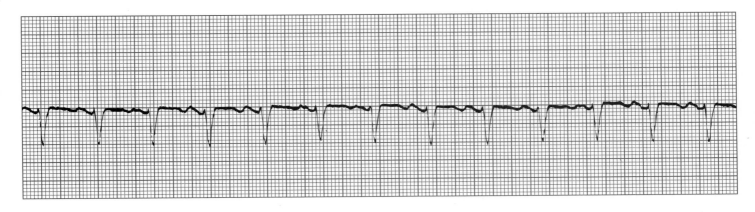

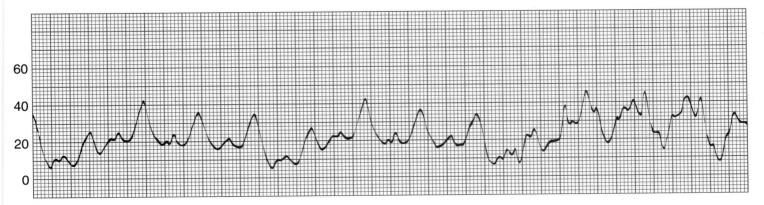

CLINICAL SCENARIO 1–1. *Analysis:* The waveform is a PCWP tracing changing to a pulmonary artery (PA) wave. The PCWP wave has large V waves and small A waves. The mean of the A wave is the closest approximation of ventricular end-diastolic pressure and is used to obtain the venous pressure. Obtaining the mean of the A wave gives a PCWP value of about 19 mm Hg. In this case the catheter does obtain a PCWP value, and this value should be used to aid in assessing the hemodynamic picture. (To learn more about this situation, see Chapter 3.)

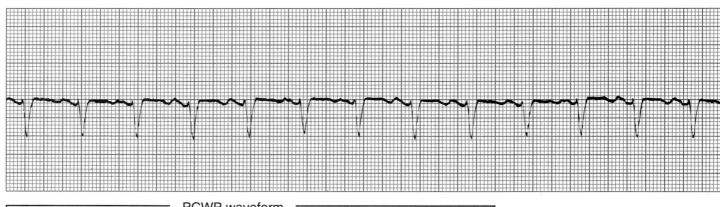

PCWP waveform

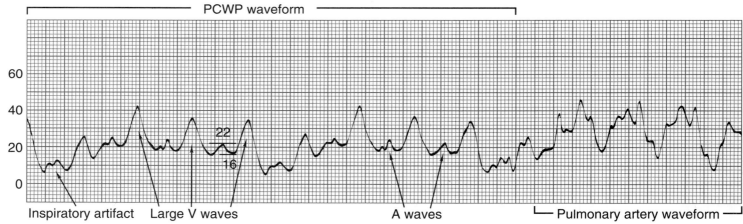

Inspiratory artifact   Large V waves   A waves   Pulmonary artery waveform

Mean PCWP = $\frac{22}{16}$ or, 19 mm Hg

CLINICAL SCENARIO 1–2. The following waveform is obtained from the proximal port of the PA catheter (right atrial or CVP port). The patient is on assist/control ventilation (assisted mandatory ventilation [AMV]) at a rate of 18 breaths per minute (bpm). No spontaneous breaths are present. What is your analysis of the waveform?

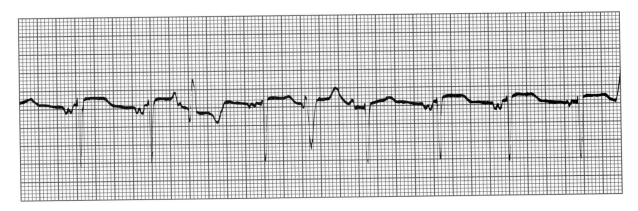

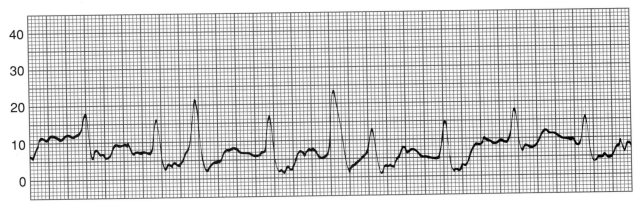

CLINICAL SCENARIO 1–2. *Analysis:* The waveform is a CVP tracing with dominant (clear) A waves. The A waves are further enlarged during ectopic beats, owing to simultaneous atrial and ventricular contraction. The CVP value in this case is about 9 mm Hg (8–10 mm Hg) after correcting for ventilator artifact. (To learn more about this situation, see Chapters 2 and 6.)

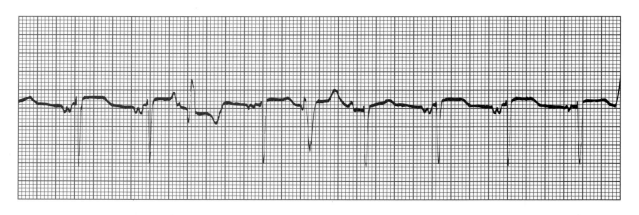

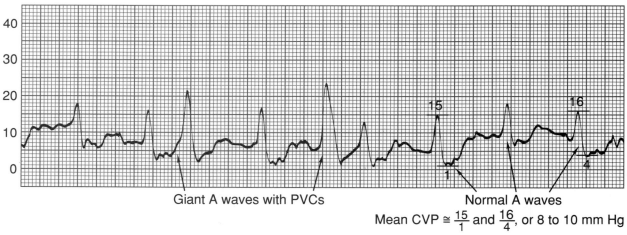

Giant A waves with PVCs   Normal A waves

Mean CVP $\cong \dfrac{15}{1}$ and $\dfrac{16}{4}$, or 8 to 10 mm Hg

CLINICAL SCENARIO 1–3. In a postoperative patient who has had an aortic aneurysm repair, you note the following waveform. The patient is not intubated. The physician states that the catheter is intermittently entering the right ventricle and wants to pull the catheter back. What is your analysis of the waveform?

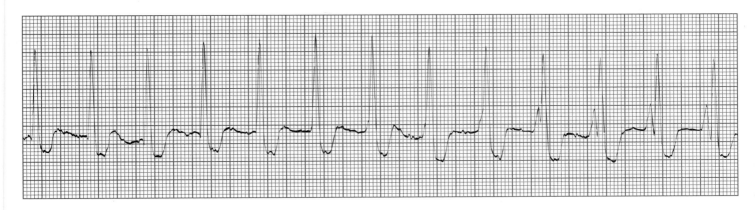

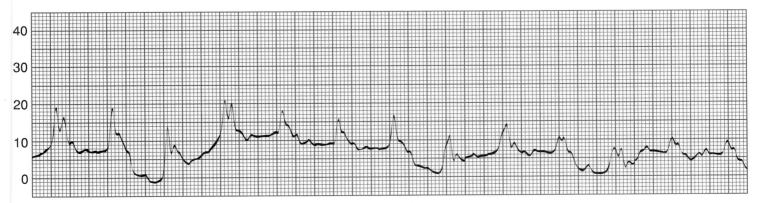

CLINICAL SCENARIO 1–3. *Analysis:* The waveform represents giant A waves secondary to the loss of atrioventricular synchrony. The catheter is not slipping into the right ventricle and should not be manipulated. The waveform reflects the hemodynamic effects of the dysrhythmia. The CVP value is read during normal atrioventricular synchrony or at the end of the QRS and is about 7–8 mm Hg. (To learn more about this situation, see Chapters 2 and 3.)

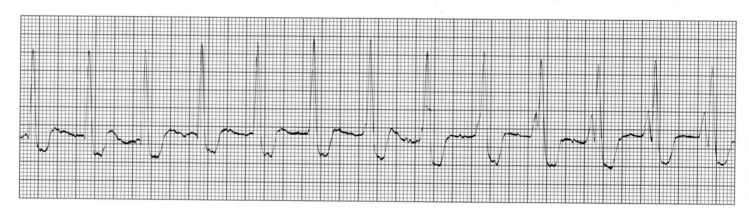

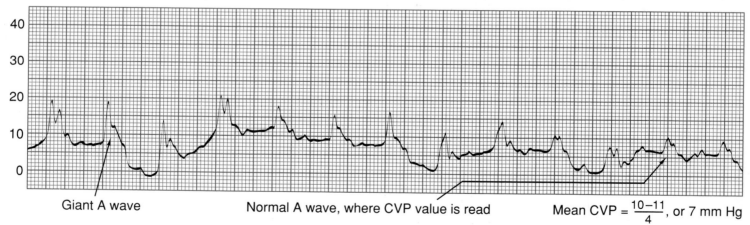

Giant A wave   Normal A wave, where CVP value is read   Mean CVP = $\frac{10-11}{4}$, or 7 mm Hg

CLINICAL SCENARIO 1–4. Your unit uses one-channel strip recorders. While obtaining a set of hemodynamic readings, you note the following waveforms. One of your colleagues states that the monitor reveals a wedge picture. What is your analysis of the waveform?

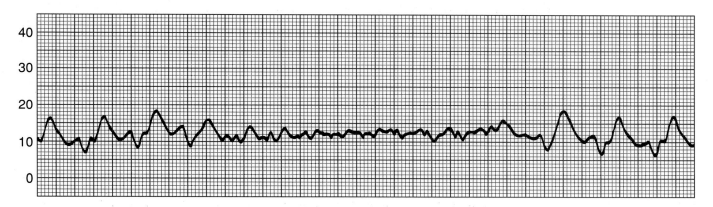

CLINICAL SCENARIO 1–4. *Analysis:* With a one-channel strip recorder, the waveform could be mistaken for a wedge, although the wedge is higher than the PA diastolic (PAD) pressure, an unlikely event. However, the real reason for the change in the pressure is a burst of paroxysmal supraventricular atrial tachycardia (PSAT). The change in waveform is not due to a wedge, but to a loss of arterial pressure because of the dysrhythmia. A two-channel strip recorder readily identifies this situation. (To learn more about this situation, see Chapter 4.)

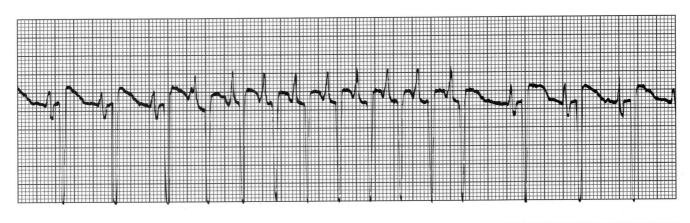

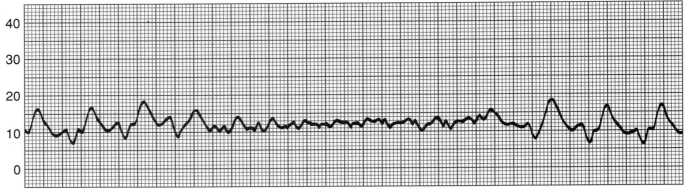

CLINICAL SCENARIO 1–5. While obtaining a PCWP value, you note the following waveform. The monitor indicates that the wedge pressure is 21 mm Hg. Do you agree with the monitor value?

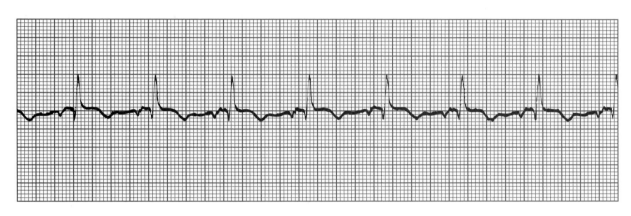

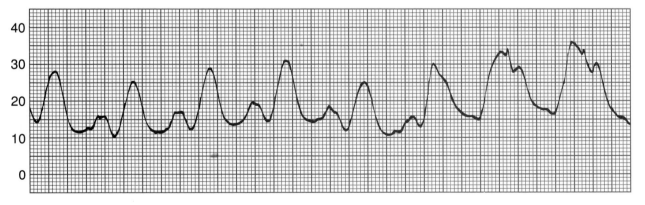

CLINICAL SCENARIO 1–5. *Analysis:* The waveform shows a PCWP changing to a PA wave. Large V waves in the PCWP tracing make it difficult for the monitor to read the wave correctly. The monitor is reading the V wave, not the A wave. The correct PCWP is about 17 mm Hg. Unfortunately, at this time, monitoring systems do not differentiate between types of waves. This is one reason why the clinician must either obtain a two-channel strip recorder tracing or obtain a freeze function on the monitor. (To learn more about this situation, see Chapter 3.)

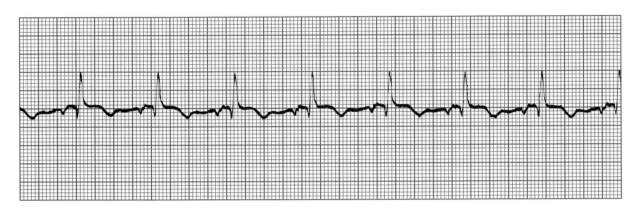

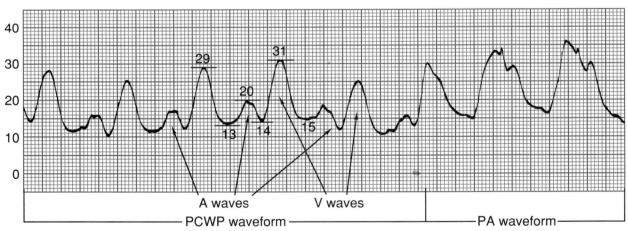

Mean "wedge" pressure = $\frac{20}{14}$, or 17 mm Hg

Mean abnormal V wave pressure = $\frac{29}{13}$ or $\frac{31}{15}$, or 21 – 23 mm Hg

CLINICAL SCENARIO 1–6. A patient is receiving mechanical ventilation in the assist/control mode at a rate of 12 bpm and a tidal volume of 800 cc. She is currently triggering the ventilator above the set rate, for a total respiratory rate of 22 bpm. Based on the waveform below, what is the correct PA pressure?

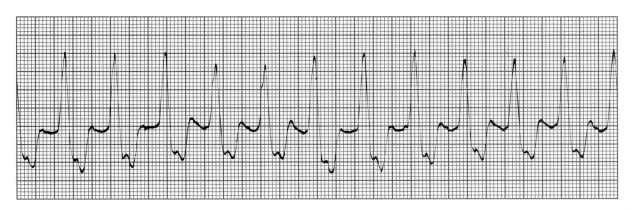

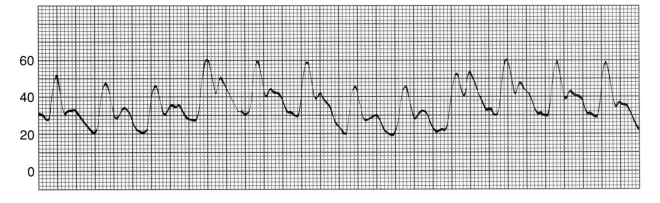

CLINICAL SCENARIO 1–6. *Analysis:* End expiration pressures are about 60/30 mm Hg. Spontaneous breathing (or triggering) creates most of the artifact in the waveform. Reading the waveform before the sudden inspiratory dip will produce the closest approximation of end expiration. End expiration readings are necessary to obtain the closest approximation of intrapleural pressures. (To learn more about this situation, see Chapter 6.)

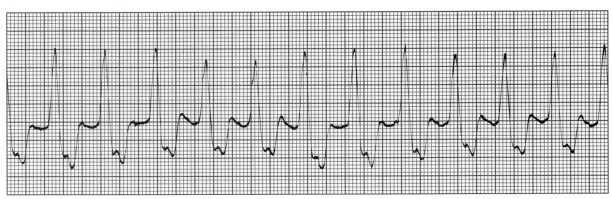

End expiration

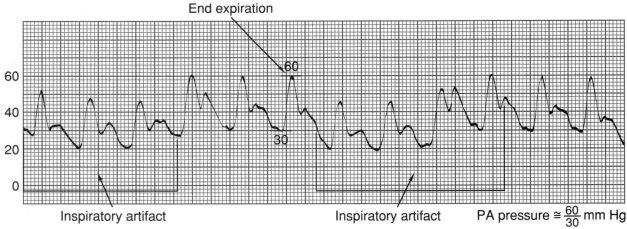

Inspiratory artifact   Inspiratory artifact   PA pressure $\cong \frac{60}{30}$ mm Hg

CLINICAL SCENARIO 1–7. A 73-year-old man is admitted with a diagnosis of congestive heart failure, requiring a PA catheter for management of cardiac output. He has a DVI pacemaker in place. You need to obtain a PA pressure reading based on the following waveform. The monitor displays a pressure of 46/12 mm Hg. Is it safe to trust the monitor value for this waveform?

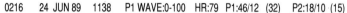

0216   24 JUN 89   1138   P1 WAVE:0-100   HR:79   P1:46/12 (32)   P2:18/10 (15)

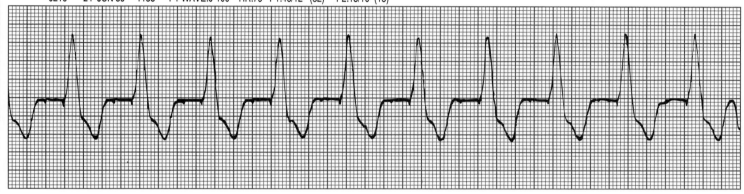

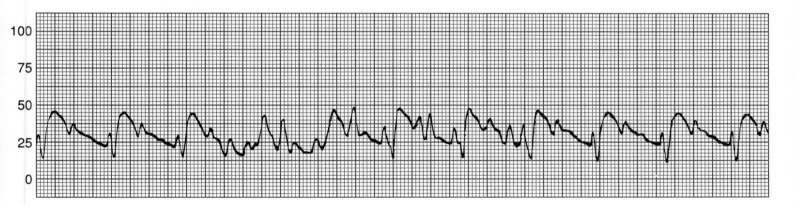

CLINICAL SCENARIO 1–7. *Analysis:* Based on the appearance of the waveform, the monitor reading is probably inaccurate. A presystolic artifact interferes with the reading of diastolic pressure, which is actually about 23 mm Hg. The monitor is unable to identify the artifact. (To learn more about this situation, see Chapters 5 and 7.)

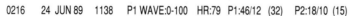

0216   24 JUN 89   1138   P1 WAVE:0-100   HR:79   P1:46/12   (32)   P2:18/10   (15)

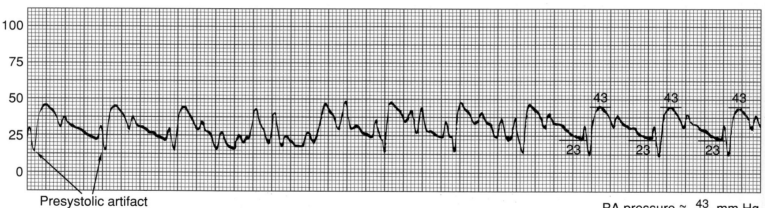

Presystolic artifact

PA pressure $\cong \dfrac{43}{23}$ mm Hg

CLINICAL SCENARIO 1–8. A 59-year-old man is admitted to the unit following coronary artery bypass surgery. At 12 hr postoperatively (0600), he is extubated and is in no respiratory distress. His catheter is unable to wedge at this time, and the physician requests that the PAD be used to estimate the PCWP value. The physician leaves orders to start dobutamine at 3 mcg/mg/min and to notify the surgeon if the PAD increases to greater than 20 mm Hg. At 0800 the patient begins to complain of shortness of breath, and his respiratory rate increases to 36 bpm. His ECG shows intermittent dependence on a pacemaker. Based on the following waveform, what is his current PA pressure? Should you notify the physician at this point?

RICU 4_ 27 MAR 90 0735 AVF PAP_ SCALE 0/20/40/60 HR 29 PAP _58/27/(38) CVP (13) ABP -?- RESP 37 PULSE 68 SAO2 98 MBP 152/70(96) C. O. _4. 12 5:28

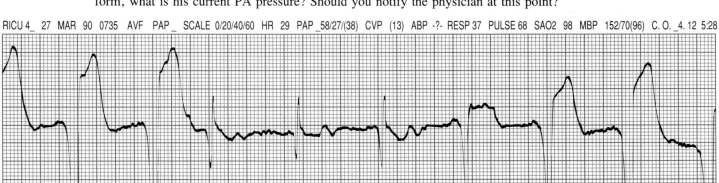

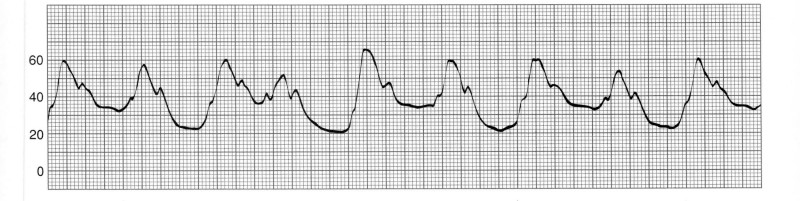

CLINICAL SCENARIO 1–8. *Analysis:* The physician should be notified and dobutamine started (provided that the cardiac and stroke volumes have decreased), inasmuch as the PA reading is about 58/32 mm Hg. The rapid respiratory rate pulls the waveform down at points, and reading the diastolic value can be difficult. The change in the ECG rhythm has little effect on the hemodynamic values. (To learn more about this situation, see Chapter 6.)

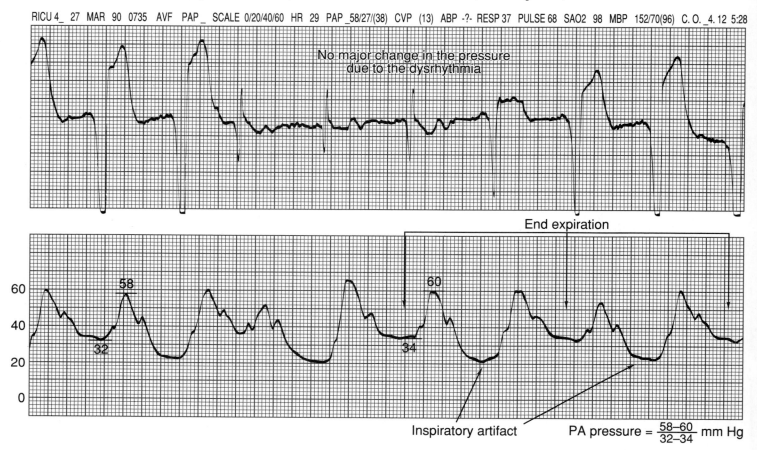

RICU 4_ 27 MAR 90 0735 AVF PAP_ SCALE 0/20/40/60 HR 29 PAP_58/27//(38) CVP (13) ABP -?- RESP 37 PULSE 68 SAO2 98 MBP 152/70(96) C.O._4.12 5:28

No major change in the pressure due to the dysrhythmia

End expiration

Inspiratory artifact

$$\text{PA pressure} = \frac{58-60}{32-34} \text{ mm Hg}$$

How did you do? Those who were able to correctly interpret the waveforms are to be congratulated. Although each of the Practice Waveforms represents a common clinical scenario, many clinicians will find interpretation difficult because their education and clinical practice had not stressed the importance of waveform analysis. Waveform analysis takes specialized training and practice. To avoid misreading waveforms, you must understand the principles of waveform analysis and learn to apply them to your clinical practice.

SUMMARY

The chapters that follow will teach you the principles of waveform analysis, provide ample opportunity for practice, and suggest clinical applications. However, accurate waveform analysis centers around employing the correct equipment. If your unit does not have two-channel strip recorders or simultaneous ECG and waveform freeze functions, your clinical application of waveform analysis will be limited. The chance of error is increased if the correct equipment is not available. The cost of proper equipment, such as easy-to-use two-channel strip recorders for waveform analysis, is a small price to pay in the face of the potential for incorrect therapies.

II PRINCIPLES OF WAVEFORM ANALYSIS

2 Normal Pulmonary Capillary Wedge and Central Venous Pressure Waveforms

Although central venous pressure (CVP) and pulmonary capillary wedge pressure (PCWP) waveforms are similar in appearance, they generally can be distinguished by the waves created during atrial contraction. CVP and PCWP waves are also called venous or atrial waveforms because the waves are generated from the right (CVP) and left (PCWP) atria. When the clinician is using a pulmonary artery catheter to obtain CVP and PCWP values, a slight difference between CVP and PCWP appearance exists owing to the difference in atrial impulse transmission between the left and right atria. This difference will be presented later. For instructional purposes, at this time assume that CVP and PCWP waveforms are similar in appearance.

Before proceeding, remember that the reason to read the CVP value is to estimate the right ventricular end-diastolic pressure (RVEDP). Similarly, the PCWP approximates and thus allows you to estimate left ventricular end-diastolic pressure (LVEDP) (Fig. 2–1). If the RVEDP is available, CVP pressures should not be used. If the LVEDP is available, the PCWP should not be used. For example, some pulmonary artery catheters have right ventricular (RV) ports, which allow for direct measurement of RVEDP. In such situations, you should measure the right ventricular pressure rather than estimate RVEDP values through CVP readings.

Central venous waves, created by right atrial contraction, and PCWP waves, created by left atrial contraction, each have three components.[13] The components of atrial waves are labeled A, C, and V waves (Fig. 2–2).

After the A wave has peaked, the downstroke following the A is termed the X descent. The location at which the C wave starts (on the downstroke of the A wave) is termed the Z point. The Z point is potentially useful because it marks end-diastolic pressure in the atrium.[14] The descent after the C wave is the remainder of the X descent (may be termed X_2 or X'). The mean of the peak of the A wave and the bottom of the X descent is the numerical value obtained for CVP and PCWP readings. The significance of the mean A wave will be presented shortly.

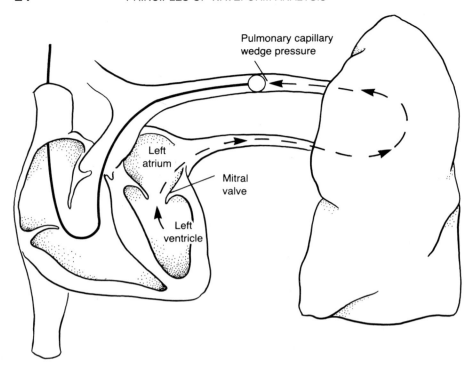

Figure 2–1. PCWP is approximately equal to LVEDP when blood flow through the lungs is unobstructed.

The descent following the V wave is termed the Y descent. The Y descent is a result of the opening of the atrioventricular (A-V) valves, essentially creating one chamber between the atria and ventricles. The equilibration of pressure between the ventricles and atria allows for atrial waves (pressures) to approximate ventricular pressures. The equilibration is complete at the end of diastole, a point marked on the ECG near the end of the QRS complex.

A slight rise in pressure may occur after the Y descent. Such a rise after the Y descent and prior to the beginning of the A wave is termed the H wave (diasthesis wave).[15]

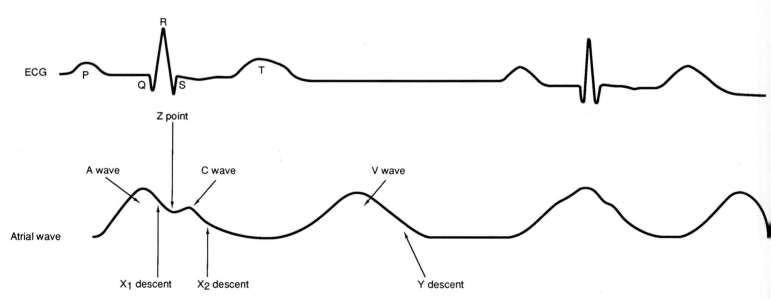

Figure 2–2. Components of the atrial waves.

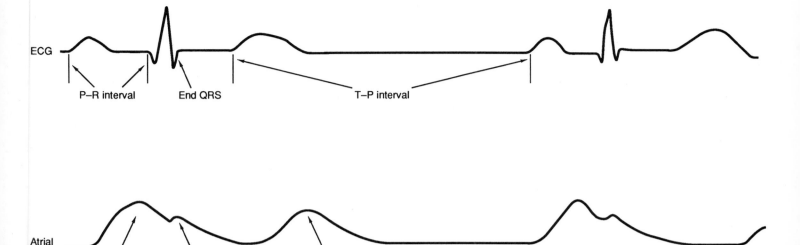

Figure 2–3. Correlation of the ECG with atrial waves.

ELECTROCARDIOGRAM CORRELATION WITH HEMODYNAMIC WAVES

Each component of the atrial wave can be identified through correlation with the (ECG) electrical activities that stimulate formation of the mechanical events generating waves (Fig. 2–3). As a practical aid, use a straight edge, such as a ruler, to help align electrocardiogram (ECG) components with the waveforms. On the ECG, the P wave generates the electrical activity that causes atrial contraction. Inasmuch as the mechanical event of atrial contraction must follow the electrical event, atrial waves will start immediately after the P wave. The first mechanical wave generated is the A wave, which represents atrial contraction (Fig. 2–4).

Immediately after atrial contraction, ventricular contraction is initiated. The first phase of ventricular contraction (isometric contraction) immediately follows ventricular depolarization. At the end of the QRS, the isometric ventricular contraction produces enough pressure to close

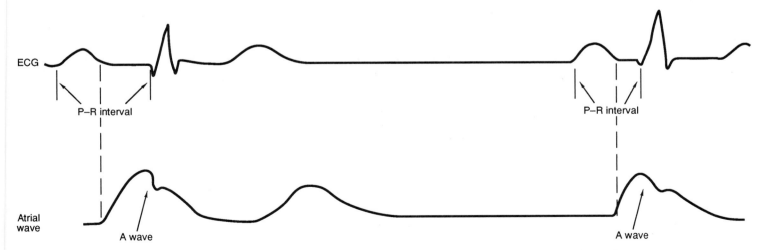

Figure 2–4. Correlation of the A wave with the ECG. The A wave starts during the P–R interval.

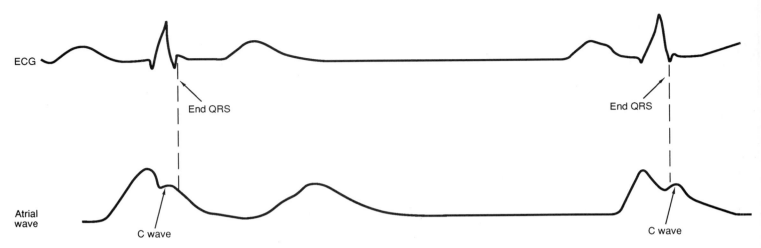

Figure 2–5. Correlation of the ECG with the C wave. The C wave starts during or at the end of the QRS complex.

the mitral and tricuspid valves. The closure of these valves produces the next wave, the C wave (Fig. 2–5). The C wave is found near the end of the QRS and is seen as a deflection in the downstroke of the A wave. The C wave is not always distinct or clearly visible, particularly in a PCWP tracing.

As ventricular systole proceeds, the mitral and tricuspid valves remain closed. Blood from the superior and inferior vena cava continues to empty into the right atrium, and blood from the pulmonary veins empties into the left atrium. The entry of blood into the atria while the mitral and tricuspid valves are closed produces a rise in atrial pressure. This rise in pressure produces the third atrial wave, the V wave (Fig. 2–6). The V wave begins during ventricular systole, represented on the ECG until the beginning of the T wave. The peak value of the V wave occurs after the T wave, prior to when ventricular diastole starts and the mitral and tricuspid valves reopen. As a rule, the V wave can be identified between the T wave and the next P wave. Waveforms 2–1 through 2–3 illustrate the normal venous waveform appearance.

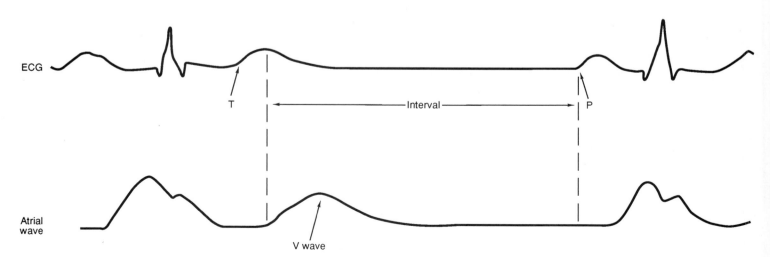

Figure 2–6. Correlation of the V wave with the ECG. The V wave starts during the T–P interval.

These waveform descriptions are generally accurate in identifying both venous (CVP and PCWP) waveforms. Practically, however, one difference should be noted, as mentioned earlier. All PCWP readings are slightly delayed (approximately 0.10 seconds). This slight delay in the PCWP reading from the CVP is partially due to two factors: one, right atrial contraction proceeds before left atrial contraction; and two, impulse transmission is delayed from the left atrium back to the pulmonary artery catheter. Figure 2–7 illustrates the difference between reading a CVP and a PCWP tracing, and Table 2–1 summarizes the difference between the CVP and PCWP ECG correlations.

Obtaining Venous Pressure Values

The CVP reading is obtained from the right atrial port (proximal lumen) of a pulmonary artery catheter (Fig. 2–8). Because the right atrial port is located in the right atrium, the waves are rapidly transmitted back to the sensing transducer. No substantial delay is noted in the ECG reading and CVP wave.

On the other hand, the distal port is used to obtain the PCWP wave. The distal port is in the pulmonary artery, however, not in the left atrium (Fig. 2–8).

A further delay may be present in the wave/ECG correlation because the pressure wave generated in the left atrium must be transmitted back through the lungs to the distal PA port. Practically, this delay is only slight, yet this difference, coupled with the difference in right

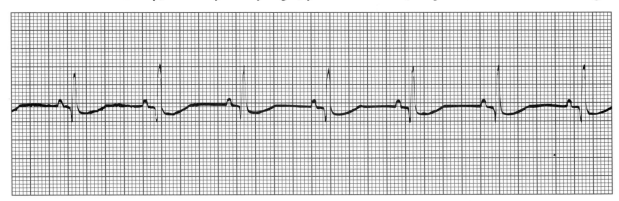

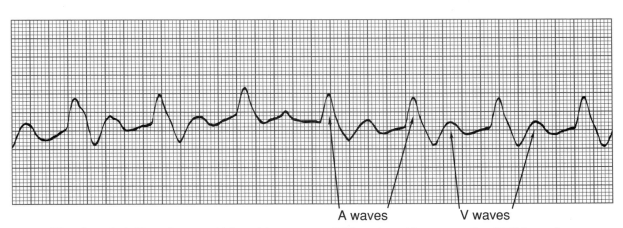

A waves   V waves

Waveform 2–1. Normal venous (right atrial pressure or CVP) tracing with corresponding ECG intervals.

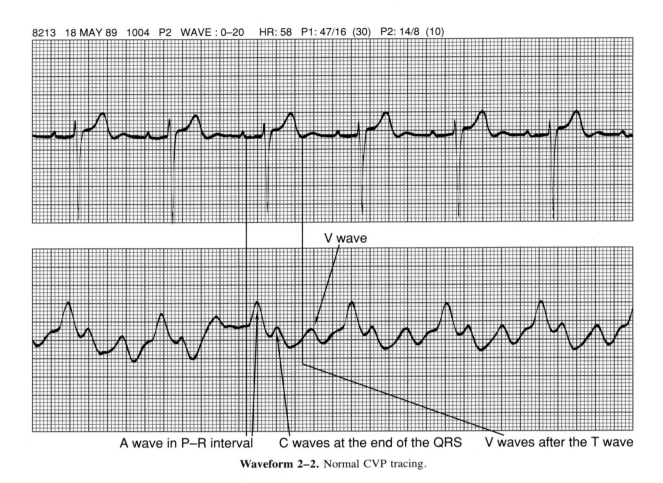

8213   18 MAY 89   1004   P2   WAVE : 0–20   HR: 58   P1: 47/16 (30)   P2: 14/8 (10)

V wave

A wave in P–R interval   C waves at the end of the QRS   V waves after the T wave

Waveform 2–2. Normal CVP tracing.

ECG

P — Interval — R   T — Interval — P

CVP

C wave

A wave starts in P–R interval   V wave starts in early T–P interval

PCWP

A wave starts in or at the end of the QRS complex   V wave starts later in T–P interval

Figure 2–7. The difference between CVP and PCWP ECG correlations.

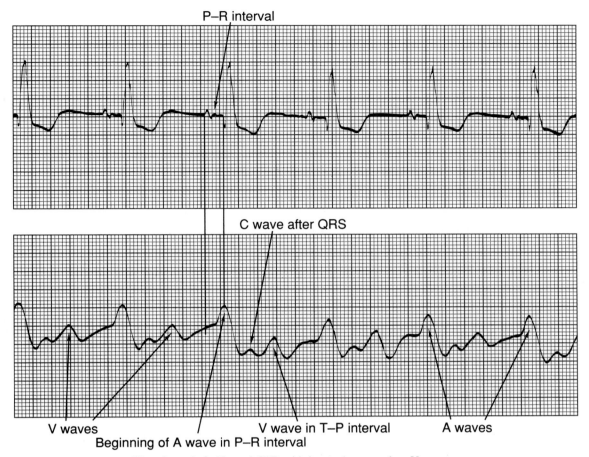

Waveform 2–3. Normal CVP with larger A waves than V waves.

and left atrial depolarization, is important to remember in order to avoid making errors in interpretation. The A wave of the PCWP reading is usually in the QRS complex rather than in the P–R interval. C waves, if present, are later in the ST segment. C waves, however, may be absent owing to loss of subtle waves during the travel through the lungs. In addition, the scale used may be too large to see the wave. V waves are delayed until later in the T–P interval, rather than closer to the T wave as in the CVP reading.

Examples of waveform differences between the CVP and the PCWP are presented in Waveforms 2–4 and 2–5.

Importance of Individual Wave Interpretation

The location of each individual wave has important implications for the identification of abnormalities as well as for the interpretation of normal hemodynamics. The location of the A wave

Table 2–1. DIFFERENCES IN CVP AND PCWP ECG CORRELATIONS

Wave	CVP	PCWP
A	In the P–R interval	End of QRS
C	End of QRS	ST segment
V	Near end of T wave	In the T–P interval

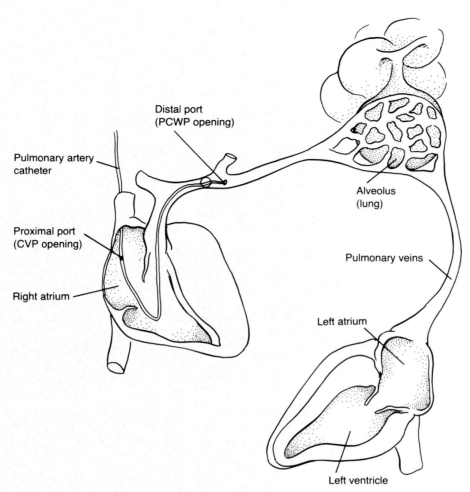

Figure 2–8. Pulmonary artery catheter with CVP lumen. Note that the CVP opening is located in the right atrium. No delay occurs in transmitting pressures to the transducer. However, the PCWP opening is located a substantial distance from the left atrium, causing a delay in pressure transmission.

is an important clinical tool owing to the correlation of the mean A wave reading with the ventricular end-diastolic pressure (Fig. 2–9). Multiple reports have appeared in the literature citing the value of the A wave in estimating LVEDP.[16,17] The mean of the A wave closely approximates the end-diastolic pressure in the ventricles for one key reason: the mean of the A wave gives a value near the end of the QRS complex, which is approximately end diastole, with systole starting immediately thereafter.

Some clinicians, when obtaining a CVP or PCWP reading, do not locate the A wave. For example, some clinicians may draw a line through all waves and take the reading from this line. Other clinicians may take the reading from the monitor without analyzing the waves. Such procedures are potentially accurate as long as the waves are of equal size and no artifact or hemodynamic abnormality exists. Under most normal circumstances, however, the A wave is slightly larger than the V wave. In addition, many variations in waveform appearance are possible, e.g., giant A or V waves or absent A waves. Therefore, inaccuracies may occur more often with techniques that do not measure the A wave directly.[18]

The primary method to ensure that all clinicians are consistently reading waveforms correctly is for all interpreters of waveforms to locate the A wave and determine its mean. An example of reading the A wave is given in Figure 2–10. Waveforms illustrating the correct reading of a CVP and PCWP are given in Waveforms 2–6, 2–7, and 2–8.

Two other locations have been suggested for reading A wave values. One is to locate the plateau immediately prior to the beginning of the A wave. This plateau is referred to as the H

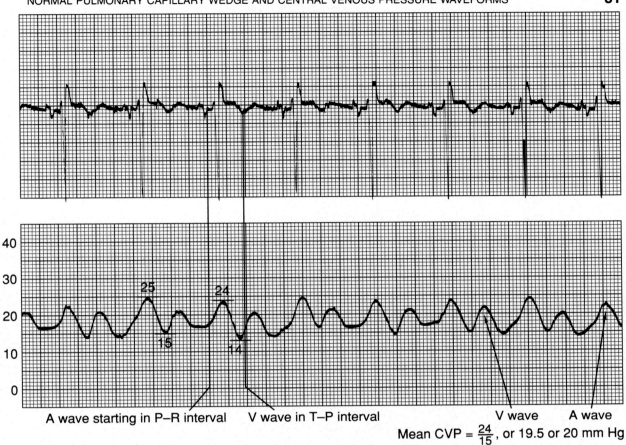

A wave starting in P–R interval   V wave in T–P interval   V wave   A wave

Mean CVP = $\frac{24}{15}$, or 19.5 or 20 mm Hg

Waveform 2–4. Normal venous tracing—CVP.

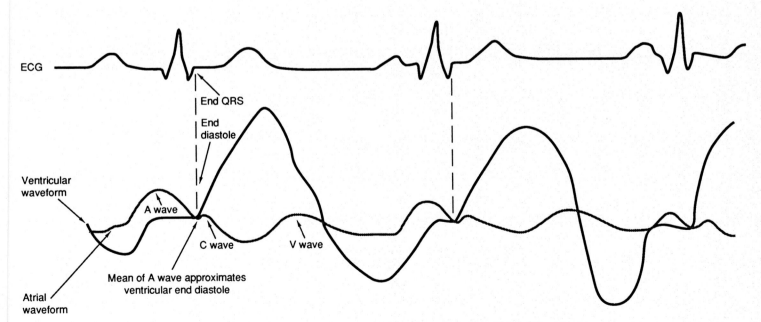

ECG

End QRS

End diastole

Ventricular waveform

A wave

C wave   V wave

Mean of A wave approximates ventricular end diastole

Atrial waveform

Figure 2–9. The mean of the A wave approximates ventricular end-diastolic pressure.

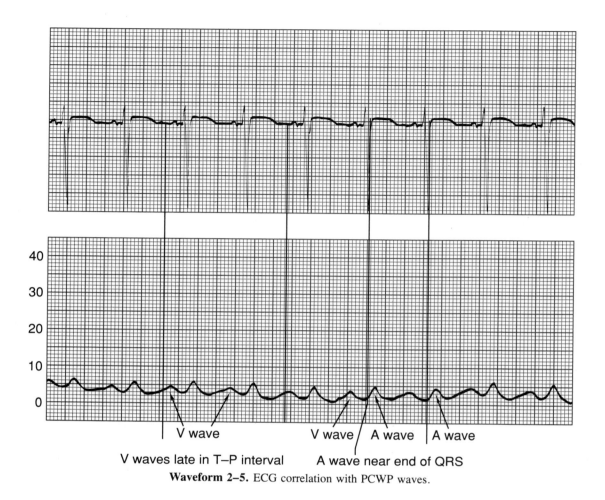

V wave   **V wave / A wave** | **A wave**

V waves late in T–P interval   **A wave near end of QRS**

Waveform 2–5. ECG correlation with PCWP waves.

wave. Unfortunately, this plateau (or H wave) is not consistently present. The same is true for the second suggested location for reading the A wave, i.e., the Z point. The Z point is located at the onset of the C wave, near the end of the QRS complex. Again, because of the inconsistency in identifying a Z point, this method is more difficult to use than finding the mean of the entire A wave.

RELATIONSHIP BETWEEN PULMONARY ARTERY DIASTOLIC VALUES AND THE PCWP

One of the most important physiologic and clinical aspects of reading a venous tracing is related to pressure and blood flow concepts. Blood essentially moves from a higher to a lower pressure, although other factors may also be present. The mean arterial pressure (MAP) must always be high enough to push blood forward. Conceptually this means that the MAP arising from the aorta must be high enough to push blood to the right atrium. In addition, the mean pulmonary artery pressure must be high enough to push blood to the left atrium (Fig. 2–11). From the perspective of waveform interpretation, pressures in the atria should never exceed mean arterial pressures. Should atrial pressures exceed mean arterial pressures, theoretically blood flow would reverse. Although this explanation presents blood flow somewhat simplistically, the concept is

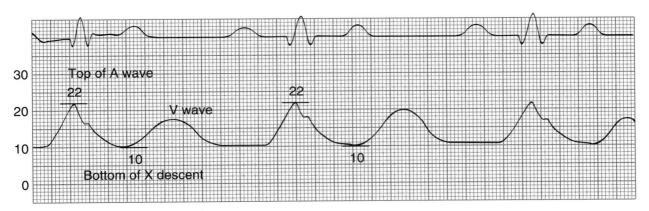

Figure 2–10. Reading the mean of an A wave. $\dfrac{22 + 10}{2} = 16$ mm Hg.

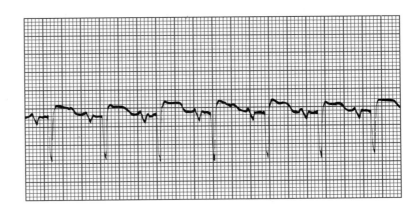

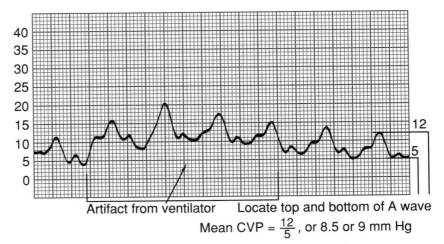

Artifact from ventilator   Locate top and bottom of A wave

Waveform 2–6. Reading a CVP tracing.

Mean CVP $= \dfrac{12}{5}$, or 8.5 or 9 mm Hg

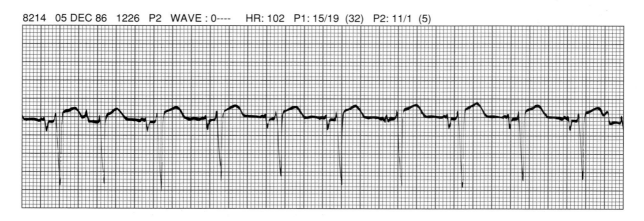

8214 05 DEC 86 1226 P2 WAVE : 0----   HR: 102 P1: 15/19 (32) P2: 11/1 (5)

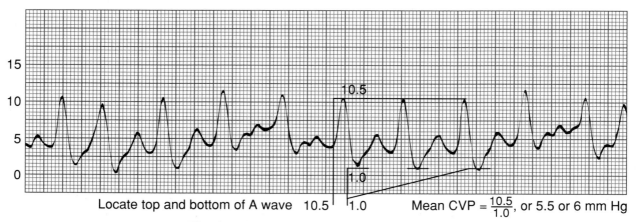

Locate top and bottom of A wave   10.5   1.0   Mean CVP = $\frac{10.5}{1.0}$, or 5.5 or 6 mm Hg

Waveform 2–7. Interpreting a normal CVP tracing.

important. Practically, when reading waveforms, specifically the PCWP, remember that the PCWP must be lower than the mean of the pulmonary artery (PA) pressure. If the PCWP is higher than the PA mean, recheck the waveform and make sure the correct points are being identified.

In addition to the mean PA being higher than the PCWP, as a rule the pulmonary arterial diastolic (PAD) pressure is usually higher than the PCWP. This is true primarily because a pressure gradient should exist between the PA mean and the PCWP. If the PCWP equals the PAD, the pressure difference necessary to move blood forward is very small. Although this situation could occur, it is not common. Practically, one can assume that the PAD is also higher than the PCWP.

Determining the trend of the PAD by interpreting the PCWP may be possible if the PAD-PCWP relationship has been established. Normally, the PCWP is from 1 to 4 mm Hg lower than the PAD.[19] Such a PAD-PCWP relationship is present, however, only under normal circumstances or when passive pulmonary hypertension exists. Of the three forms of pulmonary hypertension, primary, secondary active, and secondary passive, only secondary passive hypertension allows close PAD-PCWP correlation.

Primary pulmonary hypertension (no known cause) and secondary active hypertension (alteration in pulmonary blood flow secondary to obstruction, such as emboli, or loss of vasculature, such as in chronic obstructive pulmonary disease [COPD]) cause marked elevation in pulmonary artery pressures without a concurrent increase in the PCWP. Any PCWP increase

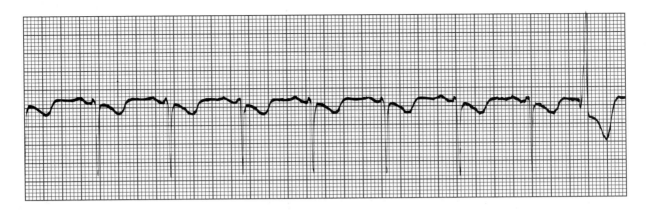

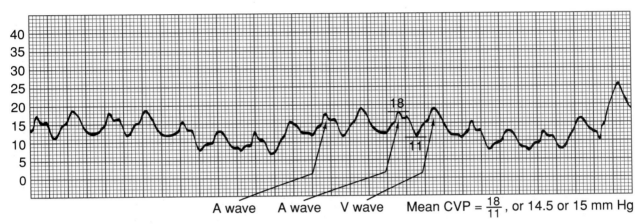

A wave   A wave   V wave   Mean CVP = $\frac{18}{11}$, or 14.5 or 15 mm Hg

Waveform 2–8. Interpreting a normal PCWP tracing. Locate the top and bottom of the A wave to obtain the value.

is usually the result of left ventricular failure; however, primary and secondary active pulmonary hypertension cause elevations in the pulmonary artery pressures without directly causing left ventricular failure. The PCWP does not increase markedly under these circumstances, thus causing a discrepancy in the PAD-PCWP relationship.

In secondary passive pulmonary hypertension, the PA pressure increases in an attempt to overcome the increasing left ventricular pressures produced by left heart failure. Only in secondary passive pulmonary hypertension is the PAD-PCWP relationship close enough to allow the PAD to correlate with the PCWP. Figure 2–12 illustrates the differences between the correlations in the types of pulmonary hypertension.

CONFIRMING A PCWP TRACING

Obtaining a PCWP tracing is possible only if an uninterrupted path exists between the distal end of the pulmonary artery and the left atrium. The best guideline for inferring the existence of a clear pathway to the left atrium is the identification of normal atrial waves. If clear waves are not present, other methods exist for potentially identifying a PCWP tracing. One method is to confirm the proper position of the PA catheter. Correct location of the catheter is necessary to ensure that an uninterrupted flow of blood exists between the end of the catheter and the left atrium. If the catheter is located improperly, an interrupted path for pressure transmission may exist.

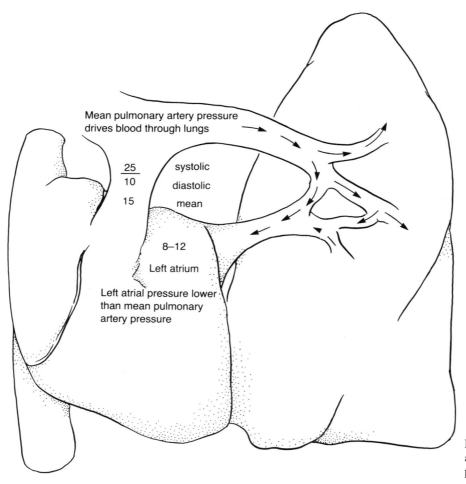

Mean pulmonary artery pressure drives blood through lungs

25 / 10
15

systolic
diastolic
mean

8–12

Left atrium

Left atrial pressure lower than mean pulmonary artery pressure

Figure 2–11. Mean pulmonary artery pressure exceeds left atrial pressures.

For example, when alveolar pressure exceeds vascular pressure, which can occur in low perfusion areas of the lung, an interrupted pathway exists. Theoretically, there exist three perfusion zones of the lung (Fig. 2–13).[20] Based on the anatomic characteristics of the lung and the effect of gravity, upper areas of the lung have less perfusion than lower regions. The lower perfusion results in a situation where alveolar pressure exceeds both arterial inflow and venous outflow pressures (zone I). If a PA catheter is placed in this first zone, no clear pathway exists to the left atrium. Alveolar pressures rather than left atrial pressures will be read by the transducer.

In zone II, arterial pressure exceeds alveolar, although alveolar exceeds venous pressure. In this zone, blood flow occurs although a constrictor effect to the flow exists due to the alveolar pressure. PA catheters in this region may not read left atrial waves accurately.

In zone III, both arterial and venous pressures exceed alveolar pressures. PA catheters in this zone will read left atrial waveforms accurately. Identifying the type of zone in which the catheter is located may be difficult because the zones can change depending on changes in alveolar pressure. For example, during mechanical ventilation or with positive end-expiratory pressure, zone I can increase in size.

As a rule, as long as the PA catheter is below the level of the left atrium, a zone III situation is likely to exist.[21] A lateral chest x-ray may help confirm the location of the PA catheter.

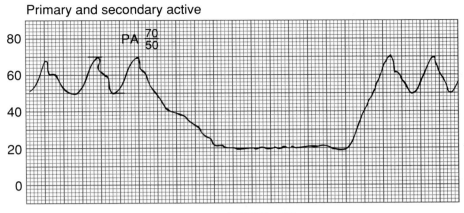

Primary and secondary active

PA $\frac{70}{50}$

PCWP – 20

Figure 2–12. Different correlations between PAD and PCWP values in various types of pulmonary hypertension. In primary and secondary active pulmonary hypertension, PAD values correlate poorly with PCWP values; however, in secondary passive pulmonary hypertension, a close correlation exists between PAD and PCWP values.

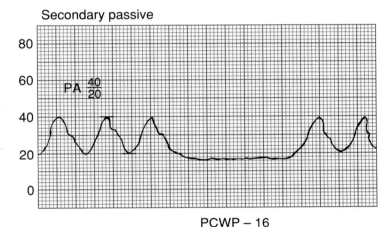

Secondary passive

PA $\frac{40}{20}$

PCWP – 16

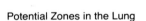

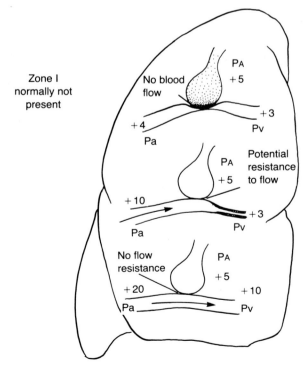

Potential Zones in the Lung

Zone I normally not present

No blood flow

PA +5

+4 Pa

+3 Pv

Potential resistance to flow

PA +5

+10 Pa

+3 Pv

No flow resistance

PA +5

+20 Pa

+10 Pv

Zone I   Pa<PA>Pv

Zone II   Pa>PA>Pv

Zone III   Pa>PA<Pv

Figure 2–13. Pulmonary zones of perfusion. In zone I, alveolar pressure (PA) exceeds both arterial inflow (Pa) and venous outflow (Pv) pressures. In zone II, arterial pressure exceeds alveolar pressure, but alveolar pressure exceeds venous pressure. In zone III, both arterial and venous pressures exceed alveolar pressures.

If distinct A and V waves are unclear, the PCWP tracing may not be accurate. The clinician should interpret PCWP values with caution in this situation.

A second method to verify a PCWP tracing is available when question exists as to the type of wave displayed. This method involves aspiration of blood from the distal port. Rapid withdrawal of about 10 cc of blood will result in arterialized blood (demonstrated by PO_2 levels near arterial levels) being withdrawn from the pulmonary capillary bed. If the catheter is not in a wedge position, the oxygen values of the blood will remain at venous levels.[22]

VARIATIONS IN WAVEFORM APPEARANCE

Normal variations in the venous waves can occur and should not mislead the clinician. For example, waves can appear large or small depending on the scale employed. A small scale will cause the waves to appear large although no abnormality exists. Waveform 2–9 illustrates a CVP tracing on a small scale, causing the A and V waves to appear large. The key point to interpreting waveforms and identifying abnormalities is the integration of other hemodynamic information at the same time. Chapter 10 addresses the integration of other data sources when interpreting the clinical significance of waveform changes.

In addition, small variations in waveform values are common and should not necessarily be considered abnormal. For example, if one nurse obtains a PCWP value of 12 mm Hg and

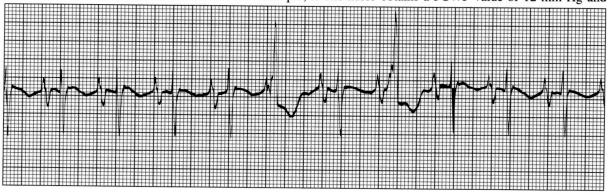

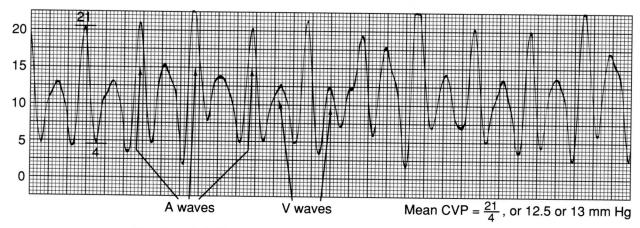

A waves   V waves   Mean CVP = $\frac{21}{4}$, or 12.5 or 13 mm Hg

Waveform 2–9. The small scale causes the A and V waves to appear large.

the next nurse obtains a value between 10 and 14 mm Hg, no real change may have occurred. Pressure fluctuations can be normal and should not be viewed in isolation.

SUMMARY

A key aspect of hemodynamic assessment is obtaining accurate values. In order to obtain accurate values, clinicians must understand how to interpret venous waveforms such as the PCWP and CVP. Correct interpretation of venous waveforms depends upon understanding normal relationships between the electrical and mechanical events in the heart. The correlation between the electrical events (reflected on the ECG) and mechanical events (waveform production) is the basis for correct interpretation of waveform analysis. From the information presented in this chapter addressing the electrical/mechanical events in the heart, clinicians should be able to develop the basis for accurate interpretation of venous waveforms.

PRACTICE WAVEFORMS

Practice your interpretation of normal venous waveforms on the Practice Waveforms that follow. Practice Waveforms 2–1 through 2–3 are CVP tracings, and 2–4 through 2–6 are PCWP tracings. Practice Waveform 2–7 requires you to identify a CVP or PCWP tracing by ECG correlation.

PRACTICE WAVEFORM 2–1. Find and determine the mean of the A wave in this CVP tracing.

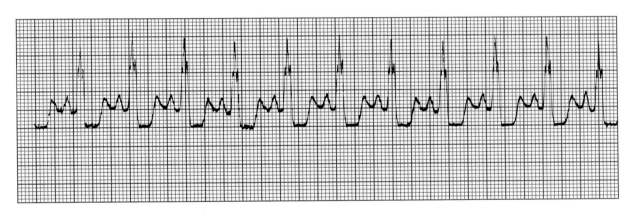

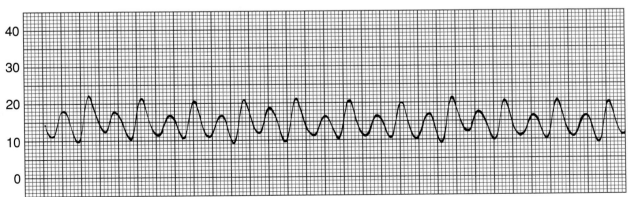

PRACTICE WAVEFORM 2–1. *Analysis:* The A wave is located in the P–R interval. Find the end of the P–R interval to locate most A waves.

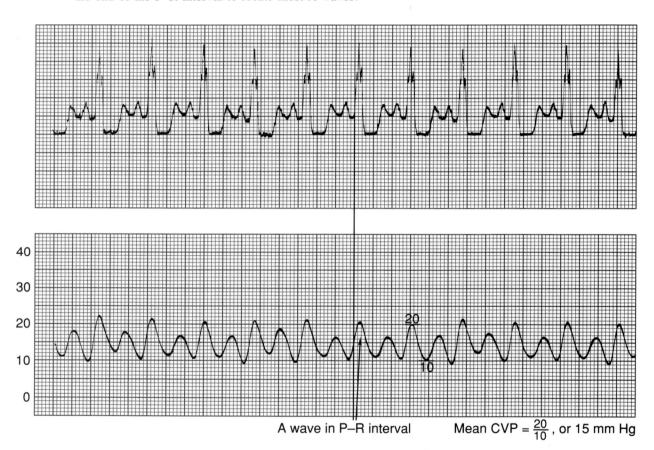

A wave in P–R interval   Mean CVP = $\frac{20}{10}$, or 15 mm Hg

PRACTICE WAVEFORM 2–2. What is the value of this CVP tracing?

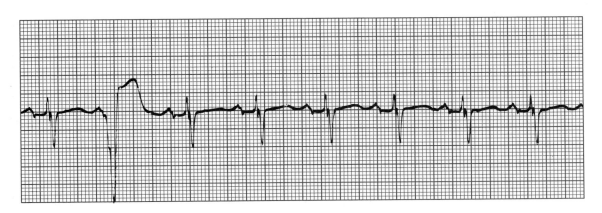

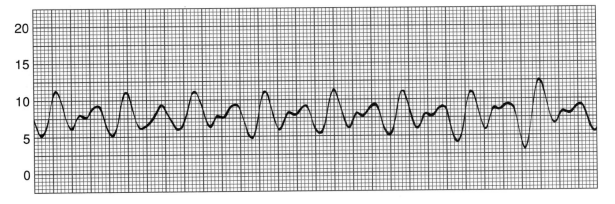

PRACTICE WAVEFORM 2–2. *Analysis:* In this normal CVP tracing, the A wave is readily found in the P–R interval.

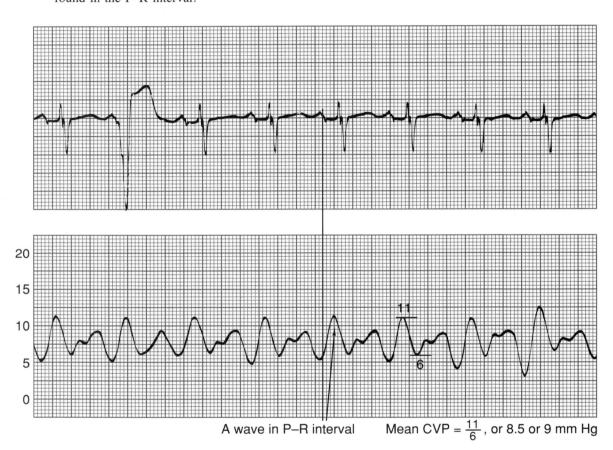

A wave in P–R interval   Mean CVP = $\frac{11}{6}$, or 8.5 or 9 mm Hg

PRACTICE WAVEFORM 2–3. Locate and determine the mean of the A wave on this CVP tracing.

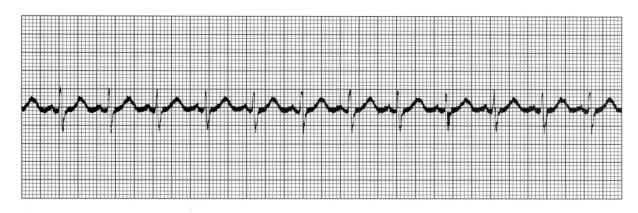

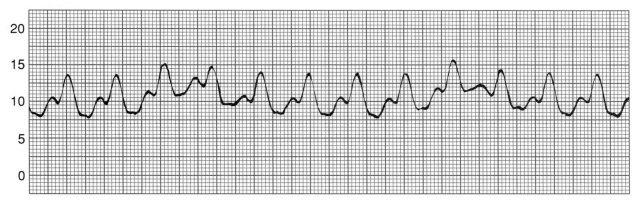

PRACTICE WAVEFORM 2–3. *Analysis:* In this normal CVP tracing, the A waves are found in the P–R interval. Note movement in the baseline, with some A waves increasing in size. This movement is due to mechanical ventilation, a concept addressed in Chapter 6. Read the A wave where the least distortion is present.

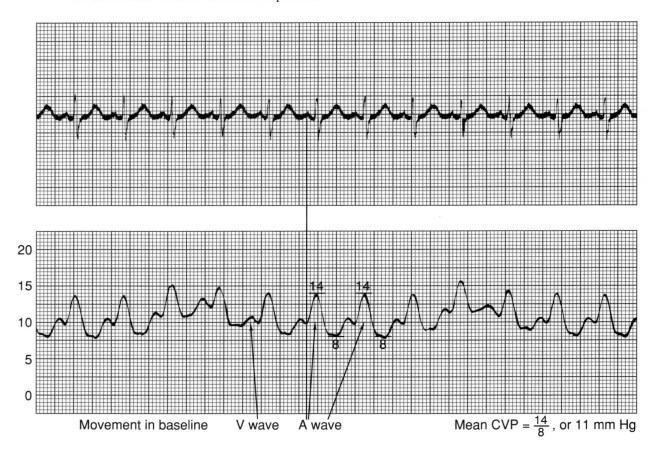

Movement in baseline   V wave   A wave   Mean CVP = $\frac{14}{8}$, or 11 mm Hg

PRACTICE WAVEFORM 2–4. Find the A and V waves in this PCWP tracing.

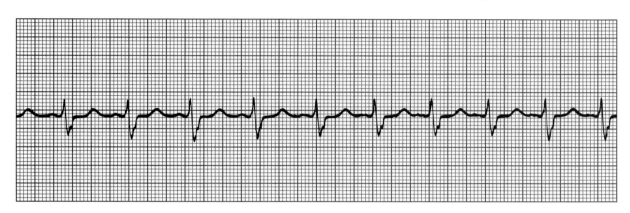

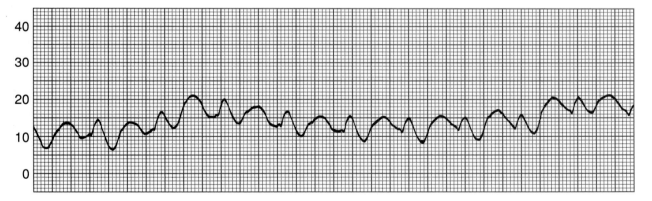

PRACTICE WAVEFORM 2–4. *Analysis:* In this PCWP tracing, the A wave is located later, near the end of the QRS complex. Also note that the V wave is near the end of the T–P interval.

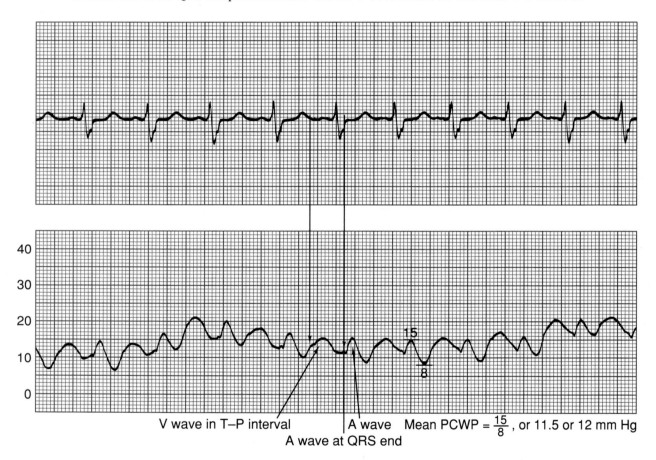

V wave in T–P interval   A wave   Mean PCWP = $\frac{15}{8}$, or 11.5 or 12 mm Hg

A wave at QRS end

PRACTICE WAVEFORM 2–5. Locate the A and V waves in this PCWP tracing.

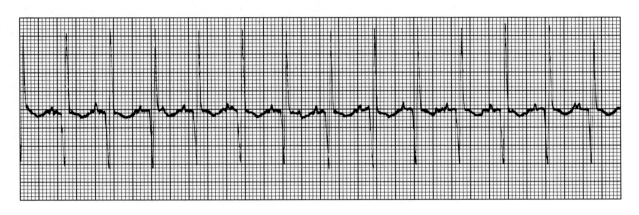

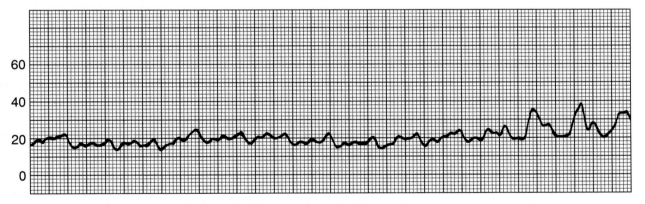

PRACTICE WAVEFORM 2–5. *Analysis:* Under normal circumstances, the A and V waves are frequently of similar size. In this case, the A and V waves are similar in size. They can be differentiated by noting the ECG intervals. The A wave is located near the end of the QRS complex, whereas the V wave is located late in the T–P interval.

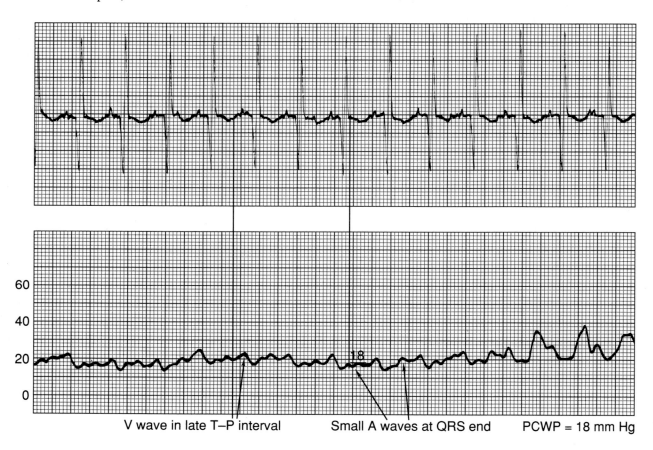

V wave in late T–P interval   Small A waves at QRS end   PCWP = 18 mm Hg

PRACTICE WAVEFORM 2–6. Normal PCWP tracing. What is the PCWP value?

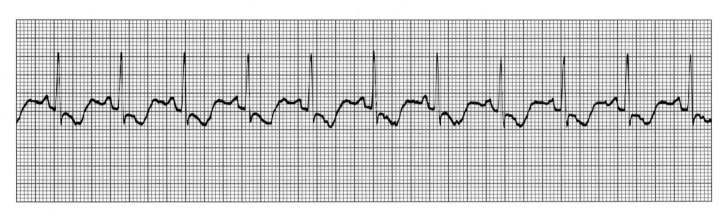

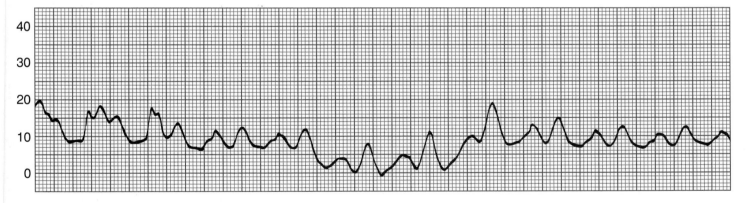

PRACTICE WAVEFORM 2–6. *Analysis:* This pulmonary artery tracing changes to a PCWP waveform. Again, note some movement in the baseline. Try to identify a stable location (consistent waveforms) to read the PCWP value. The A wave is found near the end of the QRS complex, the V wave late in the T–P interval.

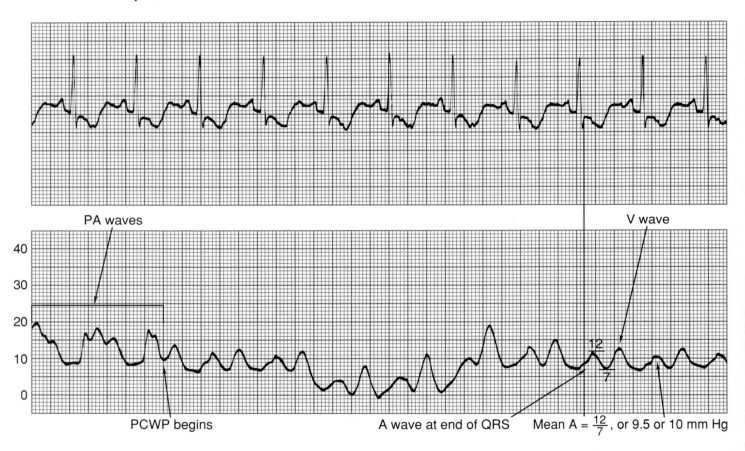

PRACTICE WAVEFORM 2–7. Identify if this tracing is a CVP or PCWP waveform.

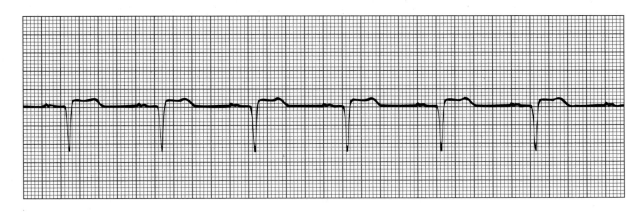

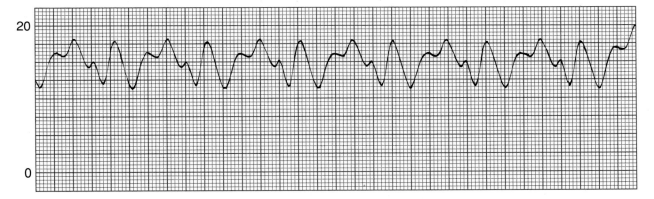

PRACTICE WAVEFORM 2–7. *Analysis:* This waveform requires you to understand the normal ECG correlation with venous waveforms. Because an A wave is found in the P–R interval, this is a normal CVP tracing. Clear C and V waves are also seen.

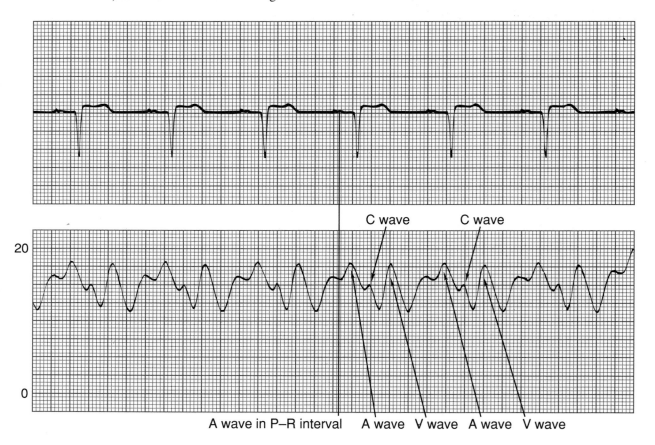

3 Abnormal Pulmonary Capillary Wedge and Central Venous Pressure Waveforms

Detecting abnormal venous waveforms (central venous pressure [CVP] and pulmonary capillary wedge pressure [PCWP] waves) has many clinical implications, including identifying (1) abnormal valve function, (2) the effect of dysrhythmias on waveform interpretation, and (3) changes in hemodynamic stability. The goal of this chapter is to illustrate the key abnormalities encountered in critical care settings relative to venous waves. Variations in A and V waves and the potential clinical implications of correct interpretation will serve as the basis for this chapter.

One important point should first be emphasized. Waveforms with abnormalities in the A, C, and V waves require correlation with the electrocardiogram (ECG). Reading waveforms directly from the monitor may be inaccurate unless simultaneous ECG and waveform freeze is possible. No monitor is capable of reading waveforms based on ECG correlation at this point. Until such a feature is available, use of a two-channel strip recorder is necessary in waveform analysis.

A WAVE VARIATIONS

Two common conditions will increase atrial pressure and make the A wave become abnormally large, subsequently failing to reflect ventricular end-diastolic pressure: (1) loss of atrioventricular (A-V) synchrony and (2) mitral or tricuspid stenosis. In addition, loss of the A wave can occur, resulting in the loss of the standard marker for estimating ventricular end-diastolic pressure. Absence of the A wave is due to dysrhythmias, e.g., atrial fibrillation, where no effective atrial contraction is present. Each of these conditions, excessively large A waves and loss of the A wave, requires correct identification in order to accurately estimate ventricular pressures.

53

Large A Waves Secondary to Loss of Atrioventricular Synchrony

The two conditions that will commonly increase atrial pressure and the size of the A wave are both related to A-V (mitral or tricuspid) valve function. When an A-V dissociation dysrhythmia exists, the loss of A-V synchrony may be present, causing the potential for giant A waves. Dysrhythmias that may cause giant A waves include second- or third-degree block, atrial premature beats or atrial tachycardias with block, premature ventricular contractions (PVCs), ventricular tachycardia, and junctional and paced rhythms. Waveforms 3–1 through 3–3 illustrate how dysrhythmias can produce large A waves.

When atrial contraction is delayed, it may occur simultaneously with ventricular contraction. The atrium cannot force blood past the now closed mitral or tricuspid valve and into the ventricle. The result is an increase in atrial pressure and the forcing of blood back into the inferior and superior vena cava. The pressure monitor sees this event as an extra large A wave (Fig. 3–1). Physically the patient may be noted to have venous pulsations, particularly in the jugular veins, during these blocked atrial contractions.[23]

Two compelling reasons for identifying large A waves exist.

1. Noting the large A wave is necessary for correct interpretation of the CVP or PCWP reading. Because the large A wave will not approximate ventricular end-diastolic volume, it should be avoided during analysis and interpretation. Waveform 3–4 illustrates the correct interpretation of tracings with large A waves. The clinician must keep in mind that the monitor cannot differentiate normal from abnormal A waves.

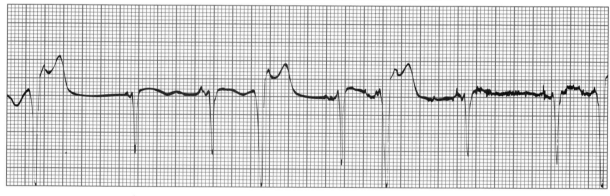

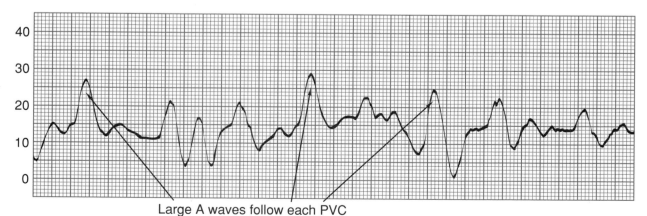

Large A waves follow each PVC

Waveform 3–1. PVCs induce large A waves in a CVP tracing.

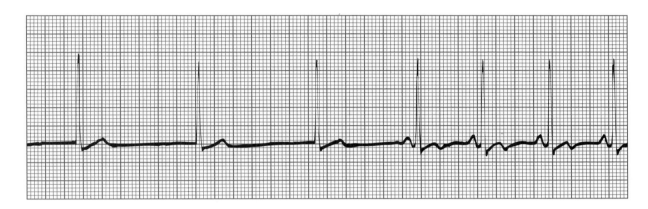

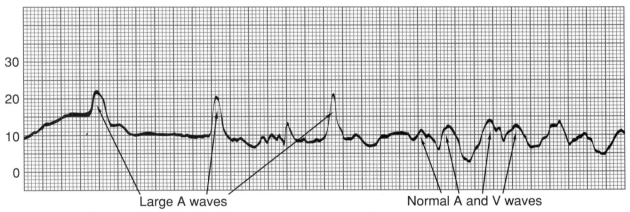

Large A waves   Normal A and V waves

Waveform 3–2. Large A waves with a junctional rhythm. Normal C waves return with return of sinus rhythm (normal A-V synchrony).

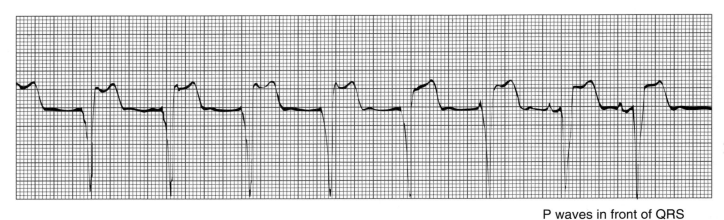

P waves in front of QRS

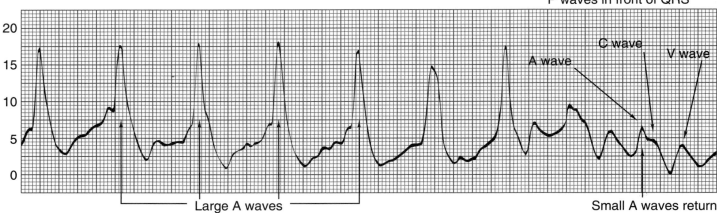

Waveform 3–3. Paced rhythm with large A waves until coincidental re-establishment of A-V synchrony.

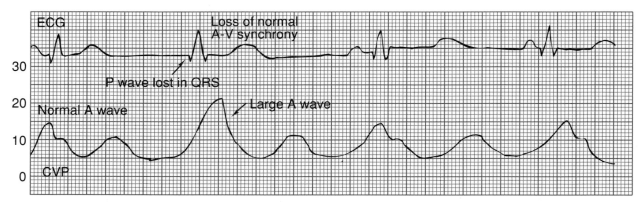

Figure 3–1. Simultaneous atrial and ventricular contraction producing a large A wave.

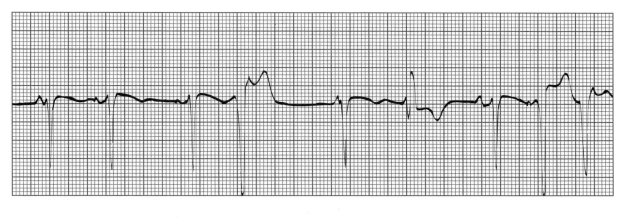

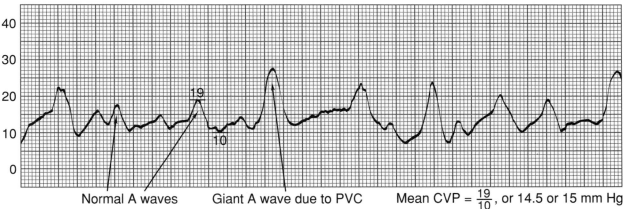

Normal A waves   Giant A wave due to PVC   Mean CVP = $\frac{19}{10}$, or 14.5 or 15 mm Hg

Waveform 3–4. Analysis of a CVP with large A wave. Identify ECG pattern with normal P-QRS relationship and read the A wave beneath the normal P–R interval.

2. The waveform can also be used to indicate the existence of a dysrhythmia as well as its potential hemodynamic implications. When a large A wave is noted, loss of atrial contribution to the cardiac output occurs.[24] An atrial tachycardia without loss of A-V synchrony can sometimes be differentiated from ventricular tachycardia by the presence of large A waves in the ventricular tachycardia pattern. In addition, the potential effect of the loss of atrial contribution is a reduction in the the cardiac output. If the effect is substantial, a reduction in blood pressure (BP) can occur (Waveform 3–5). Pacemakers in a VVI mode can produce reduced blood pressure and cardiac output because A-V synchrony may be lost.

If the effect of the dysrhythmia is not correlated with changing waveforms and the subsequent potential changes in pressures, treatment may incorrectly center on increasing the blood pressure with inotropes or vasopressors rather than on treating the A-V synchrony disturbance.

When the clinician is interpreting the PCWP, one indication that an A wave is abnormal in size is when the mean of the A wave is larger than the pulmonary artery (PA) mean pressure. Theoretically, the PA mean must be higher than the mean A wave pressure. If, when reading the A wave, you find that the mean is higher than the PA mean, it would be prudent to investigate potential causes for abnormal A waves.

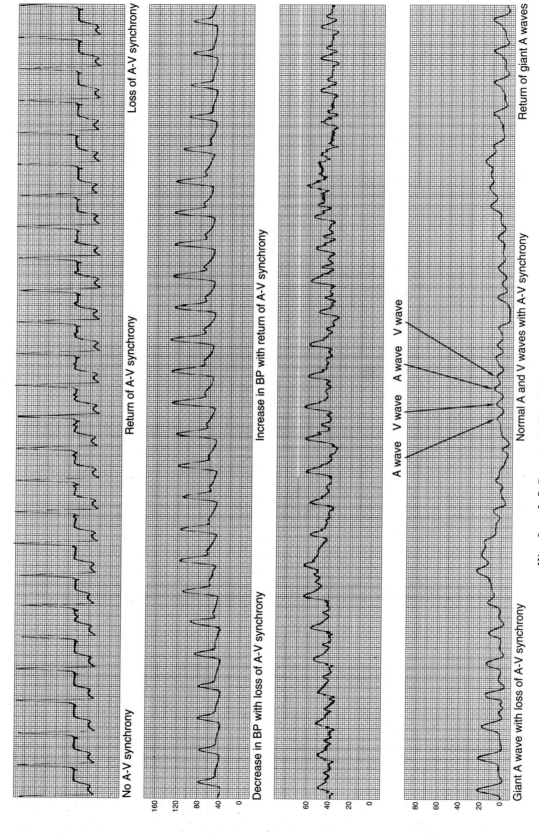

No A-V synchrony

Return of A-V synchrony

Loss of A-V synchrony

Decrease in BP with loss of A-V synchrony

Increase in BP with return of A-V synchrony

Giant A wave with loss of A-V synchrony

A wave   V wave   A wave   V wave

Normal A and V waves with A-V synchrony

Return of giant A waves

Waveform 3–5. Decrease in BP with loss of A-V synchrony.

58

Large A Waves Secondary to Mitral or Tricuspid Stenosis

Circumstances in which the A wave may be abnormally elevated, in the absence of dysrhythmias, include mitral or tricupsid valve stenosis. If the atrium has difficulty pushing blood past either valve, atrial pressure facing the involved valve will increase, resulting in a large A wave. Interpretation is the same as mentioned above. Clues that mitral or tricuspid stenosis might exist include physical assessment indicating a diastolic murmur. Echocardiography, due to its ability to identify valvular function, is an excellent modality for indicating the potential presence of an abnormal A wave. Another method to identify when the A wave does not reflect end-diastolic pressure is possible if the patient has had a cardiac catheterization. Note the catheterization pressures and observe if atrial pressures are correlating with ventricular end-diastolic pressures. If mitral or tricuspid stenosis exists, reading the mean of the A wave may not accurately represent ventricular pressures.

The problem faced in mitral or tricuspid stenosis centers on the inability to use PCWP or CVP readings to estimate pressures. If the large A wave associated with stenosis is present, do not use the PCWP or CVP for treatment decisions. Keep in mind that the A wave now reveals only that the ventricular end-diastolic pressure is lower than the mean A wave. How much lower is unknown without ventricular catheterization. If primary or secondary active pulmonary hypertension does not exist, the diastolic pulmonary artery pressure may be used for estimating the LVEDP (see Chapter 2). For tricuspid stenosis, pulmonary artery catheters with right ventricular ports should be substituted for CVP readings if this is feasible.

Loss of A Waves

The most common reason for the loss of the A wave is loss of atrial contraction. Dysrhythmias producing this situation include junctional or ventricular rhythms and atrial fibrillation. If the A wave is absent, estimation of ventricular end-diastolic pressures can be attempted through ECG correlation. Considering that end diastole occurs near the end of the QRS complex, noting the pressure at the end of the QRS should give an approximate value of ventricular pressure (Fig. 3–2). This is referred to as a pre–V wave interpretation.[25]

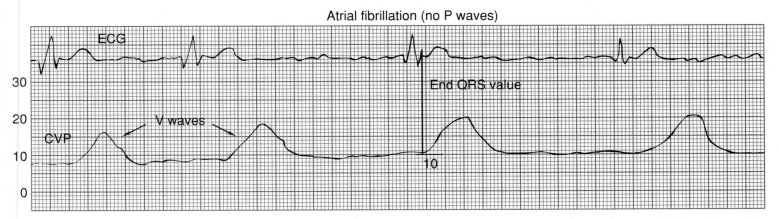

Figure 3–2. When both P and A waves are absent, end QRS most closely approximates ventricular end-diastolic pressure.

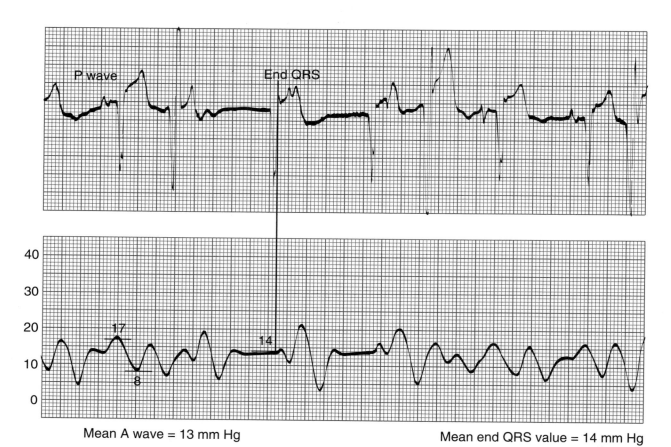

Mean A wave = 13 mm Hg   Mean end QRS value = 14 mm Hg

Waveform 3–6. Reading CVP tracing with frequent ectopic beats. Read beneath sinus beats that have abnormal A-V relationship. Alternatively, read at the end of the QRS in junctional beats. Values will be approximately the same.

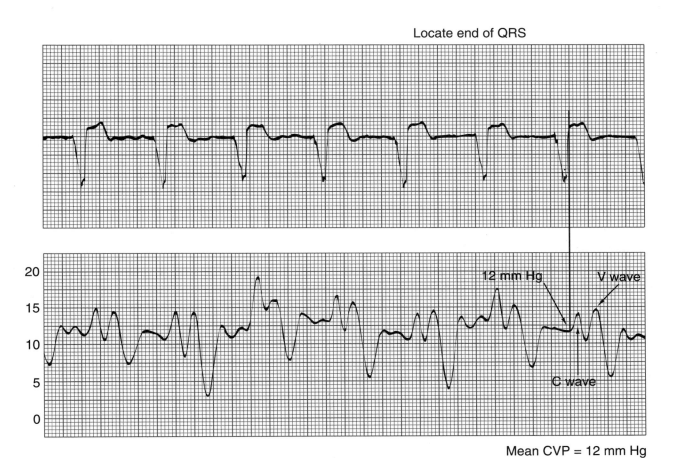

Waveform 3–7. Reading a CVP in a paced rhythm. End-QRS values give best approximation of ventricular end-diastolic value.

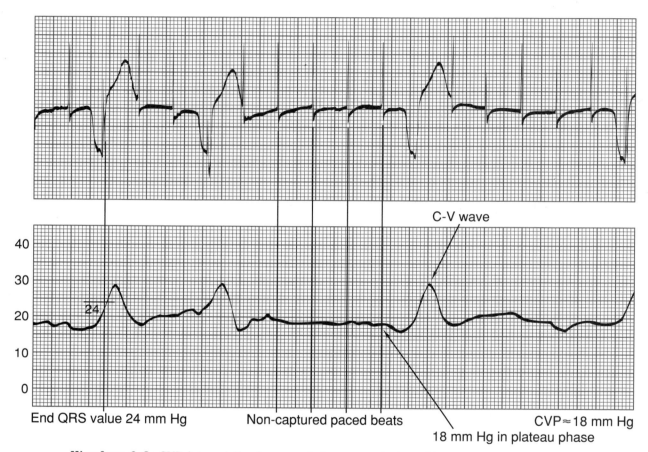

Waveform 3–8. CVP interpretation in a ventricular escape rhythm with a noncapturing pacemaker. Prolonged plateau between beats generates a value of about 18 mm Hg. End QRS value is about 25 mm Hg. Plateau value is probably more accurate owing to increased equilibration time between atria and ventricles from the slow rate.

During the above dysrhythmias, care must be taken not to read incorrect waves, such as V or large C waves. As long as the ECG is used as the guide, inappropriate waves, e.g., C and V waves, can be avoided and correct interpretation is still possible. Waveforms 3–6 through 3–8 illustrate clinical conditions that may produce loss of A waves and demonstrate methods of interpretation.

LARGE V WAVES

Large or "giant" V waves are not uncommon in clinical settings. Perhaps the most common cause is mitral (for PCWP readings) or tricuspid (for CVP readings) incompetence, although noncompliant atria are also likely causes (Fig. 3–3). Large V waves may be due to actual valvular injury or valves that have become incompetent through left ventricular (LV) stretching as LV failure develops. Clinically, one sees large V waves at the onset of LV failure. The appearance of the large V waves may occur before clinical symptoms present.

One point that makes utilizing the V wave as a marker of valvular incompetence or LV failure difficult is the inconsistency with which the giant V wave occurs in these conditions.[26] However, if the V wave appears to increase in the patient with LV failure, an acute episode of failure may be imminent. The absence of giant V waves does not mean failure is absent. The likely reason for the inconsistency in variations is atrial compliance, which will be presented in more depth later in this chapter.

The key to identifying abnormal V waves is locating the waves in the T–P interval. With CVP readings, the V wave is closer to the T wave, whereas with PCWP tracings, the V is closer to the P wave. Figure 3–4 illustrates the ECG and V wave correlations with CVP and PCWP tracings. Waveforms 3–9 through 3–11 illustrate identification and mapping of giant V waves.

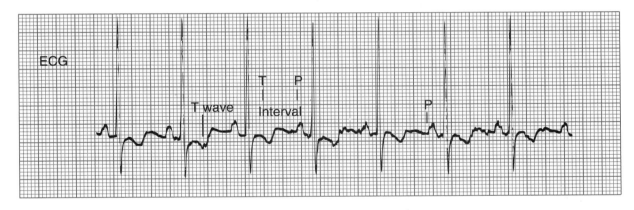

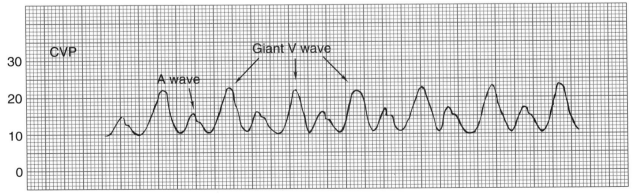

Figure 3–3. Giant V waves, possibly due to mitral regurgitation or a noncompliant (stiff) atrium.

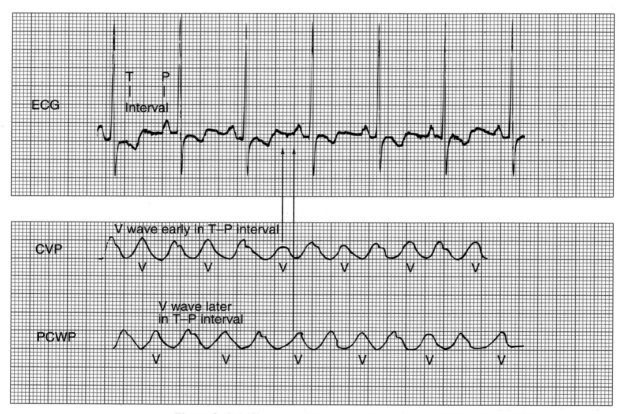

Figure 3–4. Difference in V wave location between a CVP and a PCWP tracing.

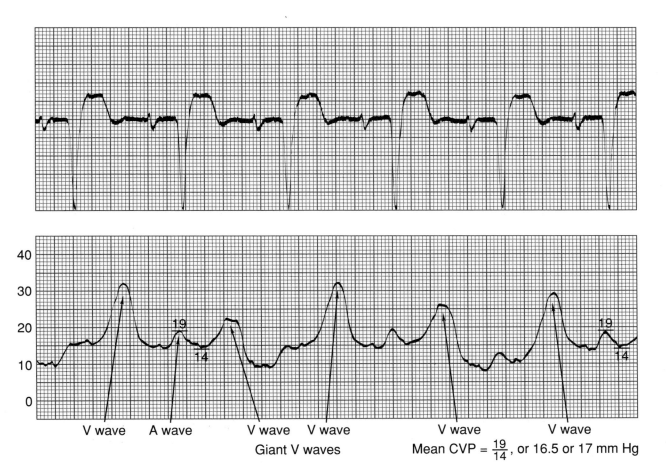

Waveform 3–9. Giant V waves in a PCWP tracing. Avoid reading V waves in the PCWP interpretation.

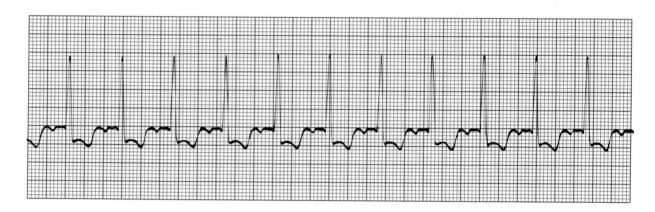

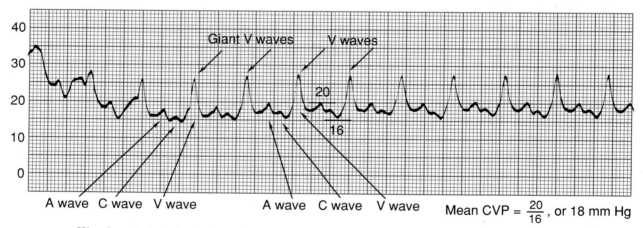

Waveform 3–10. Giant V waves in a CVP tracing. Locate and determine the mean of the A wave.

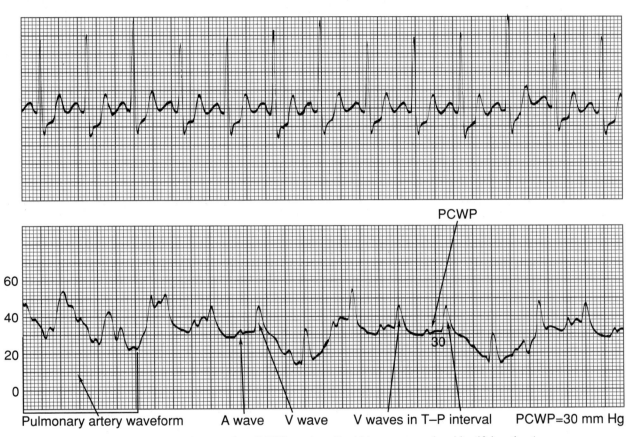

Waveform 3–11. Large V waves in a PCWP tracing. Rapid heart rate makes identifying the A wave more difficult.

Large V waves are not, however, present only with valvular incompetence. Several studies have demonstrated the presence of large V waves in the absence of mitral or tricuspid dysfunction.[27–29] Clinically one can note the absence of systolic murmurs when V waves are present on the venous waveform. If mitral or tricuspid dysfunction were present, a systolic murmur should be present. The likely mechanism of large V waves in the absence of A-V valve dysfunction is differences in atrial compliance. In a chronically distended atrium, such as in patients with repeated bouts of congestive heart failure, large volume changes may not produce substantial pressure changes. This is due to the highly compliant atrium, already stretched due to chronic volume overload. In an acutely distended atrium, the atrial muscle is unaccustomed to distention, and small increases in volume may produce large pressure changes. A condition in which one may find an acutely distended atrium would be acute myocardial infarction with accompanying left ventricular failure in patients without prior heart disease.

The exact reason for all V wave abnormalities is not always clear. Under most circumstances, however, the regurgitation of blood into the atrium during ventricular systole or a noncompliant atrium will account for most of the large V waves.

Waveforms 3–12A and B were generated by a patient with a normal PCWP tracing who, with the onset of chest pain, developed large V waves. This patient had no evidence, either with physical assessment or with echocardiography, of mitral dysfunction. In this case, the large V wave heralded the onset of left ventricular failure.

The large V wave can present several types of clinical problems. Most commonly, the large V will generate erroneously high venous pressures if it is used in the CVP or PCWP interpretation. The V wave has less correlation with the end-diastolic ventricular pressures than the A wave and to use it when measuring the venous pressures will lead to incorrect values.[30]

The large V wave can manifest itself in the PA tracing as well as in the PCWP or CVP. Waveform 3–13 indicates how a large V can give the PA tracing an M appearance. If the V to V distance is plotted, one can trace the V in the PA into the PCWP. Noting this reflected V in the PA tracing will prevent erroneous readings of systolic PA values when the V is very large.

In the clinical setting, when the V is very large, masking of the PA tracing can occur. In Waveform 3–14, the tracing was interpreted as being unable to wedge. On closer inspection of the tracing, however, one can note the large V in the T–P interval, near the beginning of the P wave. The systolic of the PA is after the QRS and not in the T–P interval. Recognizing the large V can forestall the assumption that the catheter was unable to wedge and the subsequent manipulation of the PA catheter. Note the inability of the monitor value to coincide with the accurate PCWP value (mean of 34 from the monitor vs 19 from the paper).

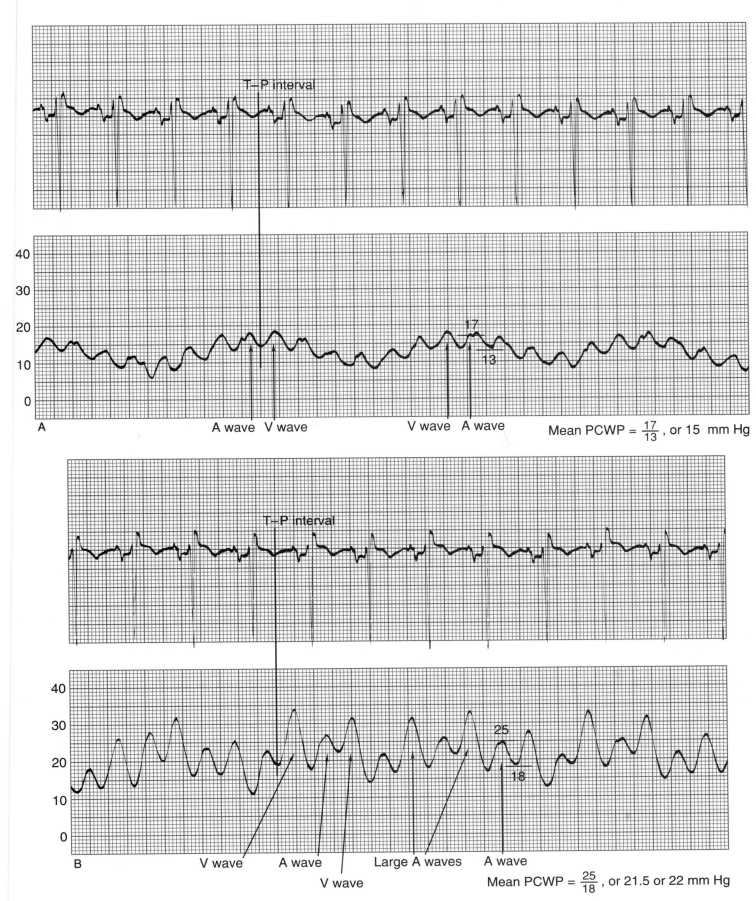

Waveform 3–12. Changes in PCWP tracing with the development of chest pain. *A*, The PCWP when the patient is free of pain. *B*, The PCWP when chest pain develops.

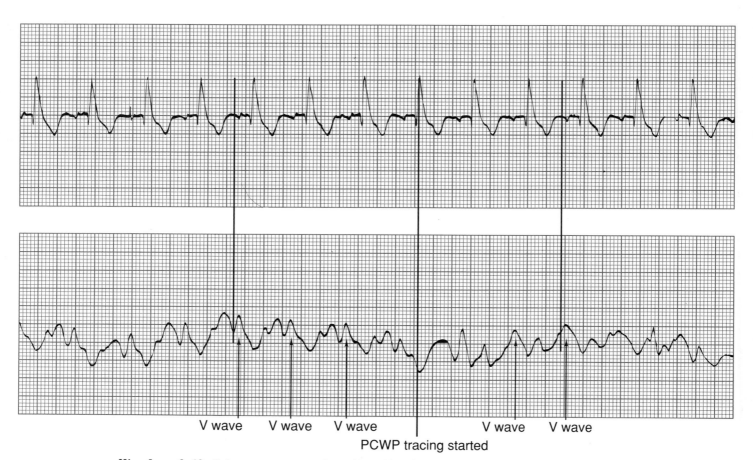

V wave   V wave   V wave   V wave   V wave

PCWP tracing started

Waveform 3–13. Pulmonary artery tracing with artifact from large V waves. Note large V waves corresponding to beginning of P wave (end of T–P interval) on both PA and PCWP tracings.

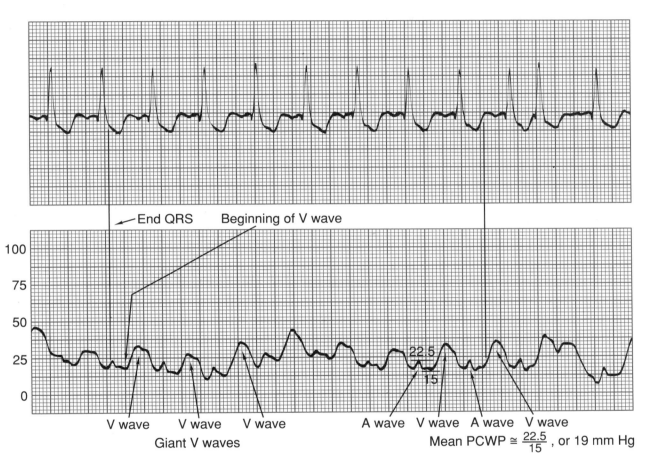

Waveform 3–14. A giant V wave that was mistaken to be a pulmonary artery waveform. Note the large V wave starts too late after the end of the QRS complex to be an arterial wave.

SUMMARY

Variations seen in venous tracings, i.e., CVP and PCWP, are a potential source of error. Only with careful interpretation of the venous tracings can accurate data be obtained for the assessment of hemodynamics. Correct interpretation centers on identifying abnormal waves and avoiding using inappropriate waveform values. Abnormalities in both A and V waves were presented in this chapter, with the emphasis on identification of abnormal waves. Through identification of abnormal waves, a better approximation of accurate assessment of ventricular function is likely through venous waveform analysis.

PRACTICE WAVEFORMS

Practice Waveforms 3–1 through 3–9 present examples of abnormal waveforms introduced in this chapter. Practice interpreting these waveforms to assist your ability to identify abnormal venous (CVP and PCWP) tracings.

PRACTICE WAVEFORM 3–1. Waveform from the distal port. Is this a pulmonary arterial waveform or a PCWP tracing?

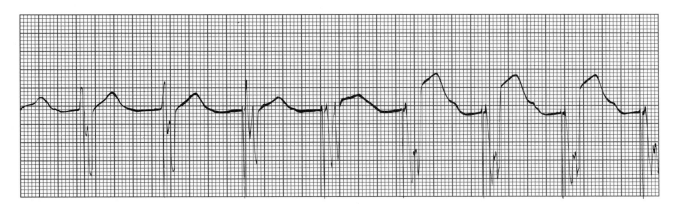

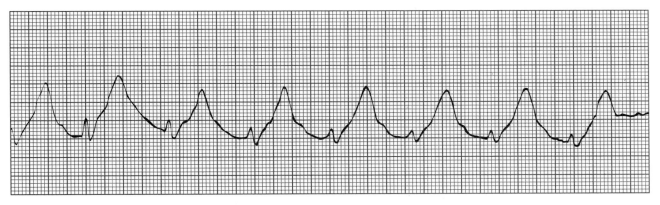

PRACTICE WAVEFORM 3–1. *Analysis:* This is a PCWP tracing. A large V wave is present late in the T–P interval, suggesting a PCWP rather than a PA waveform. The PCWP value is read near the end of the QRS complex due to the absence of an A wave (no P wave is present). Presystolic wave is not an A wave.

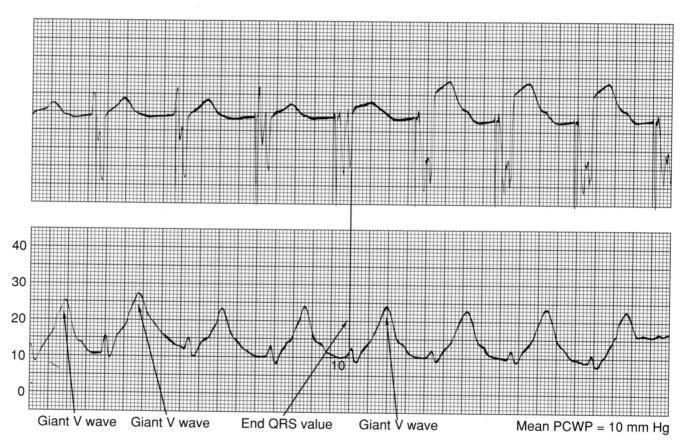

Giant V wave   Giant V wave   End QRS value   Giant V wave   Mean PCWP = 10 mm Hg

PRACTICE WAVEFORM 3–2. Tracing from the proximal port. Where is the tracing read?

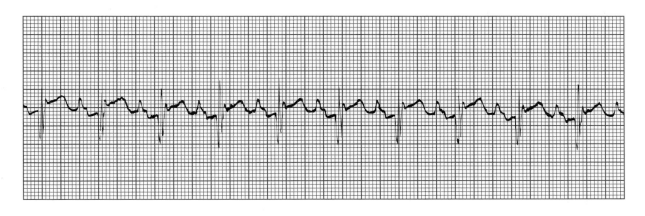

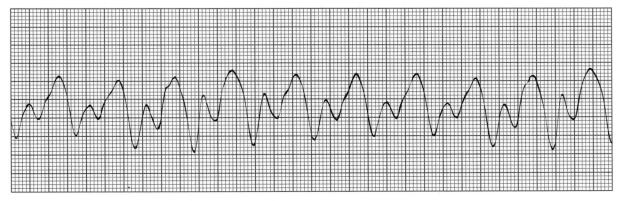

PRACTICE WAVEFORM 3–2. *Analysis:* This is a CVP tracing with large V waves. The value is obtained by finding the A wave in the P–R interval and determining the mean of the A wave.

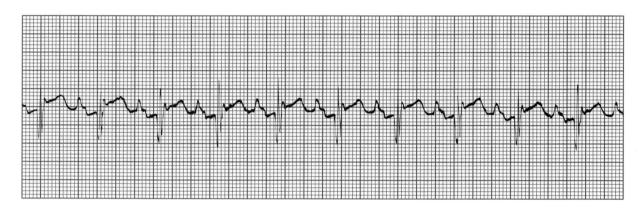

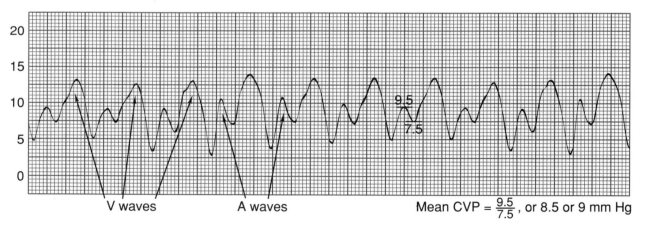

V waves   A waves   Mean CVP = $\frac{9.5}{7.5}$, or 8.5 or 9 mm Hg

PRACTICE WAVEFORM 3–3. In the PCWP tracing, where would the waveform be read inasmuch as no P wave is present?

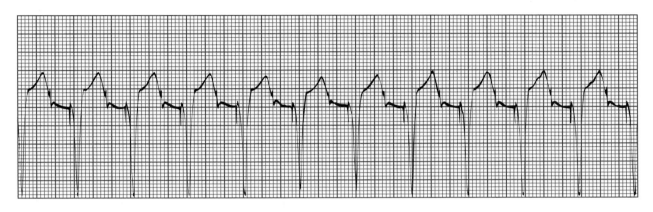

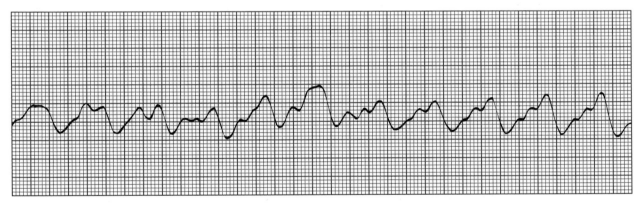

PRACTICE WAVEFORM 3–3. *Analysis:* Because no clear P wave exists, read the PCWP at the end of the QRS complex. V waves are larger than A waves in this tracing.

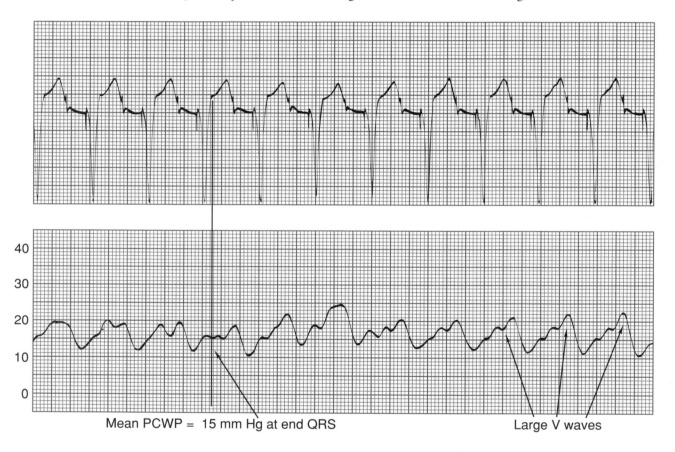

Mean PCWP = 15 mm Hg at end QRS   Large V waves

PRACTICE WAVEFORM 3–4. A large scale diminishes the waveform appearance in this tracing. Where would this CVP tracing be read?

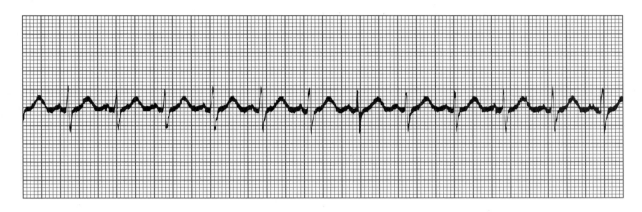

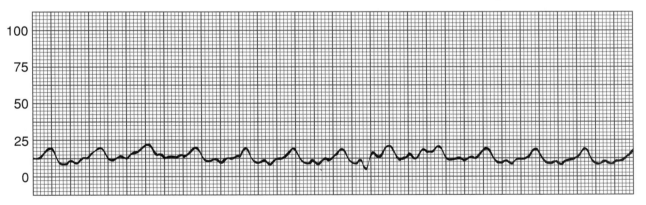

PRACTICE WAVEFORM 3–4. *Analysis:* The A wave is less clear because of the large scale. The V wave is larger than the A wave. Locate the A wave in the P–R interval.

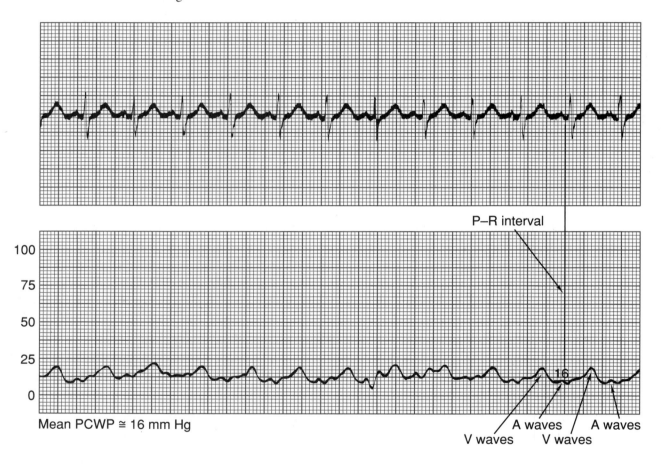

P–R interval

100
75
50
25
0

16

Mean PCWP ≅ 16 mm Hg

A waves   A waves
V waves   V waves

PRACTICE WAVEFORM 3–5. Where would this CVP tracing be interpreted? Note the ECG rhythm when assessing this rhythm.

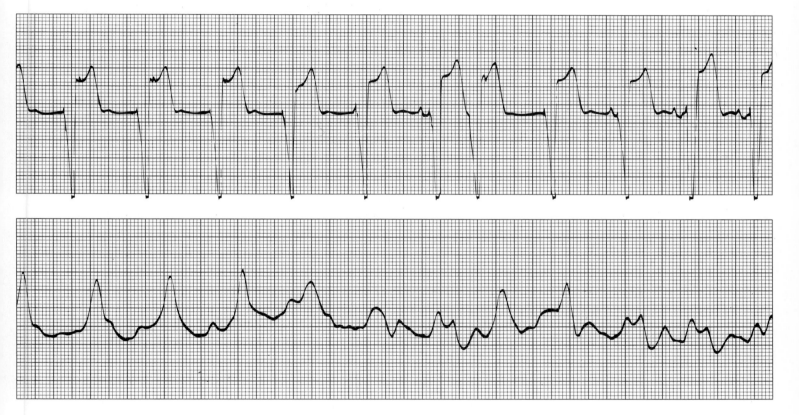

PRACTICE WAVEFORM 3–5. *Analysis:* Two methods for reading this waveform exist. (1) Find a normal A-V synchrony pattern. In this case, a normal P–R interval should be present. (2) In the paced rhythm, find the end of the QRS complex and locate the value at this point.

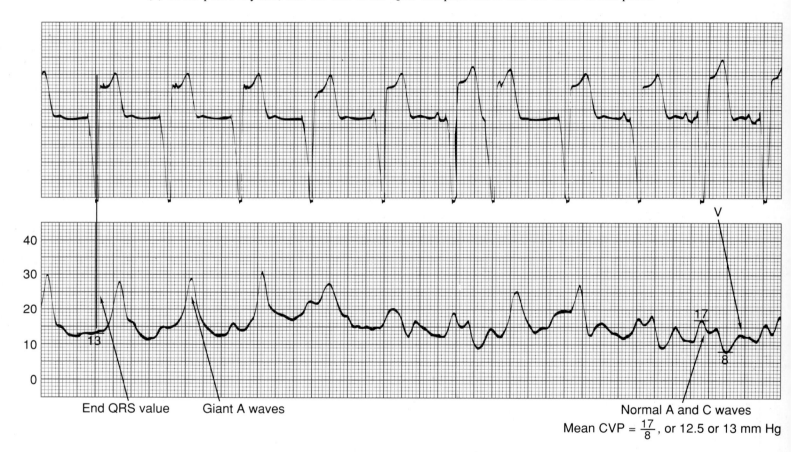

End QRS value   Giant A waves

Normal A and C waves

Mean CVP = $\frac{17}{8}$, or 12.5 or 13 mm Hg

PRACTICE WAVEFORM 3–6. Upon inflation of the balloon to obtain a PCWP tracing, the following tracing appears. Where would you read this PCWP value?

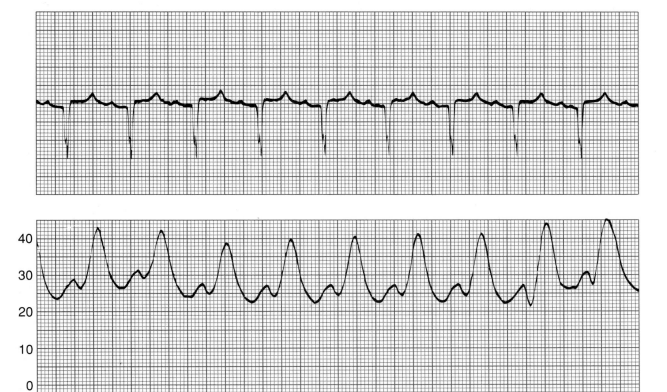

PRACTICE WAVEFORM 3–6. *Analysis:* A giant V wave exists in this tracing as noted by the large wave in the T–P interval. The smaller A wave is near the end QRS. Read this smaller A wave for the PCWP value.

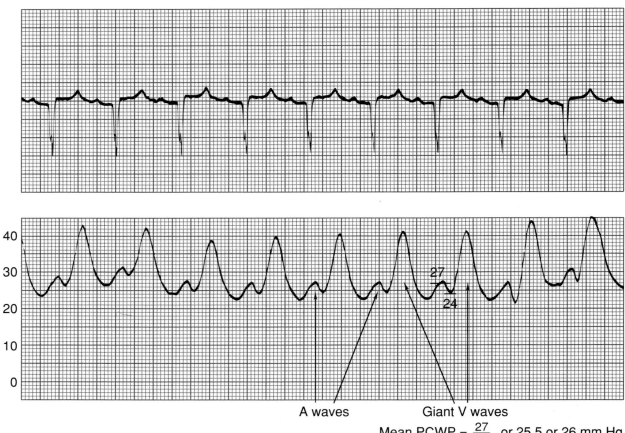

A waves   Giant V waves

Mean PCWP = $\frac{27}{24}$, or 25.5 or 26 mm Hg

PRACTICE WAVEFORM 3–7. Tracing from the distal port. What is the tracing and the value?

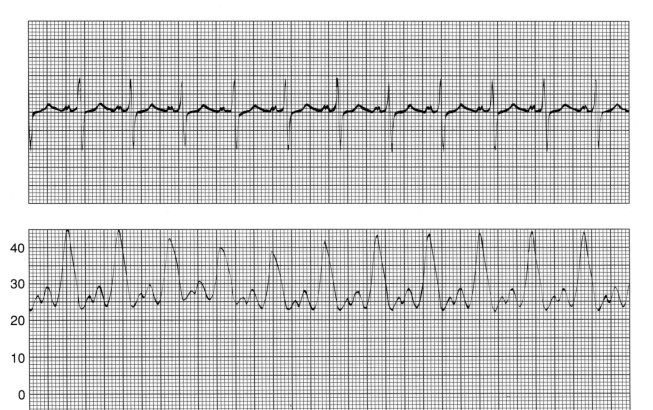

PRACTICE WAVEFORM 3–7. *Analysis:* This is a PCWP tracing with a giant V wave. The V wave starts after the T wave, too late for an arterial upstroke. The A wave is found at the end of the QRS complex.

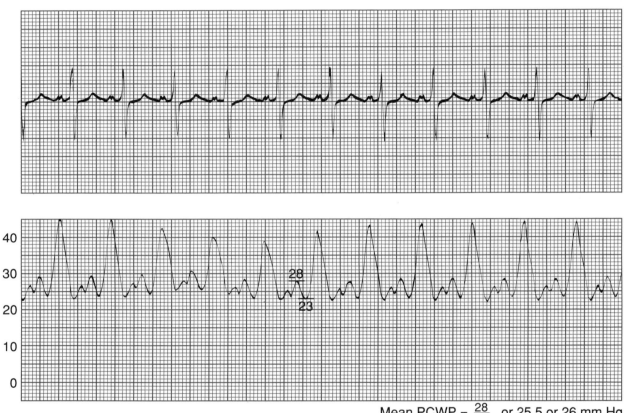

Mean PCWP = $\frac{28}{23}$, or 25.5 or 26 mm Hg

PRACTICE WAVEFORM 3–8. What is the value in this PCWP tracing?

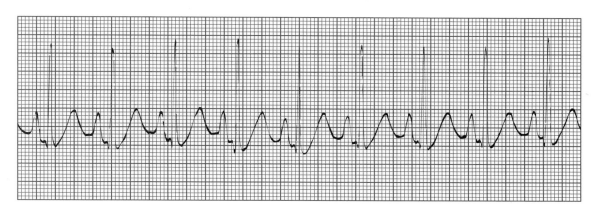

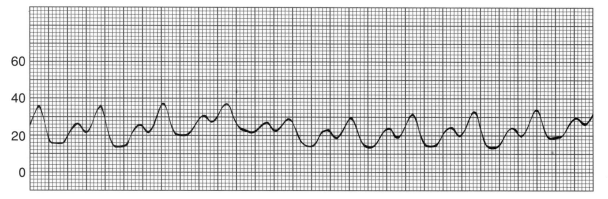

PRACTICE WAVEFORM 3–8. *Analysis:* Note the V wave is larger than the A wave in this tracing. Find the A wave at the end of the QRS complex to obtain this PCWP value.

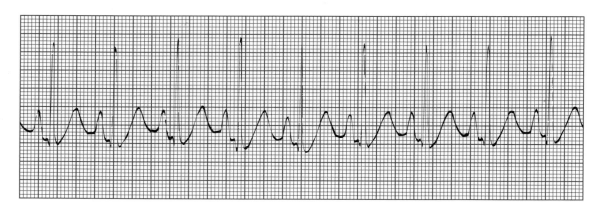

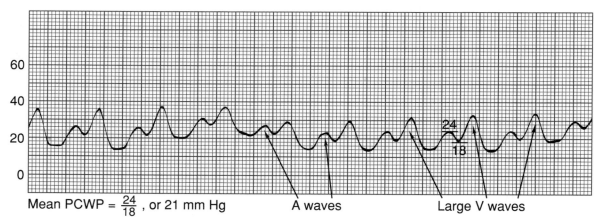

Mean PCWP = $\frac{24}{18}$, or 21 mm Hg   A waves   Large V waves

PRACTICE WAVEFORM 3–9. In this CVP tracing, multiple PVCs are present. Where would you read this CVP waveform?

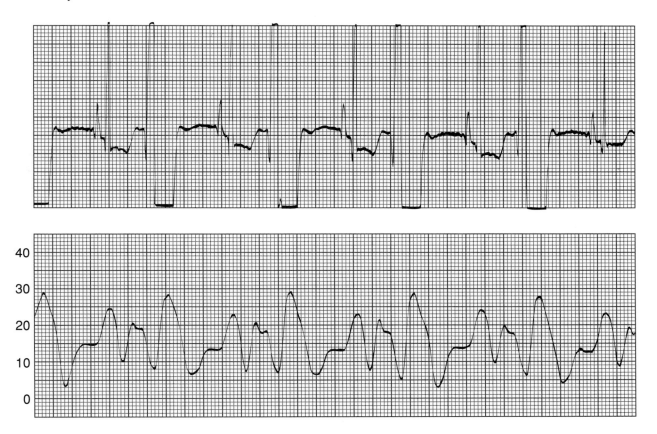

PRACTICE WAVEFORM 3–9. *Analysis:* Note the giant A waves after each PVC. Avoid these giant A waves. Note a normal P–R interval and read the A wave beneath this normal P–R interval.

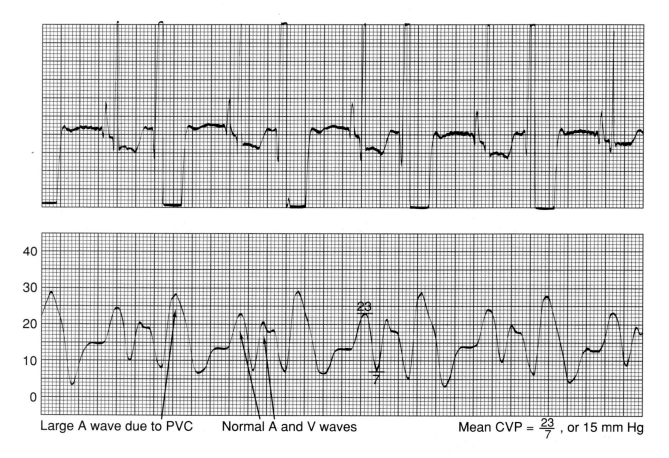

Large A wave due to PVC   Normal A and V waves   Mean CVP = $\frac{23}{7}$, or 15 mm Hg

4 : Normal Arterial Waveforms

Arterial waveforms are generated from the pulsatile changes in the left and right ventricles. Arterial waveforms can be categorized as systemic if generated from the left ventricle or pulmonary if from the right ventricle. For the purpose of this chapter, ventricular waveforms are also considered a type of arterial waveform. Interpretation of each arterial waveform, whether ventricular, systemic, or pulmonary, is similar with only a few differences. The focus of this chapter is to review principles associated with interpretation of each type of normal arterial waveform.

Three arterial pressure waveforms will be presented: pulmonary, right ventricular, and systemic (or peripheral). In general, all arterial waveforms are a result of ventricular contraction and relaxation. Because arterial waveforms have the same origin, i.e., from a ventricular contraction, each has similar components in the pressure tracing. Waveforms 4–1 and 4–2 are examples of normal pulmonary (PA) and peripheral arterial tracings. Differences exist, however, between waveforms. These differences are necessary to know in order to correctly interpret arterial waveforms.

MEASURING ARTERIAL SYSTOLIC AND DIASTOLIC VALUES

Arterial waveforms emanate from the pulse pressure created by ventricular systole and diastole. When interpreting arterial tracings, the clinician measures two pressures, the peak systolic and end-diastolic pressure.

Just as with venous waveforms, arterial waveforms should be interpreted in conjunction with the electrocardiogram (ECG). In respect to the ECG tracing, the arterial diastolic pressure correlates with the end of the QRS complex for pulmonary and ventricular waveforms; for the systemic waveforms, it correlates with the end of the T wave or about 0.2 second after the end of the QRS.[31] A slight difference is noted between systemic (or peripheral) and pulmonary arterial pressures in regard to the onset of diastole, due to the location of the sensing catheters.

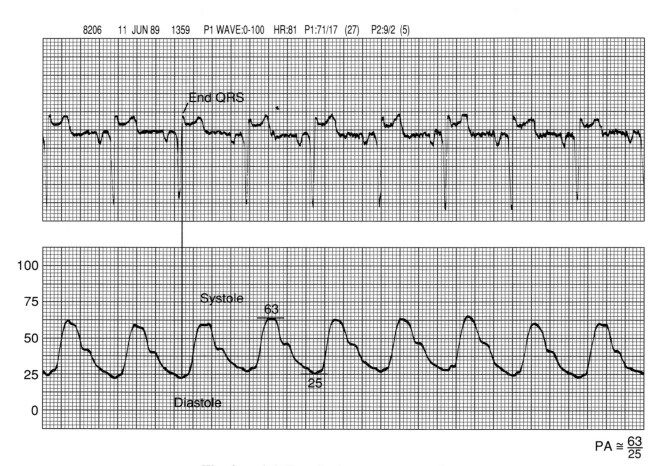

Waveform 4–1. Normal pulmonary artery waveform.

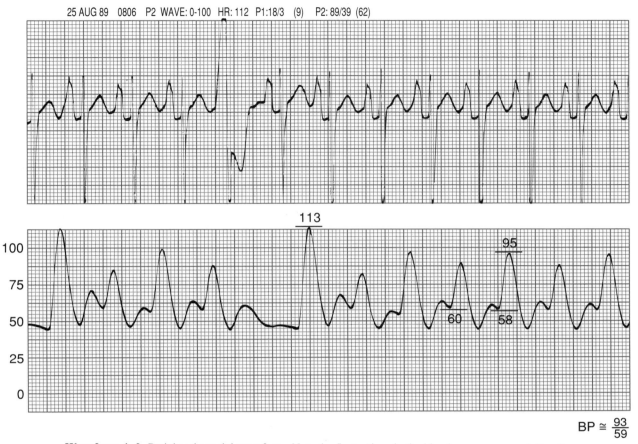

25 AUG 89   0806   P2 WAVE: 0-100   HR: 112   P1:18/3   (9)   P2: 89/39 (62)

$$BP \cong \frac{93}{59}$$

Waveform 4–2. Peripheral arterial waveform. Note the fluctuations in the blood pressure, especially after a premature ventricular contraction. These values are real, not artifact, and should be included in the blood pressure determination.

The pulmonary arterial waveform is sensed from a catheter immediately inside the pulmonary artery. Impulse transmission to the transducer is rapid with a pulmonary artery catheter. Systemic catheters, with the exception of intra-aortic catheters, are more distal from the heart, causing a delay in impulse transmission (Fig. 4–1). The difference in catheter-sensed pressures will be presented in more depth later in the chapter.

The QRS complex, representing ventricular depolarization, occurs prior to ventricular contraction. Ventricular systole, the period of the cardiac cycle between the closure of the atrioventricular valves and the closure of the semilunar valves, causes a sharp upstroke in the pulse pressure tracing. The upstroke occurs as blood is ejected into the aorta and pulmonary artery. This upstroke is noted to begin immediately after the end of the QRS complex (Fig. 4–2).

Ventricular diastole, the period of the cardiac cycle between the opening and the closure of the atrioventricular valves, is signified by ventricular relaxation. Upon ventricular relaxation, the waveform shows a fall in intraventricular pressure to levels at or below the atrial pressure.[32] On the downslope of this pressure curve is an incisura, notably the dicrotic notch (Waveform 4–3).[33]

The dicrotic notch on the pulmonary and aortic waveforms is the result of pulmonic and aortic valve closure, respectively. The dicrotic notch may or may not be present on the arterial tracing. Waveform 4–4 demonstrates an arterial waveform without a dicrotic notch.

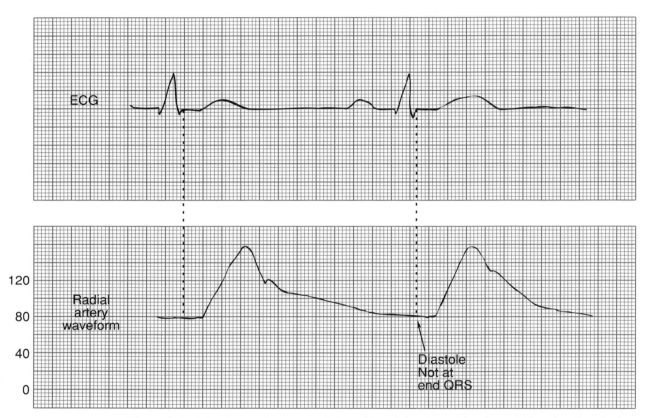

Figure 4–1. Delay in waveform transmission with peripheral arterial catheters. Note that diastole does not immediately follow the end of the QRS complex (delays of about 0.2 sec are common).

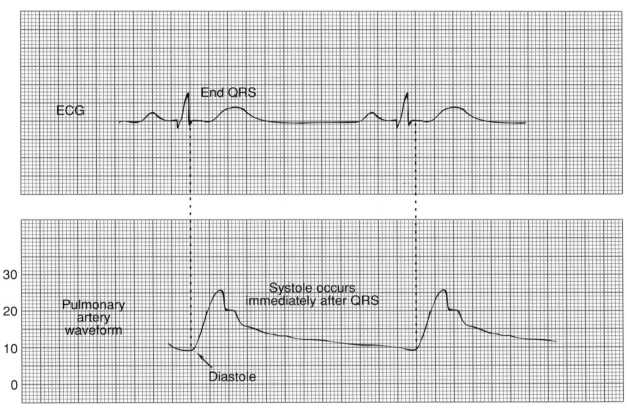

Figure 4–2. How to read a PA waveform. Note that diastole is immediately below the end of the QRS complex.

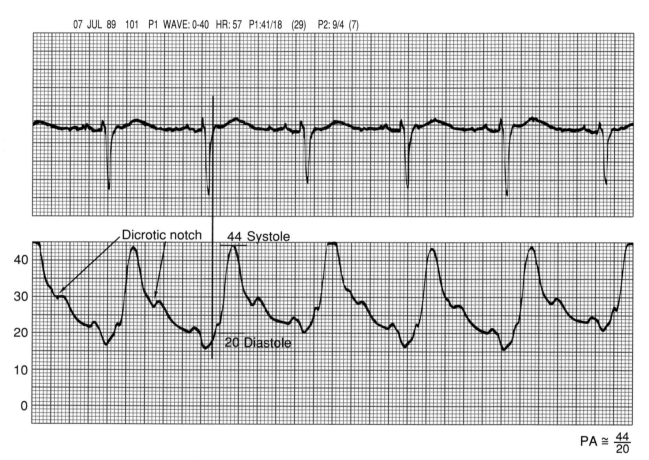

Dicrotic notch   44 Systole

20 Diastole

$$PA \cong \frac{44}{20}$$

Waveform 4–3. Dicrotic notch in the PA waveform.

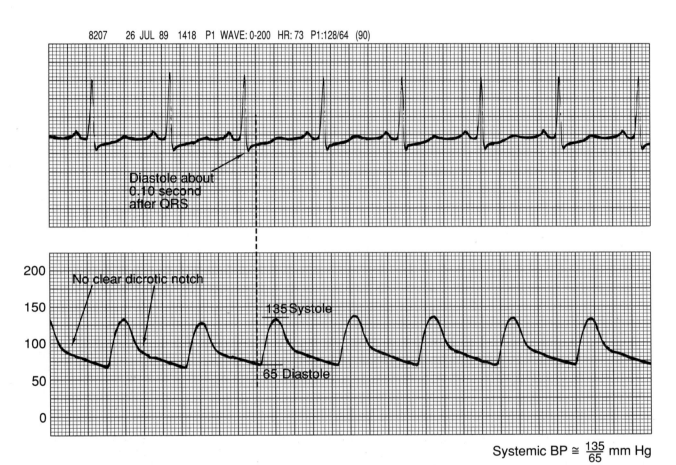

8207   26 JUL 89   1418   P1 WAVE: 0-200   HR: 73   P1:128/64 (90)

Diastole about
0.10 second
after QRS

200

No clear dicrotic notch

150   135 Systole

100

65 Diastole

50

0

Systemic BP ≅ $\frac{135}{65}$ mm Hg

Waveform 4–4. Radial arterial waveform without a clear dicrotic notch.

Aortic and systemic arterial pulse pressures are measured by intra-aortic catheters and peripheral arterial catheters, respectively. Pulmonary arterial and right ventricular (RV) pulse pressures are measured via the pulmonary artery (PA) catheter. The pulmonary arterial pressure is usually monitored continuously, whereas the RV pressure is measured during PA catheter placement as the distal tip passes through the right ventricle. RV pressures can be monitored continuously with right ventricular ports normally utilized for pacemaking features.

VENTRICULAR WAVEFORMS

The RV pressure tracing reflects RV diastolic and systolic pressures (Waveform 4–5). Approximately 60% of the right ventricle is filled during early rapid filling, causing a rapid upstroke in the pulse pressure tracing. A slow period follows, with 25% of RV filling occurring.[34] The slow period results in a rise in pressure at the end of diastole. This rise in pressure helps distinguish a ventricular from a pulmonary artery waveform.

When the RV pressure drops below the pulmonary pressure, the pulmonic valve closes, ending RV emptying. As blood flows through the pulmonary artery and veins into the left atrium and ventricle, pressures in the pulmonary artery gradually decrease. The pulse pressure tracing falls to the end-diastolic pressure at this point. The systolic and diastolic pulmonary artery (PAS and PAD) pressure and mean pulmonary artery pressure are usually measured in clinical settings.

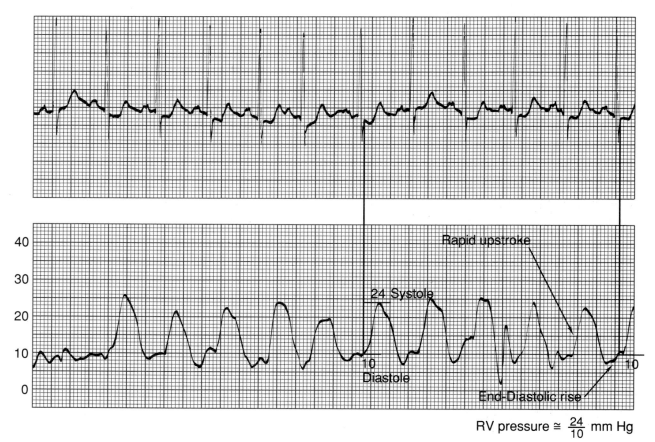

$$RV \text{ pressure} \cong \frac{24}{10} \text{ mm Hg}$$

Waveform 4–5. RV waveform.

NORMAL ARTERIAL PRESSURES AND CONFIGURATIONS

In the clinical setting, correct catheter location is essential. Determining if the catheter tip is resting in the pulmonary artery, for example, or in the right ventricle, is an important clinical issue. A PA catheter tip left to rest in the right ventricle could stimulate life-threatening ectopy. If the catheter is in the ventricle, it would be necessary to either advance the catheter to the pulmonary artery, or remove the catheter. Knowing normal chamber pressures can be helpful in differentiating the RV tracing from the PA tracing. Normal arterial pressure values are listed in Table 4–1.

The RV systolic pressure is about 15–25 mm Hg, with a diastolic pressure of 0–8 mm Hg. Normal systolic PA pressure is 15–25 mm Hg, with a diastolic pressure of about 8–15 mm Hg. The right ventricle will generally display a wider pulse pressure variation and thus, a greater range between systolic and diastolic pressures. However, in the diseased myocardium, normal pressures often cannot be used as a guide in determining catheter position, and waveform configuration may be more valuable. Because RV wall tension is greater than that of the PA, the RV pulse pressure will create a sharper upstroke followed by a rapid decrease to diastole. In contrast to the ventricular waveform, the PA pressure tracing will have a gradual runoff to diastole. Note the difference in waveform configuration between the RV tracing and the PA tracing (Waveform 4–6).

Systolic, diastolic, and mean pressures are also measured when monitoring aortic or systemic arterial pressures. Once again, end diastole is correlated with end QRS. However, with peripheral arterial catheters, a slight time delay between end QRS and onset of end diastole is consistently noted. The time delay is due to the distance between the myocardial activity and the peripheral catheter. Generally, diastole is noted to occur about 0.2 second after end QRS, depending on the location of the catheter (Waveforms 4–7 and 4–8).

This time delay would not be noted when interpreting arterial pressures monitored directly by a catheter in the aorta. In Waveform 4–9, which is obtained from an intra-aortic balloon pump, the diastolic blood pressure correlates directly with end QRS.

PROBLEMS IN READING DIASTOLE

Diastole in PA waveforms can have some interference from artifact and waveform variations. One of the most common examples is the extra waveform noted just in front of the arterial wave (Waveform 4–10).

This wave may arise from isometric ventricular contraction, although the exact origin is unclear. Some authors refer to this as a reflected A wave from the left atrium.[35] This explanation is unlikely, however, considering that the waveform is present even in the absence of P waves, which are necessary to generate A waves, such as with junctional and atrial fibrillation rhythms (Waveform 4–11).

When this presystolic wave is present, read the diastolic value as if the wave was not present. End diastole, if measured from the end of the QRS, may land in the middle of this wave. Try to plot a continued diastolic runoff through the extra wave (Fig. 4–3).

Table 4–1. NORMAL ARTERIAL
PRESSURES*

Pressure Location	Normal Values
Right ventricle	25/0–5
Pulmonary artery	25/10
Left ventricle	110/10
Aorta	120/80

*All values are approximate—individual variations are common.

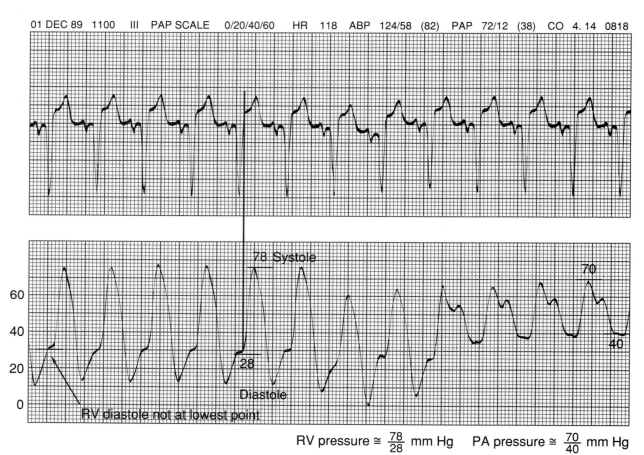

RV pressure ≅ $\frac{78}{28}$ mm Hg   PA pressure ≅ $\frac{70}{40}$ mm Hg

Waveform 4–6. RV waveform changing to a PA wave.

14 FEB 91   2026   AVF   ABP SCALE   0/40/80/120   HR 88   PAP 36/21(25)   CVP (12)   ABP 109/51(73)   PULSE 88 SA02 97

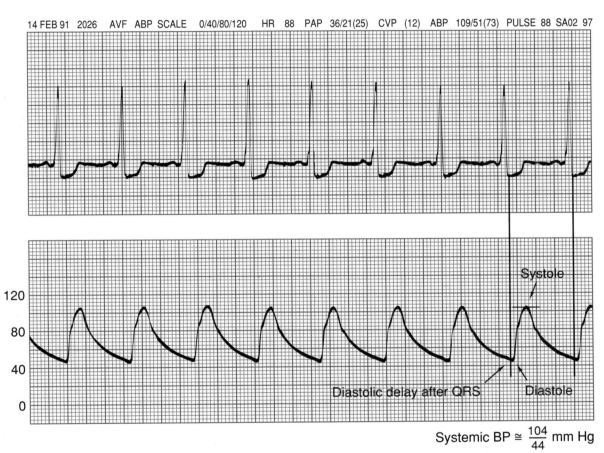

Systole

Diastolic delay after QRS   Diastole

Systemic BP ≅ $\frac{104}{44}$ mm Hg

Waveform 4–7. ECG relationship with a peripheral arterial waveform.

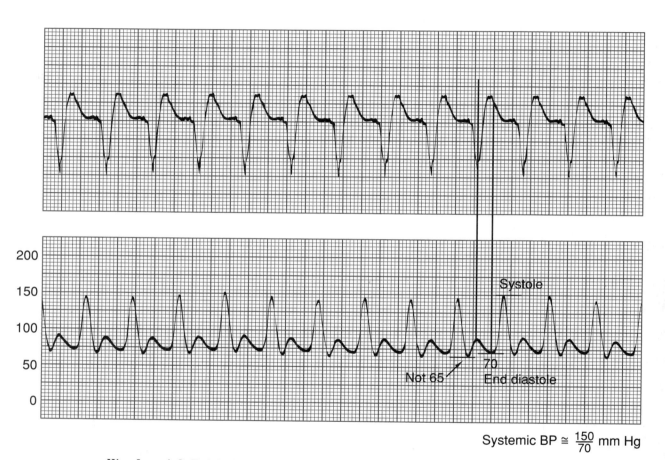

Systemic BP ≅ $\frac{150}{70}$ mm Hg

Waveform 4–8. End QRS does not align with diastole in the peripheral arterial waveform.

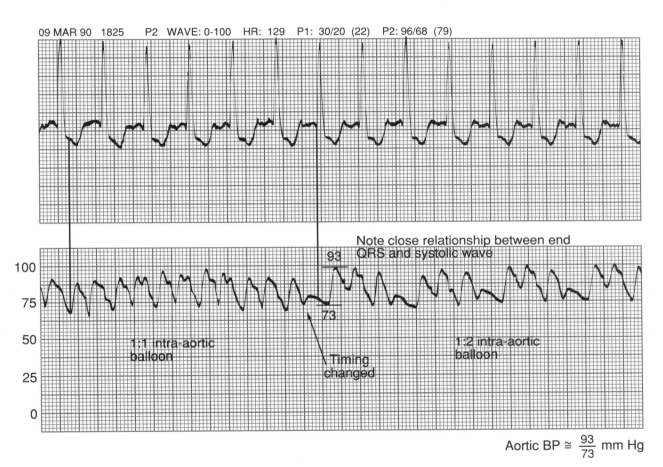

09 MAR 90 1825   P2 WAVE: 0-100   HR: 129   P1: 30/20 (22)   P2: 96/68 (79)

Note close relationship between end
QRS and systolic wave

93

73

1:1 intra-aortic
balloon

Timing
changed

1:2 intra-aortic
balloon

Aortic BP ≅ $\frac{93}{73}$ mm Hg

Waveform 4–9. ECG correlation with aortic arterial waveform. Note close relationship of end QRS to
diastole.

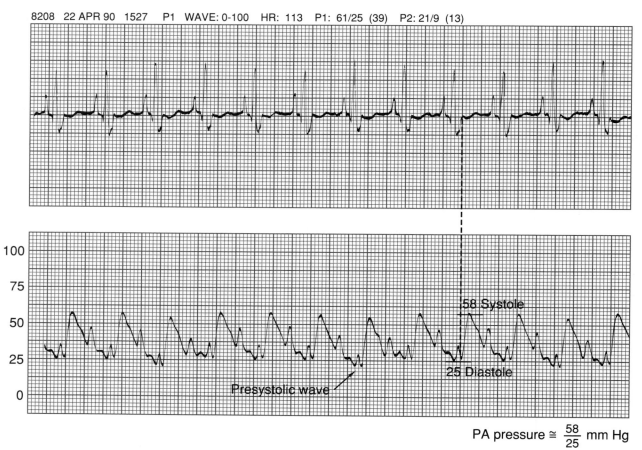

Waveform 4–10. Presystolic wave can interfere with diastolic value.

02 AUG 89   0908   P1   WAVE: 0-100   HR: 101   P1: 43/17 (30)   P2: 20/9 (13)

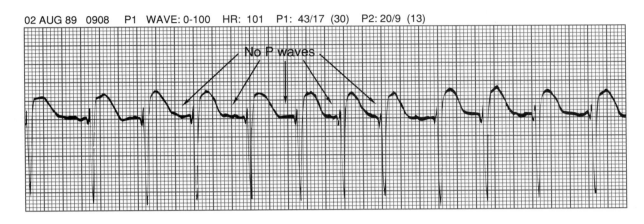

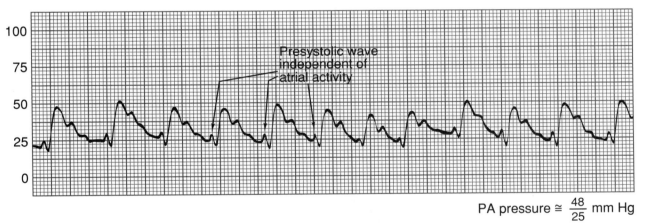

PA pressure $\cong \dfrac{48}{25}$ mm Hg

Waveform 4–11. Presystolic wave is unrelated to atrial activity. Note that in the junctional rhythm (no P waves), the presystolic wave remains.

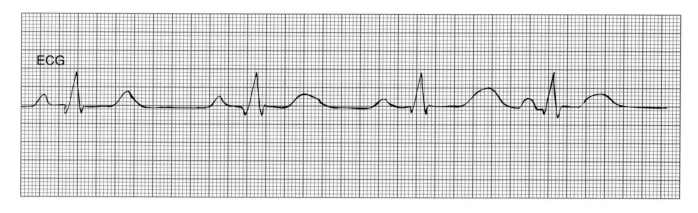

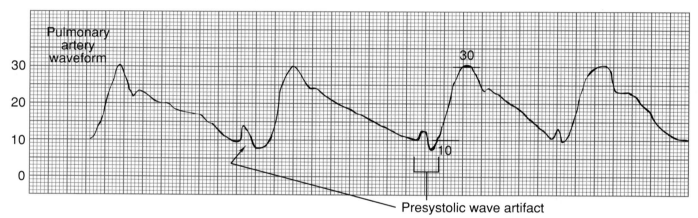

Figure 4–3. Presystolic waves in the PA tracing. The presystolic wave can interfere with reading diastole. Attempt to estimate the diastolic value by following the diastolic slope through the presystolic wave.

SUMMARY

The three arterial waveforms commonly seen in critical care settings are right ventricular, pulmonary arterial, and systemic arterial waveforms. Each has slightly different configurations and alignments with the ECG. Understanding these differences allows for differentiating between waveforms as well as indicating the correct location to read each waveform.

PRACTICE WAVEFORMS

Practice Waveforms 4–1 to 4–5 give examples of the waveforms presented in this chapter. Practice your interpretation of normal arterial waveforms with these examples.

PRACTICE WAVEFORM 4–1. What is the reason for the beat-to-beat variation in the arterial pressures?

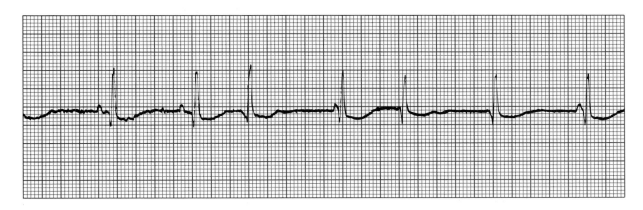

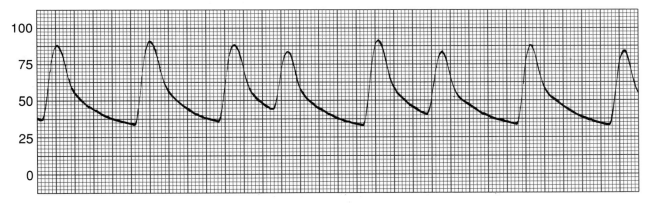

PRACTICE WAVEFORM 4–1. *Analysis:* This PA waveform has a slight drop in pressure with each premature atrial contraction. The decreases in pressure are real and need to be accounted for during blood pressure determination.

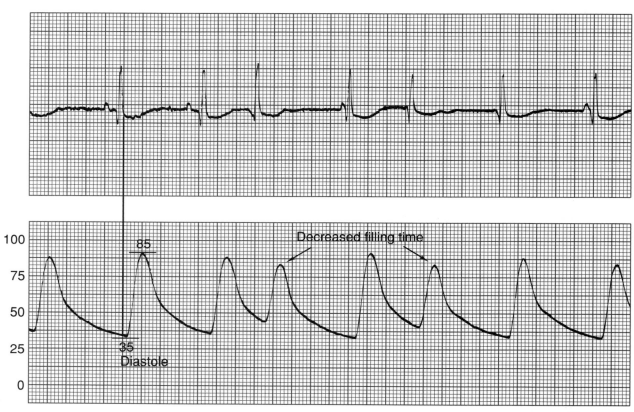

PA pressure = $\frac{85}{35}$ mm Hg

PRACTICE WAVEFORM 4–2. When you first observe the PA waveform during your shift, you note the following tracing. What is your interpretation of this waveform?

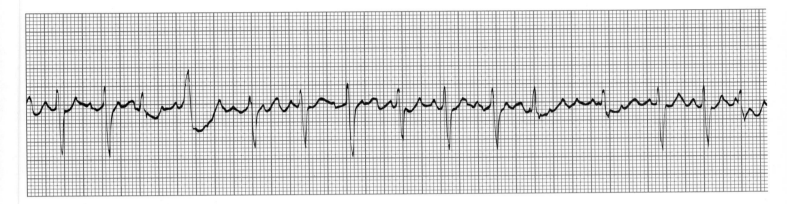

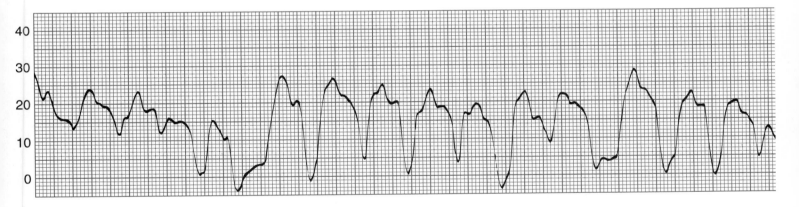

PRACTICE WAVEFORM 4–2. *Analysis:* This is a PA waveform that changes to a RV waveform.

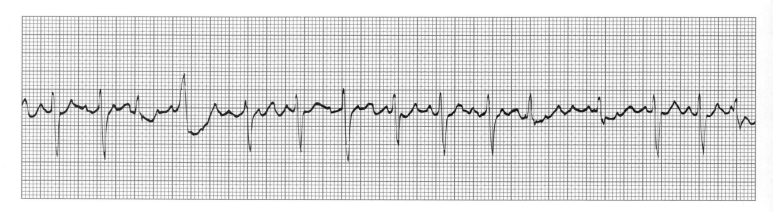

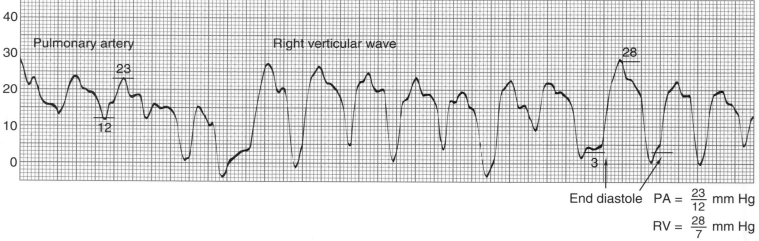

Pulmonary artery

Right verticular wave

23

12

28

3

End diastole   PA = $\frac{23}{12}$ mm Hg

RV = $\frac{28}{7}$ mm Hg

PRACTICE WAVEFORM 4–3. What is the value associated with the following PA waveform?

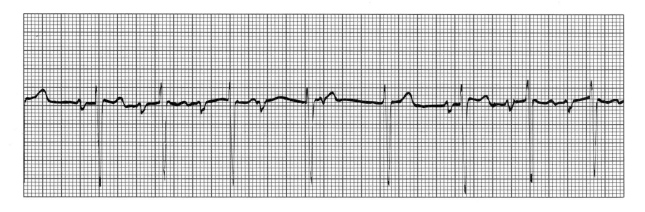

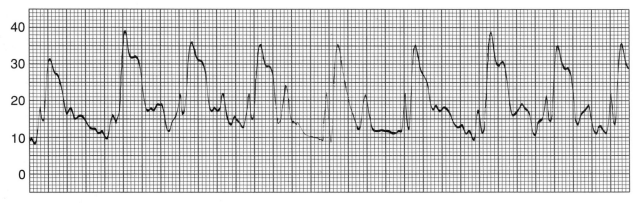

PRACTICE WAVEFORM 4–3. *Analysis:* The PA value fluctuates between systolic values of 32–39 and diastolic values of 10–15. The fluctuation is partially caused by inconsistent atrioventricular synchrony due to the second-degree type I heart block.

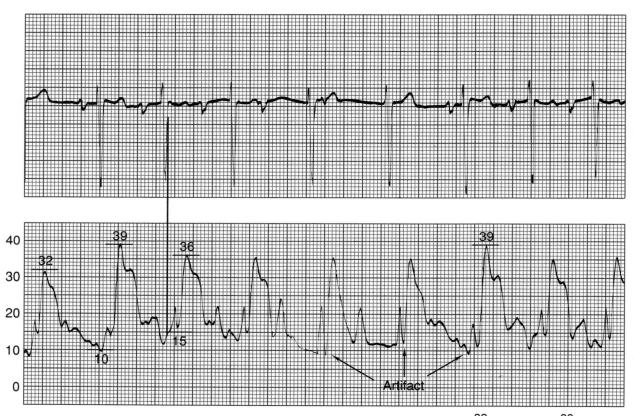

PA pressure = $\dfrac{32}{10}$ mm Hg to $\dfrac{39}{15}$ mm Hg

PRACTICE WAVEFORM 4–4. What is the value associated with this radial artery waveform?

8215   09 MAR 90   2000   P2 WAVE:0-100   HR:129   P1:25/15 (25)   P2:100/57 (81)

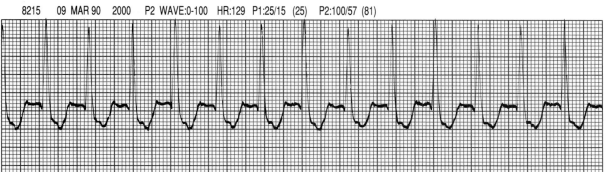

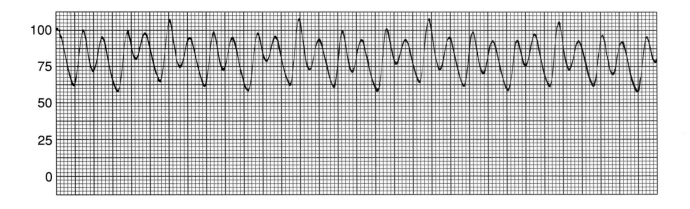

PRACTICE WAVEFORM 4–4. *Analysis:* Systemic blood pressure is about 100/62 mm Hg. Note that diastole occurs about 0.14 sec after the end of the QRS.

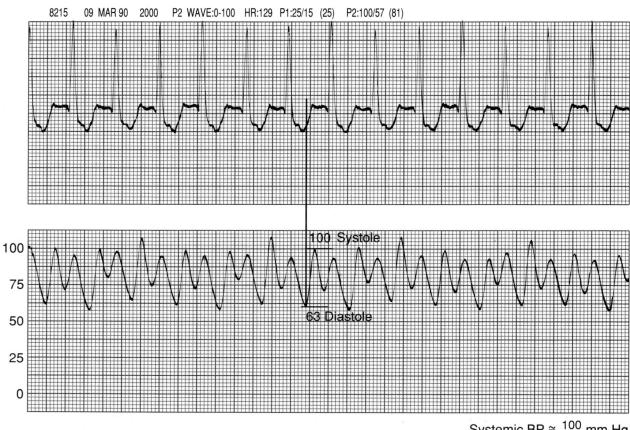

8215   09 MAR 90   2000   P2 WAVE:0-100   HR:129 P1:25/15 (25)   P2:100/57 (81)

100 Systole

63 Diastole

Systemic BP $\cong \dfrac{100}{63}$ mm Hg

PRACTICE WAVEFORM 4–5. What is the value associated with this PA waveform?

8283   04 MAR 90   1735   P1 WAVE:0-100 HR:93 P1:60/26 (39)   P2:279/278 (278)

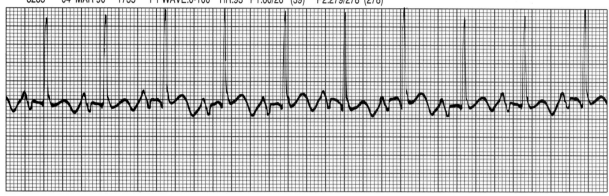

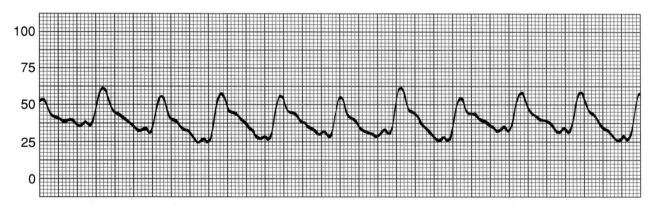

PRACTICE WAVEFORM 4–5. *Analysis:* The PA value is about 55/28 mm Hg. The tracing represents a normal PA waveform.

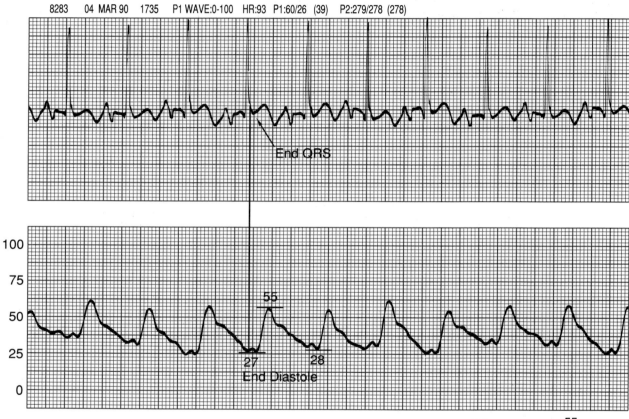

8283   04 MAR 90   1735   P1 WAVE:0-100   HR:93   P1:60/26 (39)   P2:279/278 (278)

End QRS

End Diastole

$$\text{PA pressure} \cong \frac{55}{28} \text{ mm Hg}$$

PRACTICE WAVEFORM 4–6. Identify the blood pressure from this radial artery waveform.

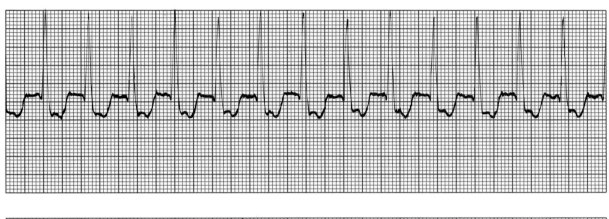

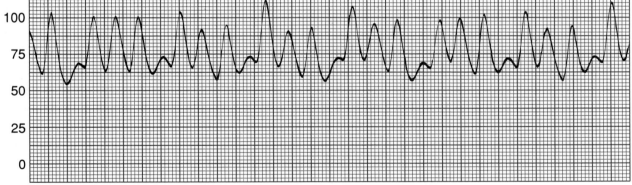

PRACTICE WAVEFORM 4–6. *Analysis:* Identifying the systolic and diastolic values can be accomplished if the ECG is used for correlation. About 0.14 sec after the end of the QRS, we find a diastolic value of about 63 mm Hg. Systolic values immediately follow this, with a value of about 98 mm Hg.

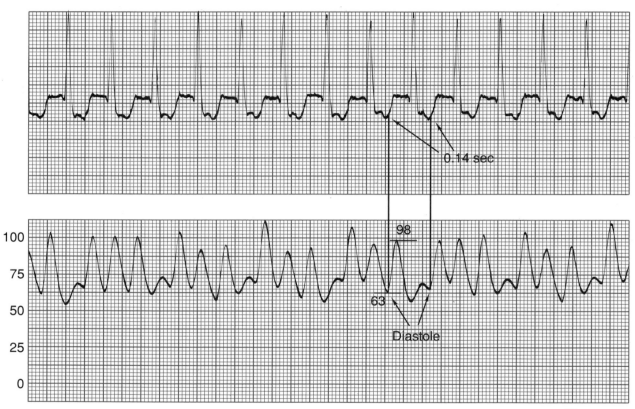

Systemic PB = $\frac{98}{63}$ mm Hg

PRACTICE WAVEFORM 4–7. As the physician attempts to place a PA catheter into the "wedge" position, you obtain the following waveform. What is your interpretation of what is occurring in this tracing?

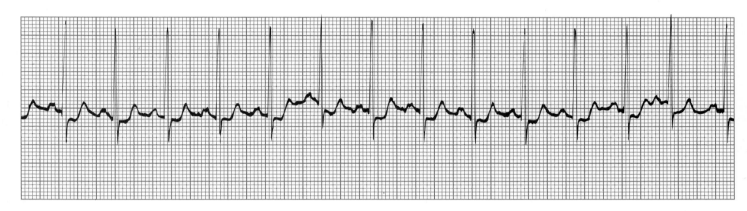

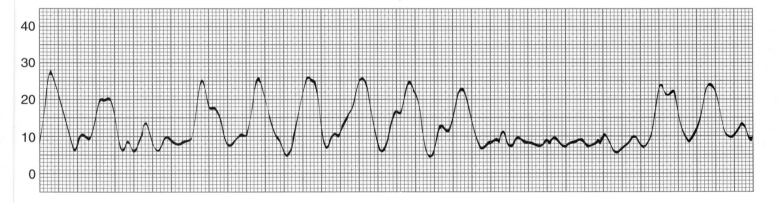

PRACTICE WAVEFORM 4–7. *Analysis:* This waveform represents a right ventricular waveform that fluctuates between right atrial and ventricular waves. The catheter is not advancing properly into the pulmonary artery.

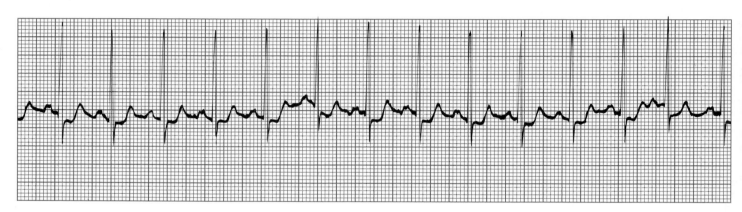

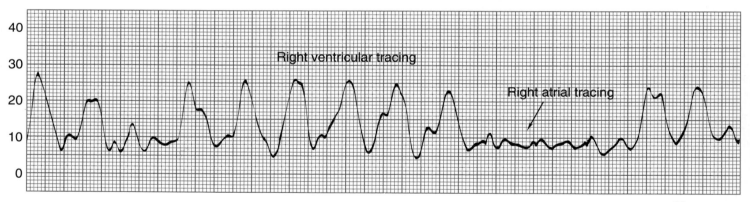

Right ventricular tracing

Right atrial tracing

$$RV = \frac{26}{7} \text{ mm Hg}$$

$$RA = 9 \text{ mm Hg}$$

5 : Abnormal Arterial Waveforms

Arterial waveforms can be divided into two types: waves with left ventricular origin, e.g., radial or femoral waveforms; and those with right ventricular origin, i.e., pulmonary arterial waveforms. For the sake of clarity, left ventricular–generated waveforms will be referred to simply as arterial waveforms. Most of the waveforms that are clinically difficult to interpret are in the pulmonary artery but each type has its own variations. This chapter will address the variations seen in both left and right ventricular–generated arterial waveforms. Abnormalities in the pressure waves due to technical problems, such as "catheter fling," will not be addressed in this chapter but are addressed in Chapter 7.

Variations seen in arterial waveforms can usually be traced to actual hemodynamic disturbances.[36] For example, hypovolemia will produce low amplitude pressure waves, making the waveform appear smaller than normal. Hypervolemia may cause the opposite effect, i.e., an increased pressure wave. However, variations in the actual appearance of the arterial waveform can usually be attributed to a dysrhythmia, intrathoracic pressure changes altering stroke volume, and aortic or pulmonic valve dysfunction. Hypo- and hypervolemia are discussed in Chapter 11. This chapter will focus on factors that can change the arterial waveform appearance unrelated to blood volume alterations.

DYSRHYTHMIAS

Loss of Atrioventricular Synchrony

As a normal mechanism of maintaining adequate stroke volumes, atrial contraction adds to the volume filling the ventricle before each ventricular contraction. Because atrial contraction contributes up to 25% of each stroke volume, loss of atrial contraction (reflected by loss of the P wave) can reduce stroke volume (Fig. 5–1).

Loss of atrioventricular (A-V) synchrony will cause loss of atrial contribution to the cardiac output. If this loss is clinically significant, the arterial waveform will reflect a reduced stroke volume (Waveform 5–1).

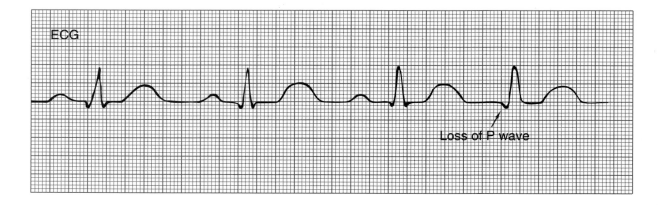

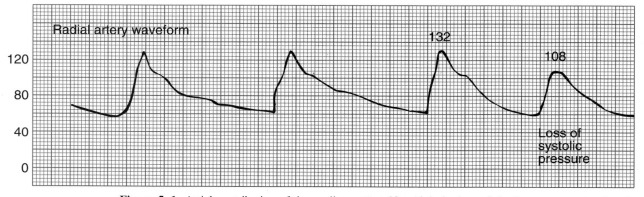

Figure 5–1. Atrial contribution of the cardiac output. Note that the loss of the P wave causes reduced stroke volume and systolic pressure.

Waveform 5–1. Loss of A-V synchrony produces a loss of stroke volume and systolic blood pressure. *See waveform on facing page.*

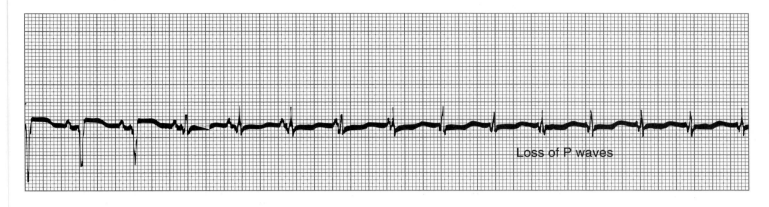

Loss of P waves

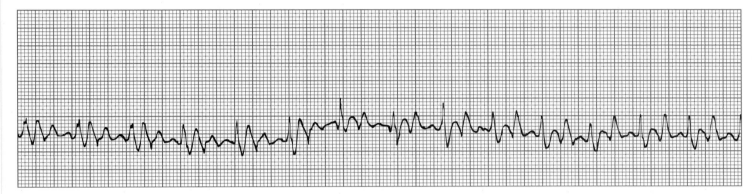

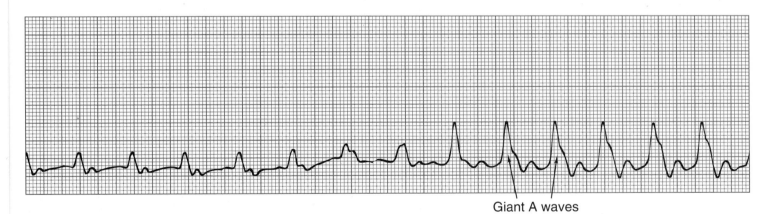

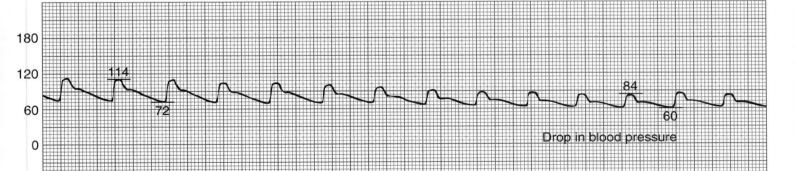

Giant A waves

Drop in blood pressure

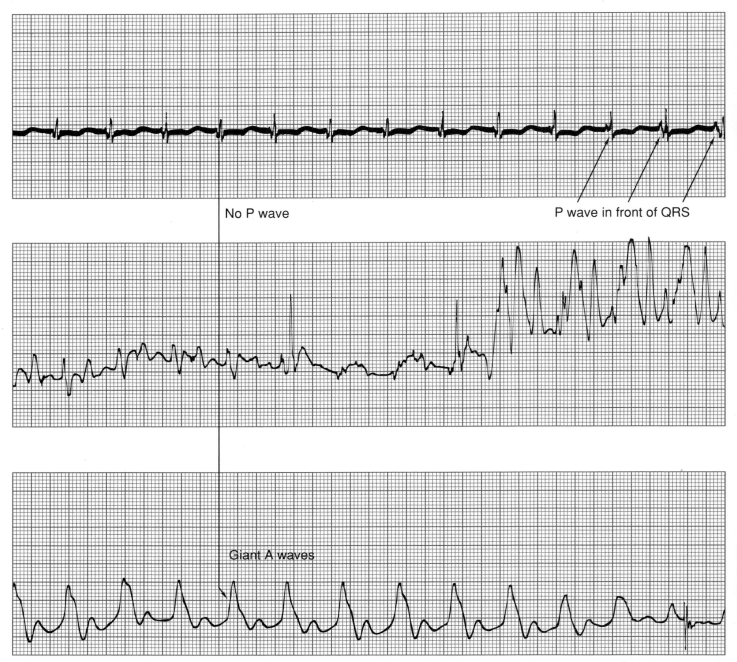

No P wave

P wave in front of QRS

Giant A waves

Return of normal
A waves

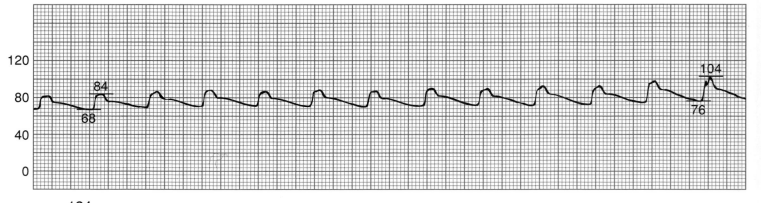

120

84

80

68

104

76

40

0

124

The loss of A-V synchrony can cause a substantial reduction in stroke volume, enough to warrant institution of vasopressor agents in order to maintain the cardiac output. Such a treatment may be avoided, however, if the waveform is observed with the dysrhythmia. Treatment of the dysrhythmia may change the focus of therapy to correction of the dysrhythmia as opposed to use of vasoactive agents. As an example, in Waveform 5–2, simultaneous comparison of the electrocardiogram (ECG) and waveform makes it clear that an A-V sequential pacemaker rather than vasopressors or preload manipulation is the treatment of choice in this transiently hypotensive patient.

Ectopic Beats

Ventricular ectopic beats will generally cause a marked reduction in stroke volume because of shortened diastolic filling time and dyscoordinated ventricular contraction. The effect of the ectopic beat can be noted in the arterial waveform (Waveform 5–3).

Atrial ectopic beats can also cause reduced stroke volume owing to shortened ventricular filling time (Waveforms 5–4 and 5–5). The clinical significance of any individual ectopic beat can be determined by the effect on the arterial waveform. Atrial premature contractions, for example, can cause variations in the effect on the arterial waveform. The more significant the disturbance, the more likely treatment is necessary (Waveforms 5–6 and 5–7). Although the waveform cannot predict deterioration of a dysrhythmia, the wave can reveal important characteristics regarding the seriousness of the rhythm disturbance. For example, if a patient was having frequent short bursts of premature ventricular contractions (PVCs), the clinical significance of each burst could be identified by noting the pressure associated with each group of PVCs (Waveform 5–8).

If the pressure was maintained during the burst, pharmacologic treatment is more likely to be instituted first. If the pressure is markedly reduced, electrical treatment should be a higher priority and kept in readiness as well as pharmacologic therapy.

Whenever ventricular response becomes irregular, the arterial waveform reflects the variations in diastolic filling time. In Waveforms 5–9 and 5–10, notice how the waveforms are higher when longer diastolic filling is present. If blood pressure is measured noninvasively (by sphygmomanometer), the auscultated value may be the larger one produced by the beat with increased diastolic filling time. Unfortunately, the real mean pressure may not be this high. The problem with interpreting tracings affected by dysrhythmias is that the variation in values is not artifact. The variations noted are physiologic and all variations should be accounted. One patient may be more susceptible to hemodynamic disturbances from the same dysrhythmia than another. Reading the waveforms will give the best possibility of obtaining accurate mean pressures and ascertaining the dysrhythmic effect on each patient.

Waveform 5–2. Loss of P waves causes giant A waves and a reduced blood pressure. As the P wave returns, the giant A wave disappears and blood pressure increases. *See waveform on facing page.*

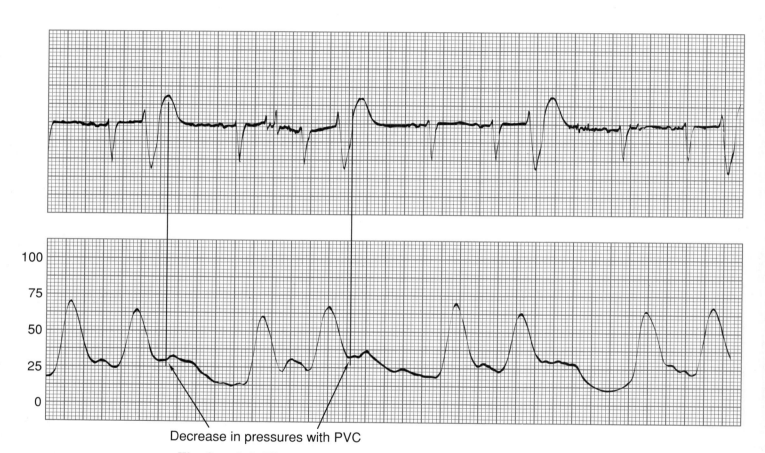

Decrease in pressures with PVC

Waveform 5–3. Effect of premature ventricular contractions on arterial waveform.

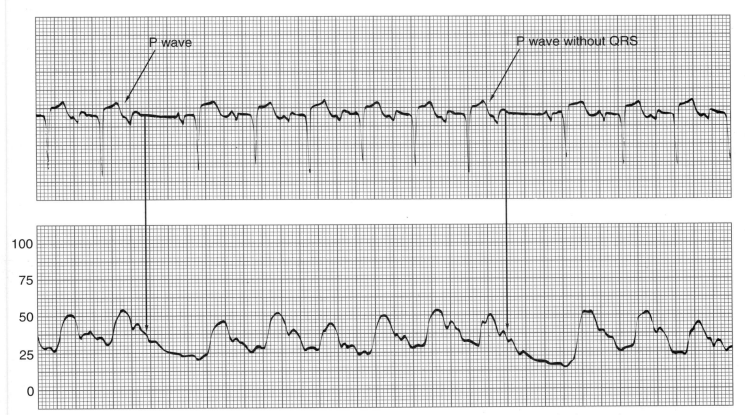

P wave

P wave without QRS

Waveform 5–4. Effect on arterial pressure of second-degree type I heart block. Note the decrease in blood pressure after the blocked atrial impulse.

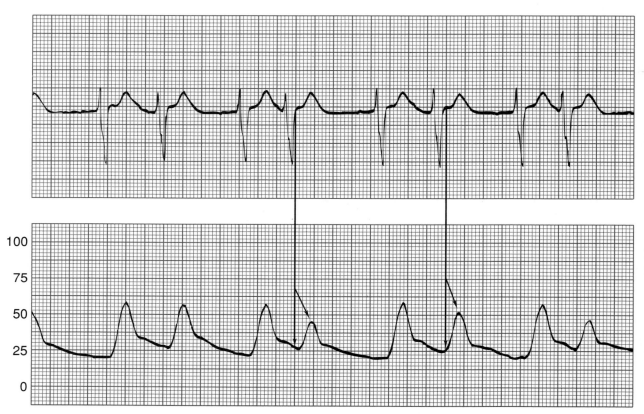

Waveform 5–5. Effect of atrial premature contractions on arterial blood pressure. In this example, the change in blood pressure is slight.

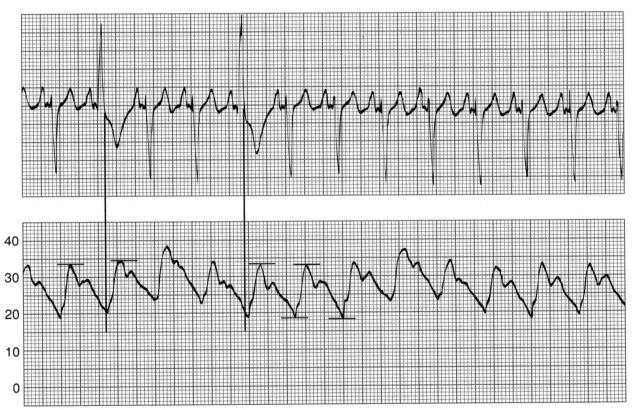

Waveform 5–6. Ectopic beat without effect on stroke volume or blood pressure.

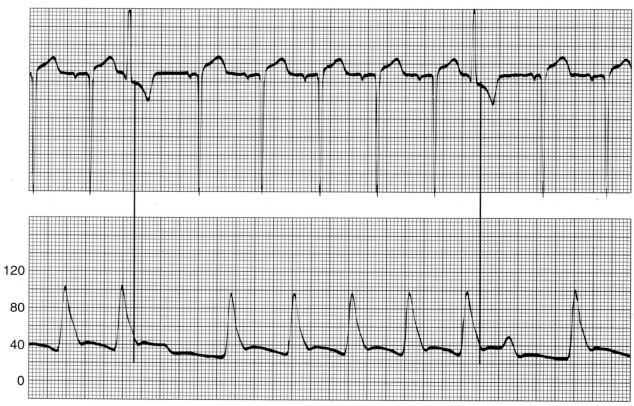

Waveform 5–7. Ectopic beat producing significant loss of blood pressure. The seriousness of ectopic beats, either atrial or ventricular, can be further assessed through the effect present on the blood pressure.

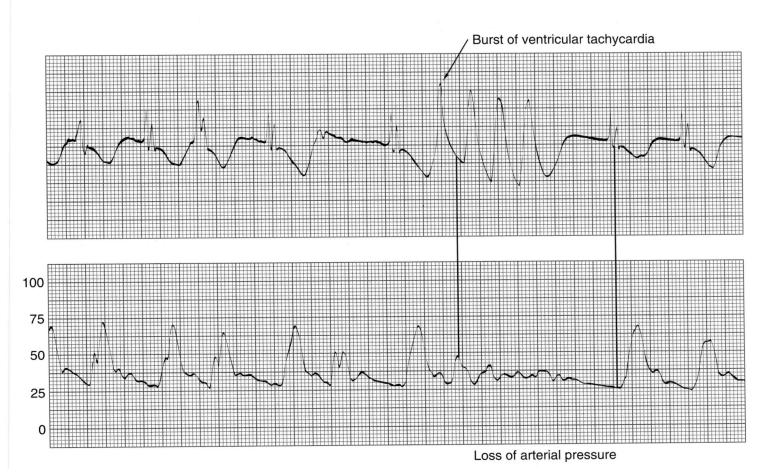

Burst of ventricular tachycardia

Loss of arterial pressure

Waveform 5–8. Effect of ventricular tachycardia on arterial waveforms.

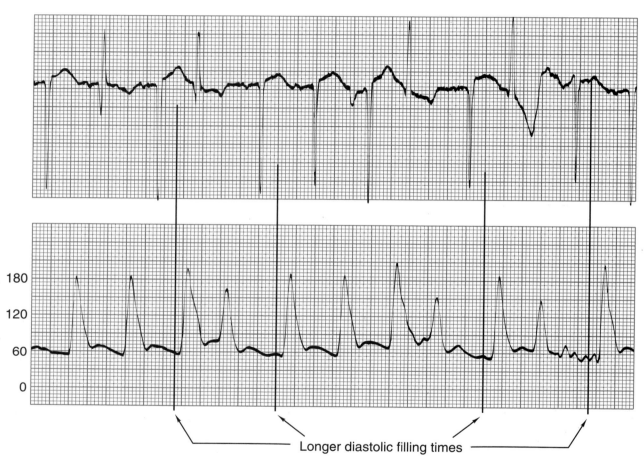

Waveform 5–9. Variations in arterial pressure with changes in diastolic filling times. Note how the blood pressure is higher following a delay in ventricular filling.

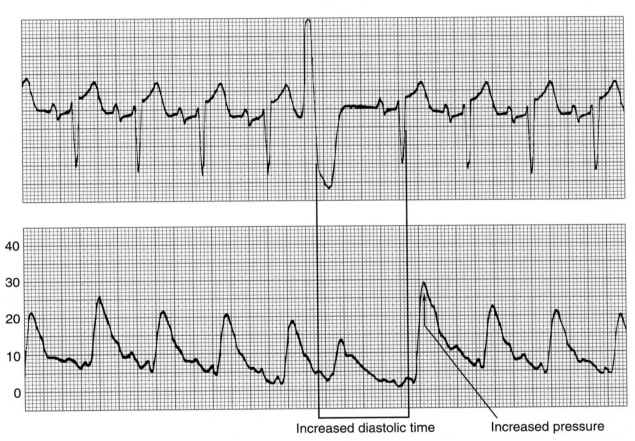

Increased diastolic time   Increased pressure

Waveform 5–10. Prolonged filling time after a PVC.

Reading Waveforms with Multiple Dysrhythmias

Because of the difficulty posed by adding all the variations produced by a dysrhythmia encountered in an arterial tracing, we recommend that you measure the waveforms by one of the following methods:

1. The most accurate method would be to measure all waveforms in a specified and representative time period, e.g., measuring all values in a 6-second strip that is characteristic of the dysrhythmia (Fig. 5–2).
2. A second method is to note the most commonly occurring values, both high and low, and average these two.
3. The third method is to read the values from the monitor. The monitor reading method has problems but generally uses an averaging technique over a short time period.[37] Averaging values over a 6-second strip recorded reading and comparing the values with the monitor values will reveal if the monitor readings are consistent and accurate.

The peripheral waveform can be used to obtain information regarding the effectiveness of perfusion. For example, when a patient goes into ventricular tachycardia or fibrillation, the effect is readily seen on the waveforms (Waveforms 5–11 and 5–12).

Arterial waves can also be used if question exists as to the origin of a rhythm. If it is unclear whether the rhythm is of ventricular origin or due to aberrantly conducted atrial beats, the waveform can indicate the effectiveness of perfusion, regardless of the rhythm.

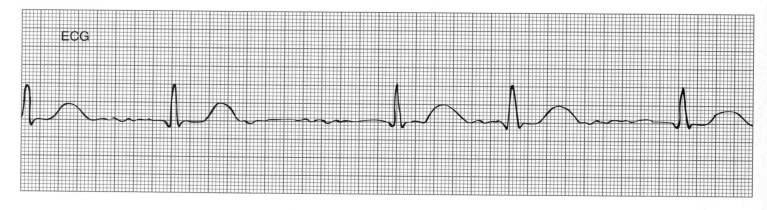

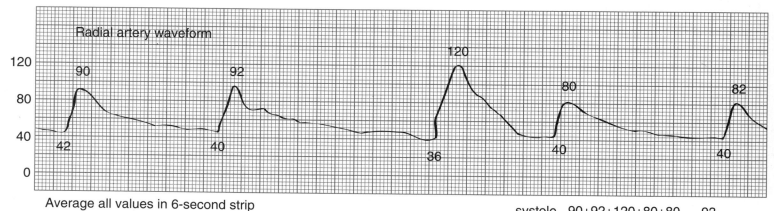

Average all values in 6-second strip

$$\frac{\text{systole}\quad 90+92+120+80+80}{\text{diastole}\quad 42+40+36+40+40} = \frac{93}{40}\ \text{mm Hg}$$

Figure 5–2. Averaging arterial pressures when variations in pressure exist.

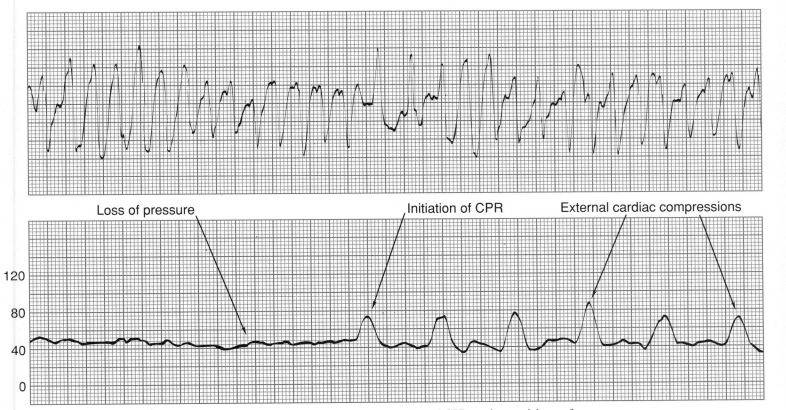

Waveform 5–11. Effect of ventricular tachycardia and CPR on the arterial waveform.

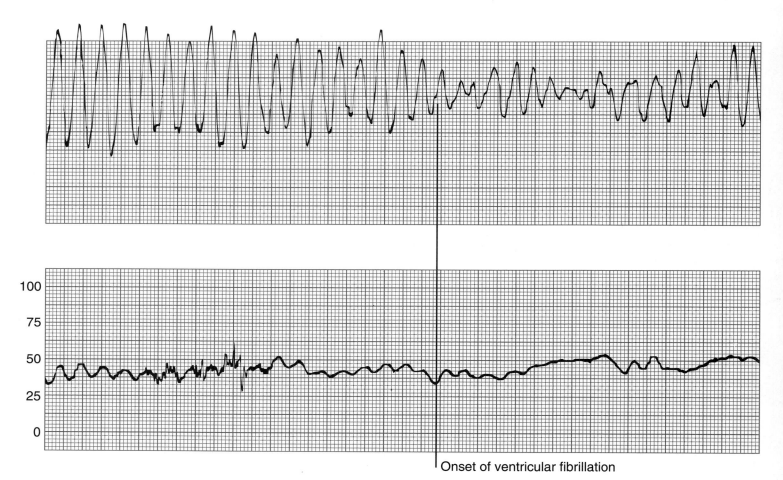

| Onset of ventricular fibrillation

Waveform 5–12. Effect of ventricular tachycardia converting to ventricular fibrillation on the arterial waveform.

One practical use of the arterial waveform is during cardiopulmonary resuscitation (CPR). Determination of effectiveness of external cardiac compression can be readily obtained by noting the waveforms generated during compression. During CPR, noting the waveforms generated during compressions is more reliable than checking for pulses. In addition, if a rhythm develops for which its ability to generate a pressure is unclear, the arterial catheter is the most accurate method of determining the pressure-generating capability of the rhythm.

The arterial waveform, due to its ability to signify perfusion, is also a useful tool in identifying electromechanical dissociation (EMD). EMD is the separation of the electrical activity in the heart from the mechanical event of muscle activity (contraction and relaxation). According to the American Heart Association, EMD can occur with severe acidosis, hypovolemia, tension pneumothorax, pericardial tamponade, hypoxia, and ventricular rupture.[38] When EMD occurs, an electrical impulse is present on the ECG but little if any pressure is generated by myocardial contraction. The arterial pressure wave quickly reflects EMD by its absence in the face of an ECG impulse (Waveform 5–13).

A related example can be seen in the use of pacemakers, particularly the external pacemaker. Because the external pacemaker has less likelihood of stimulating effective stroke volumes, it is important to identify if outputs are acceptable, and the arterial line can readily do so (Waveform 5–14).

Use of the arterial line can also help distinguish artifact from actual rhythm disturbances. Waveform 5–15 was obtained from a 71-year-old woman who knew that if she wiggled the ECG cable, she would get attention immediately. The arterial waveform demonstrates that the ECG rhythm is artifact rather than actual ventricular tachycardia.

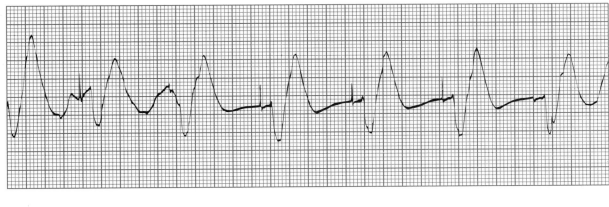

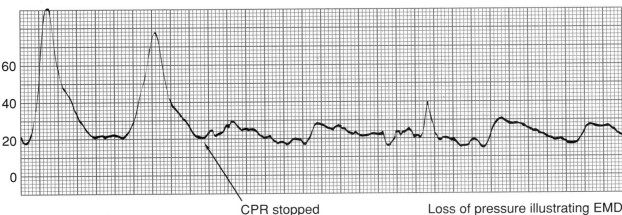

CPR stopped   Loss of pressure illustrating EMD

Waveform 5–13. Effect of CPR and paced electromechanical dissociation on the arterial waveform.

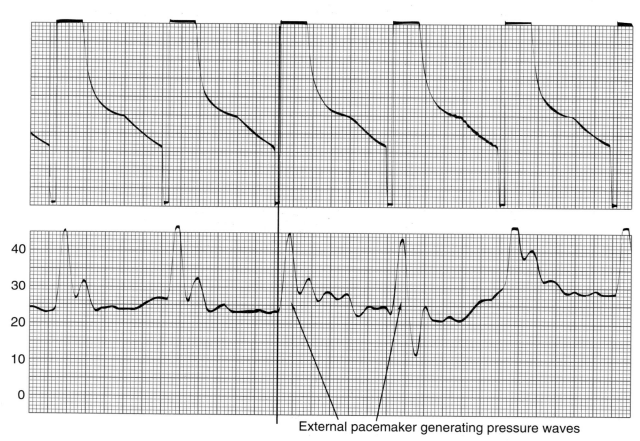

External pacemaker generating pressure waves

Waveform 5–14. Effect of external pacemaker on arterial pressure values.

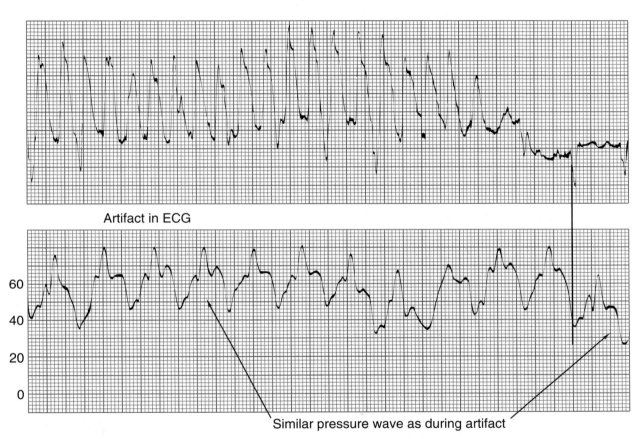

Artifact in ECG

Similar pressure wave as during artifact

Waveform 5–15. Differentiating ventricular tachycardia from artifact through the arterial pressure wave-form.

INTRATHORACIC PRESSURE CHANGES

Mechanical Ventilation–Induced Changes

As normal spontaneous inspiration (negative pressure ventilation) begins, a slight increase in right ventricular stroke volume occurs. No marked change is noted on the arterial waveform. However, during mechanical ventilation, the normal augmentation of blood return to the heart is potentially altered.[39] The degree of alteration is dependent on intrapulmonary factors such as lung compliance. The net effect of mechanical ventilation on arterial waveforms is potentially to cause transient reductions in pressure during the ventilator-delivered breath (Waveform 5–16). If the positive pressure breath from the ventilator is interfering with stroke volume, the result will be a reduced stroke volume during positive pressure–delivered inspirations.

Mechanical ventilation can also increase the stoke volume under some circumstances. As the lungs are distended during positive pressure inspiration, afterload reduction can occur due to changes in transmural pressure.[40] (Transmural pressure is discussed in Chapter 6.) If the reduction is substantial, an increase in the blood pressure may occur (Waveform 5–17).

When noting the effect of ventilation on the arterial waveform, remember that a delay in waveform transmission will occur if the catheter is not placed immediately outside the heart. The delay (normally about 0.2 sec for a radial arterial line) is the result of the time necessary for the waveform to travel to the sensing catheter (Fig. 5–3).

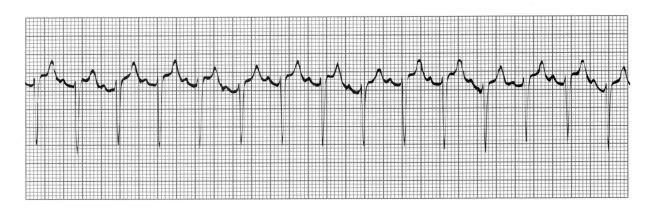

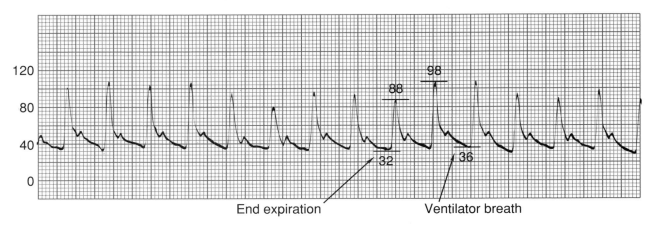

Waveform 5–16. Blood pressure can increase during mechanical ventilation.

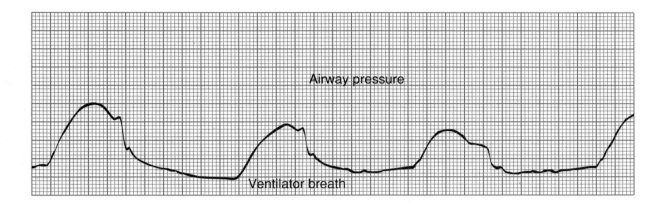

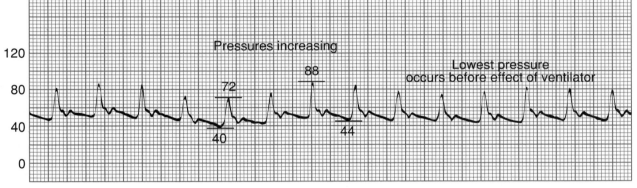

Pressure change from 72/40 to 88/44

Waveform 5–17. Augmentation of arterial pressure during mechanical ventilation.

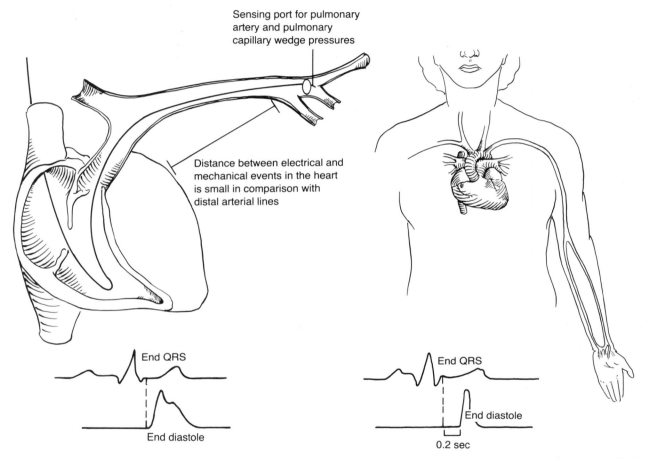

Figure 5–3. Difference in ECG intervals between pulmonary and radial artery lines. In pulmonary artery lines, end QRS approximates end diastole; however, approximately 0.2 sec after the end QRS approximates end diastole in distal (radial) arterial lines. The difference is due to the varying distance of the catheter from the cardiac contractions.

Pulsus Paradoxus

Using the arterial catheter provides the easiest assessment method to identify pulsus paradoxus (Waveform 5–18). Pulsus paradoxus, the decreasing of systolic blood pressure by more than 10 mm Hg during inspiration, is not uncommon in critical care.[41] Pulsus paradoxus is due to increased pericardial pressure, such as might be present with pericardial tamponade. As the person with increased pericardial pressure inspires, increased blood return to the right heart occurs. The increased blood return can cause increased pericardial pressure, which constricts left ventricular movement. The constricted left ventricle cannot eject as much volume, resulting in a decrease in blood pressure during inspiration. Detecting pulsus paradoxus with a noninvasive blood pressure cuff is more difficult than simply comparing inspiration with the fluctuations in the arterial pressure waveform.

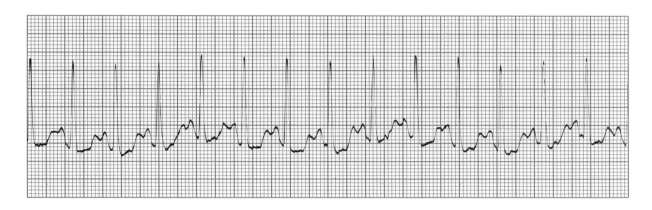

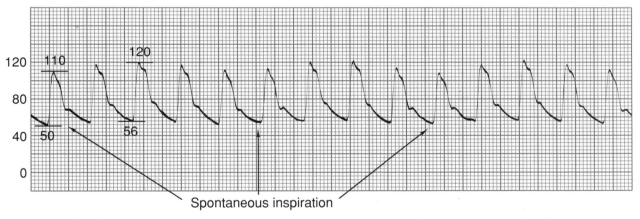

Spontaneous inspiration

Waveform 5–18. Pulsus paradoxus produces a decrease in systolic blood pressure of greater than 10 mm Hg during inspiration. Here, pressure decreases during inspiration from 120/56 to 110/50.

VALVULAR DISTURBANCES

The most prominent distortion in the arterial waveform due to a valvular defect occurs in aortic regurgitation. During aortic regurgitation, the pressure drops throughout diastole and rises again at end diastole. The potential clinical problem in aortic regurgitation is the lower mean arterial pressure. The monitor will report a diastolic value lower than the actual diastolic value due to the inability of the monitor to time where end diastole occurs. The clinician must be aware always to time end diastole with the end-QRS complex (or about 0.2 sec after the QRS in distal arterial lines) (Waveform 5–19).

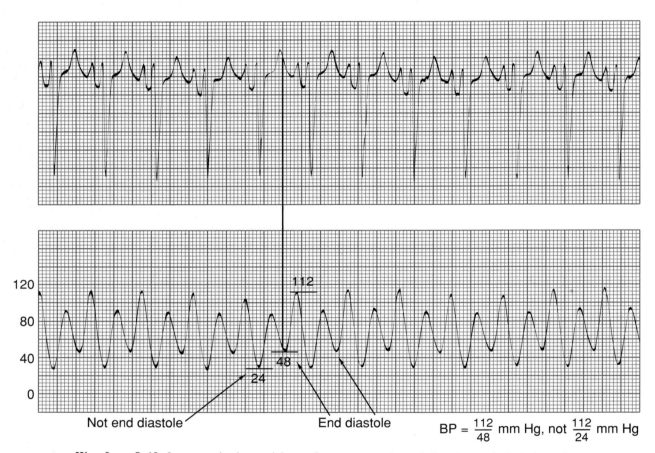

Not end diastole   End diastole   BP = $\frac{112}{48}$ mm Hg, not $\frac{112}{24}$ mm Hg

Waveform 5–19. Lowest point in arterial waveforms may not be end diastole, particularly in a distal arterial line.

Pulmonary Arterial Waveforms

Distortions in the pulmonary arterial waveform take the same pattern as presented for the arterial waveforms. A few exceptions exist, particularly in regard to reading diastolic values and valvular effects.

Several artifacts exist in pulmonary artery tracings that can make reading the correct wave difficult. One of the more common is a small wave preceding the arterial upstroke, a presystolic wave (Waveform 5–20). This wave makes identifying diastole difficult. The origin of this small wave in front of the arterial wave is unclear. Some authors have proposed that the wave is potentially the anacrotic notch, due to the opening of the pulmonic valve. Another possible explanation is that it may be a "reflected A" wave from the left atrium. This explanation is not likely, however, as illustrated in Waveforms 5–21 and 5–22, where we see that the small wave is present without a corresponding P wave (signifying no atrial contraction exists). Without a P wave, no A wave should be present.

When noting these small waves just prior to the systolic upstroke, try to avoid including the waves in identification of arterial diastolic values. The actual pulmonary arterial diastolic value is probably located beneath this wave. Read the waveform as illustrated in Figure 5–4.

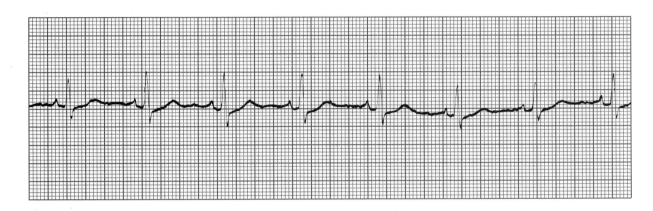

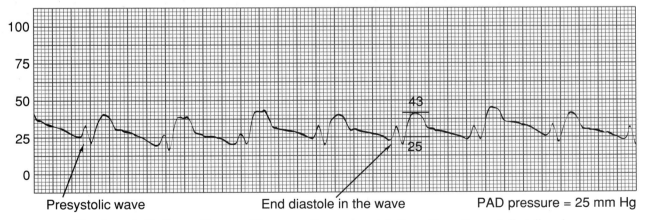

Waveform 5–20. Presystolic wave. The presystolic wave can interfere with reading end-diastolic values.

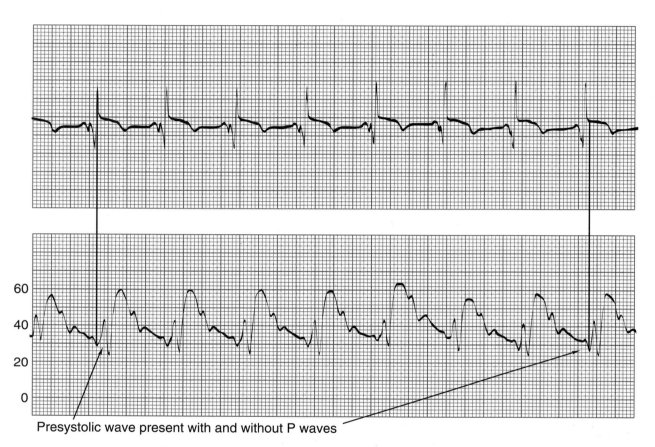

Presystolic wave present with and without P waves

Waveform 5–21. Lack of P wave correlation with presystolic wave.

No P wave

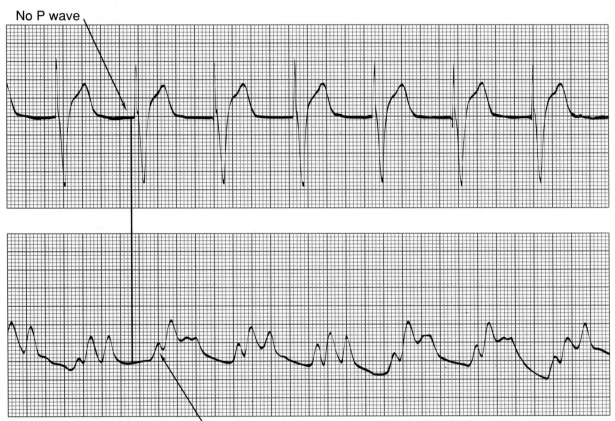

Wave preceding pressure wave in absence of P waves

Waveform 5–22. Presystolic waves exist without P waves.

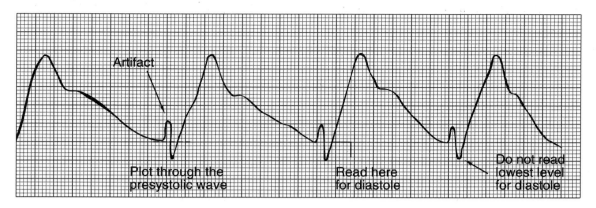

Figure 5–4. Presystolic waves. Presystolic arterial waves can make identification of diastole difficult. As a guide, plot through the wave to approximate end-diastolic values.

Valvular Effects on the Pulmonary Arterial Wave

As presented in Chapter 3, the primary valvular defect affecting pulmonary artery waveforms is mitral regurgitation. The subsequent large V can reflect on the arterial waveform. If the reflected wave is larger than the systolic arterial value, the clinician must be careful to read the correct point after the QRS complex.

ACCURACY OF ARTERIAL LINE VS SPHYGMOMANOMETER

The accuracy issue between arterial lines and noninvasive blood pressure devices is an important one in critical care. This topic is reviewed in Chapter 7.

SUMMARY

Arterial waveform interpretation is complicated by dysrhythmias, location of the sampling catheter, and presystolic waves. The influence of these complications can be isolated through application of waveform principles. For example, dysrhythmias primarily alter arterial blood pressure through the effect on diastolic filling time. The clinician must make sure to include alterations in the arterial pressure waveform in the overall pressure value in order to appropriately assess the influence of the dysrhythmia. In this chapter, key aspects of avoiding errors in reading arterial pressures have been reviewed. Given the importance of correct measurement of arterial pressures in the assessment of hemodynamics, these guidelines should prove useful to the nurse in the critical care setting.

PRACTICE WAVEFORMS

Practice Waveforms 5–1 through 5–5 provide examples of abnormal arterial waveforms described in this chapter. Employing the principles presented in this chapter has particular value because of the reliance in many institutions on arterial lines to obtain pressure values. The use of the concepts presented here will aid in the interpretation of arterial waveforms with inconsistent appearances.

PRACTICE WAVEFORM 5–1. Radial artery waveform in a 46-year-old man following aortic valve surgery. Where should this waveform be read?

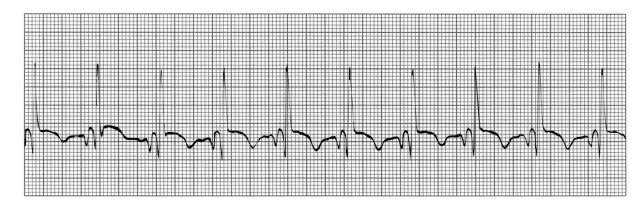

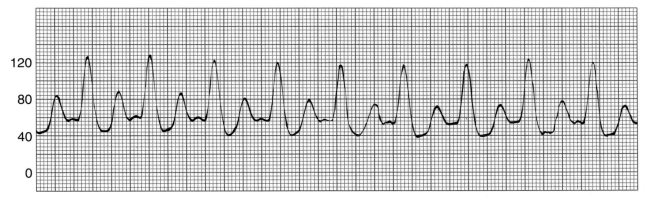

PRACTICE WAVEFORM 5–1. *Analysis:* Read end diastole about 0.2 sec after the end of the QRS complex. This would produce a value of 124/56 mm Hg. Avoid the lowest point of the waveform, which would give a diastolic value of about 42 mm Hg.

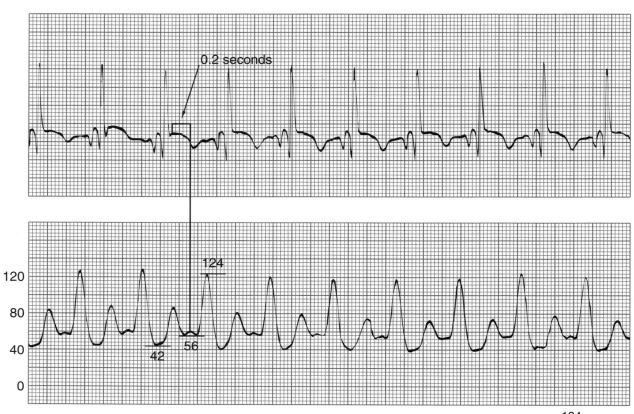

$$BP \approx \frac{124}{56} \text{ mm Hg}$$

PRACTICE WAVEFORM 5–2. Where should this pulmonary arterial tracing be read?

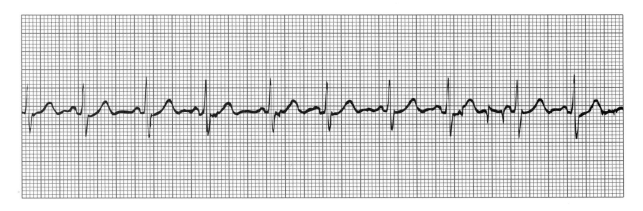

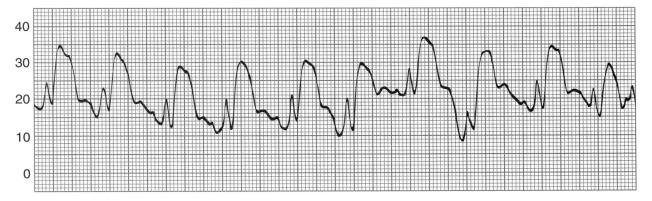

PRACTICE WAVEFORM 5–2. *Analysis:* End–QRS complex value is obtained immediately prior to the presystolic wave. PA value is about 30/11 mm Hg.

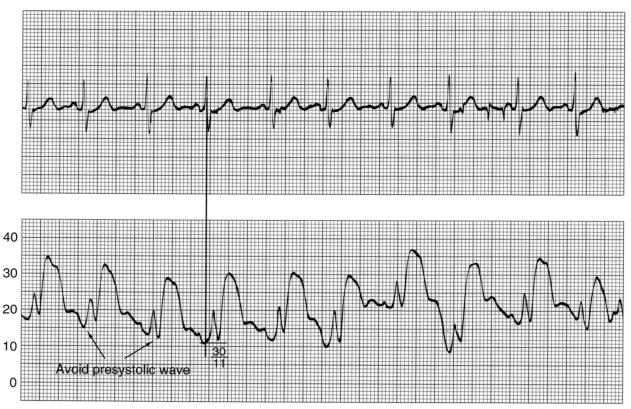

PA pressure ≈ $\frac{30}{11}$ mm Hg

PRACTICE WAVEFORM 5–3. Is this pacemaker producing an effective pulse?

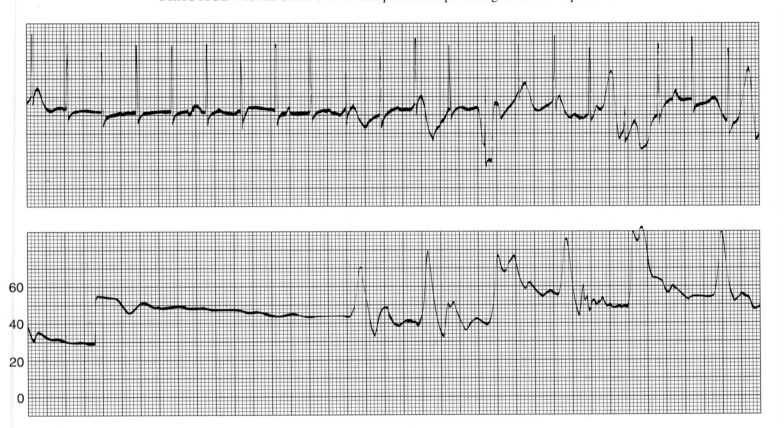

PRACTICE WAVEFORM 5–3. *Analysis:* No, with little pressure being generated except when CPR is resumed.

Paced rhythm

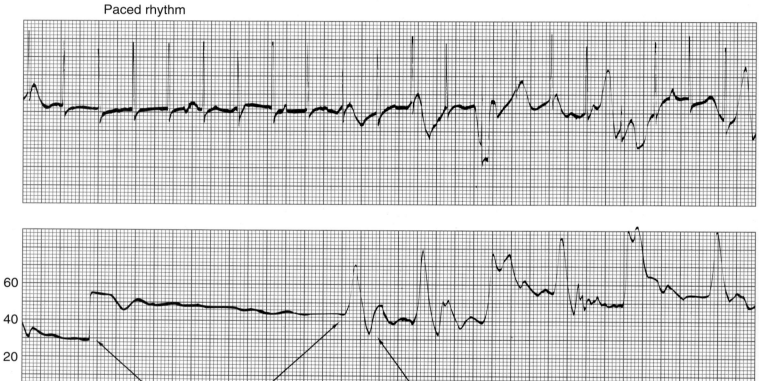

Reduced pressure with paced rhythm   CPR resumed

PRACTICE WAVEFORM 5–4. How effective is this ECG rhythm?

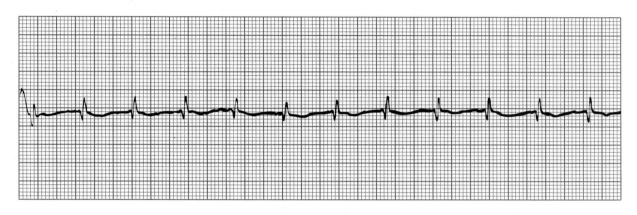

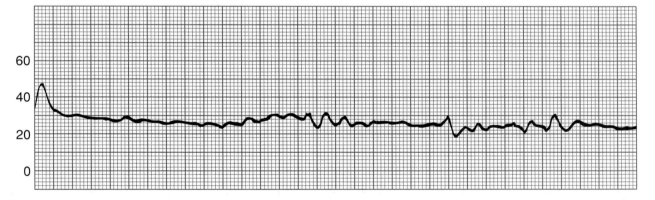

PRACTICE WAVEFORM 5–4. *Analysis:* Minimal pressure exists in this ECG rhythm. Electromechanical dissociation is present in this case.

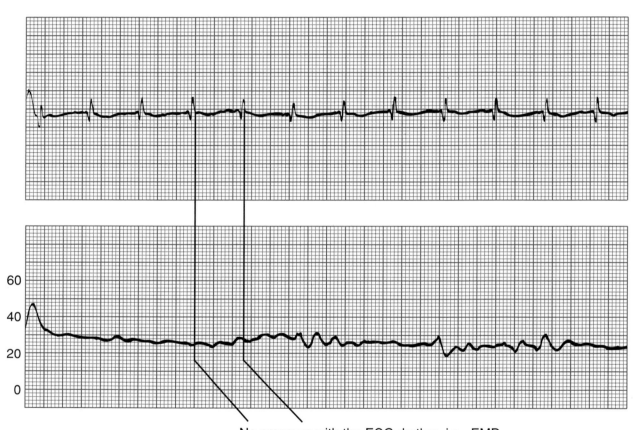

No pressure with the ECG rhythm, i.e., EMD

PRACTICE WAVEFORM 5–5. Why does the arterial pressure change in this example?

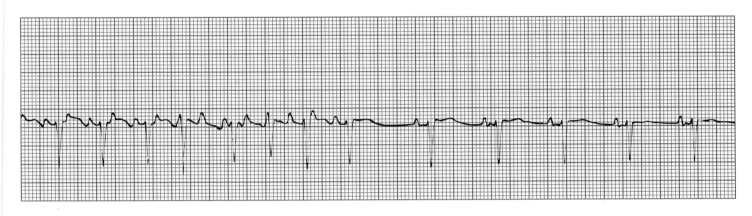

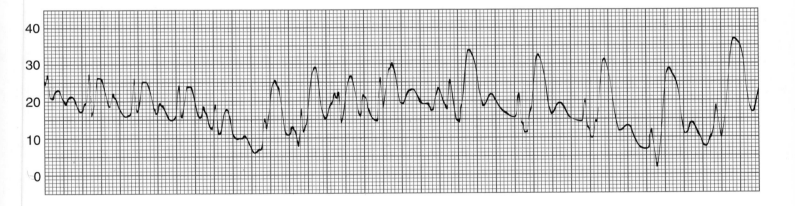

PRACTICE WAVEFORM 5–5. *Analysis:* The pressure changes because of the change in the ECG rhythm. The initial rhythm (multiform atrial tachycardia) produces a short diastolic filling time. After the development of sinus rhythm and increased diastolic filling time, the pressure increases.

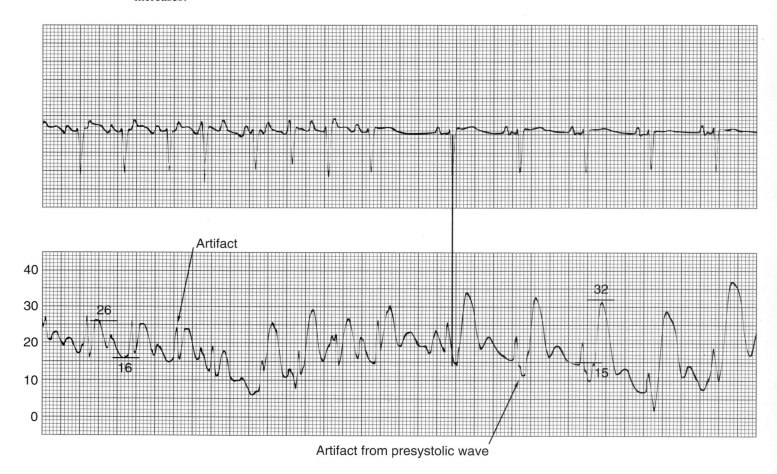

6 : Respiratory Influence on Waveforms

One of the most common and difficult to interpret variations in waveform analysis is due to respiratory artifact. Location of appropriate points to read in the waveform can be difficult, depending on the mode of mechanical ventilation and type of respiratory pattern. Monitoring companies have made major improvements in the ability of the monitor to read respiratory artifact. Unfortunately, several clinical situations still exist where reading from the monitor will result in incorrect values. The clinician must always determine if monitor-generated values are accurate before accepting their values. In order to do this, the clinician must be able to identify the correct locations of pressure waves during breathing.

In this section, samples of waveforms illustrate the influence of spontaneous breathing, mechanical ventilation respiration, and the combination of spontaneous breathing and mechanical ventilation on waveforms. Before proceeding with samples of the respiratory variations, we will provide clarification of appropriate locations to read waveforms with respiratory artifact.

ARTIFACT VERSUS ACTUAL PRESSURES

When you are reading thoracic waveforms with respiratory variation, it is extremely important to remember that the variations are artifact and not actual changes in the hemodynamic pressures. Intravascular pressures do vary with respiration but not to the extent seen with most monitoring systems. Monitoring of hemodynamics outside the thorax, such as in a radial artery, is more likely to produce actual pressures. Waveforms 6–1 and 6–2 illustrate radial arterial pressures that vary with respiration. These waveform values are actual changes in the blood pressure and should be averaged to obtain a mean arterial blood pressure.

Thoracic pressures, however, are more likely be influenced by artifact associated with breathing. The artifact arises because actual effective intravascular pressure is a function of the transmural intrathoracic pressure. Transmural pressure (PTM) is obtained by subtracting intra-pleural pressure from the hemodynamic pressure. A brief explanation of transmural pressure will help illustrate the role PTM plays in intravascular pressure interpretation.

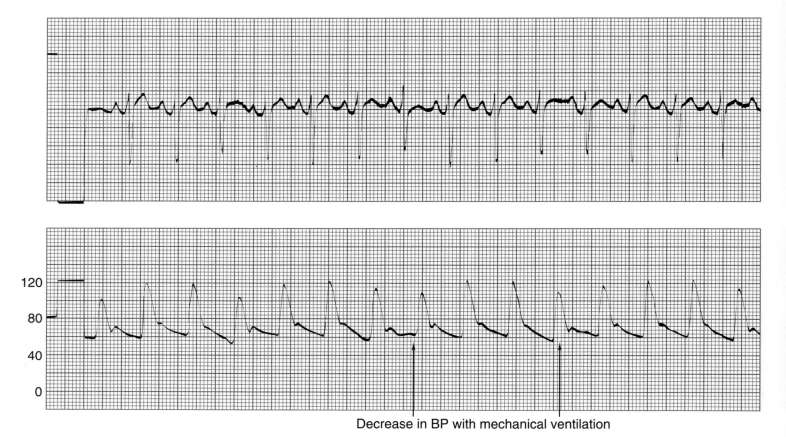

Decrease in BP with mechanical ventilation

Waveform 6–1. Decrease in blood pressure during mechanical ventilation.

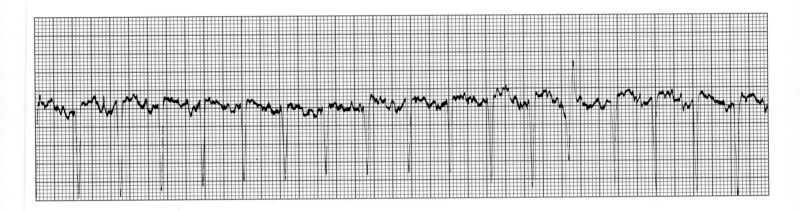

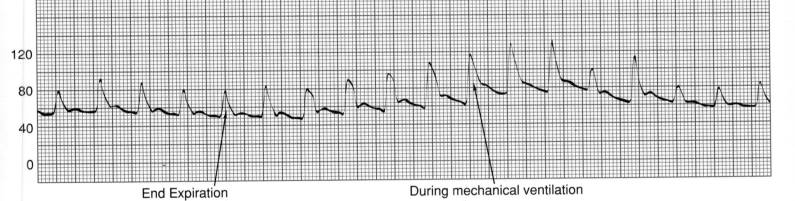

End Expiration   During mechanical ventilation

Waveform 6–2. Increase in blood pressure during mechanical ventilation. Pressure changes are real and are not artifact.

Transmural Pressure

If blood vessels were independent of forces external to their walls, only internal pressures would affect blood flow. In this case, the pressures transmitted to the transducer would be accurately reflecting all factors influencing blood flow. In the body, however, particularly in the chest, blood vessels are not independent of factors external to their walls. During inspiration, for example, the pressure outside the vessel wall decreases. The pressure outside the blood vessel is generated from intrapleural space. As inspiration occurs, the intrapleural pressure decreases, usually from -3 to -8 mm Hg (depending on the effect of gravity in the pleural space) (Fig. 6–1). The effect of the negative pressure from the intrapleural space is to pull the blood vessel outward. The pulling on the blood vessel wall acts to increase the distending pressure inside the vessel, thereby altering blood flow through the vessel. Therefore, both internal and external factors must be accounted for when you are accurately measuring the pressure affecting the blood vessel. This combination of internal and external pressures is referred to as the transmural pressure.[42] A few examples will help illustrate the effect of transmural pressure.

When the pulmonary capillary wedge pressure (PCWP) is 10 and the normal resting intrapleural pressure is -3, then the transmural PCWP is $10 - (-3) = 13$. Notice how the effective distending pressure is higher than what would be measured by the pulmonary artery catheter. Under most circumstances, this minor difference between actual transmural PCWP and measured PCWP is not a problem. Depending on the degree of changes in intrapleural pressure, however, the differences can be significant. Figure 6–2 illustrates examples of how some clinical conditions can generate erroneous readings. For example, when the inspiratory effort is strong, producing a large change in intrapleural pressure, the PCWP appears to change markedly. However, when measuring the transmural pressure, you can see that no change has occurred. The concept of transmural pressures as the true distending pressure of the blood vessel is the key to understanding why respiratory variations in waveforms are not true indicators of the distending pressures on the waveform.

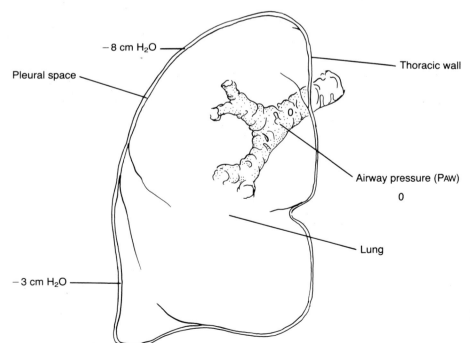

Figure 6–1. Intrapleural pressures in different regions of the lung.

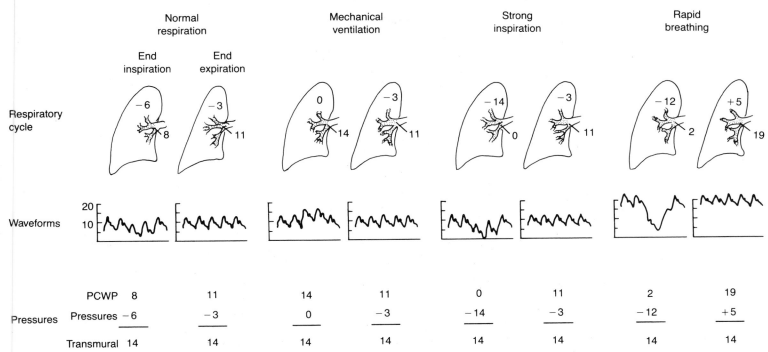

Figure 6–2. Hemodynamic vs transmural pressures associated with respiration.

The reason waveforms vary with respiration is primarily a function of the external referencing of the catheter to atmospheric pressure for a zero reading.[43] Because pressure surrounding the blood vessels in the chest is close to atmospheric but is influenced by pleural pressure, use of a transducer system referenced to atmospheric pressure and not pleural pressure will introduce error in waveform analysis. Under most circumstances, the error is small because normal intrapleural pressure (-3 mm Hg) is close to atmospheric (0). However, several circumstances exist where intrapleural pressure is no longer close to atmospheric. Identifying the conditions in which intrapleural pressure is substantially changed provides the basis for correct interpretation of hemodynamic waveforms in the presence of respiratory artifact. Before proceeding, a further review of the concept of the origin of respiratory artifact will be helpful.

Sources of Error with Respiratory Variation

Virtually all types of hemodynamic monitoring equipment employ a transducer located outside the body. The external transducer is used for convenience and approximate accuracy. In order for the transducer to read the pressure accurately, a baseline or reference point must be established. This point of reference is atmospheric pressure (see Chapter 7 for a more complete description of zeroing the transducer). From this reference point, any change of pressure in the blood vessel will be measured by the external transducer.

Unfortunately for an external measurement system, the transmural pressure is not measured because intrapleural pressure changes are not measured. Although the clinician is primarily interested in the hemodynamic changes, the intrapleural pressure change is uncontrolled and transmural pressure is not reflected. As the waveform is displayed, the true hemodynamic pressure (transmural pressure) is distorted. As a result of this distortion, the hemodynamic wave is altered, usually by a fluctuating baseline.

When the transducer is referenced to intrapleural pressure, the intrapleural pressure is accounted for and the approximate transmural pressure is read. Little respiratory artifact is displayed with pleural-referenced transducers. The problem, however, with pleural-referenced transducers is the practical difficulty in employing the technique for zeroing to the pleural pressure. One requires either an esophageal zero point, which can approximate pleural pressures, direct intrapleural measurement, or a transducer-tipped PA catheter.[44,45,46] The transducer-tipped catheter is the ideal method, eliminating the need for estimating the catheter tip (leveling) and zeroing. All three techniques are feasible but not commonly employed, primarily for technical or cost considerations, or both.

Reading of Waveforms with Respiratory Variation

In order to avoid incorrect readings, the clinician must approximate intrapleural pressures. This is most commonly done by reading pressure waves when intrapleural pressure is negligible or near normal. Intrapleural pressure is near baseline when no inspiratory or expiratory pressures are present. Gas flow at end expiration is, or should be, zero.[47] End expiration is therefore the most commonly used approximation of a stable intrapleural pressure (Fig. 6–3). Waveforms 6–3 through 6–5 provide examples illustrating end expiration in central venous pressure (CVP), PCWP, and pulmonary artery (PA) tracings.

The clinician should also keep in mind the type of distortion produced by respiratory cycles. In critical care settings, patients may be either breathing spontaneously or receiving mechanical ventilation. In any event, the most significant waveform distortion is produced by the mode that produces the most intrapleural pressure change. The respiratory component that

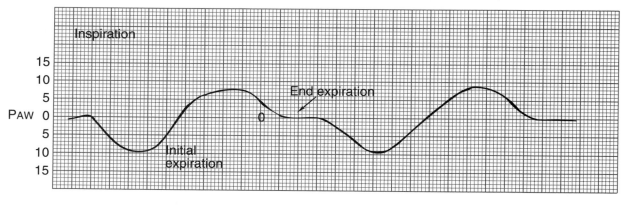

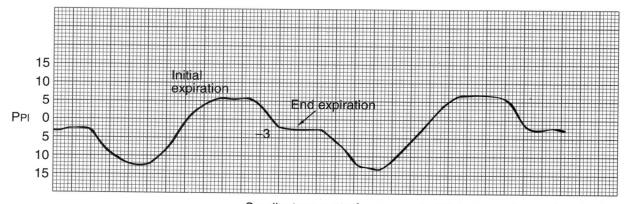

Smallest amount of unaccounted PPI changed at end expiration

Figure 6–3. Gas flow at end expiration (PAW) is approximately equal to pleural pressure (PPI).

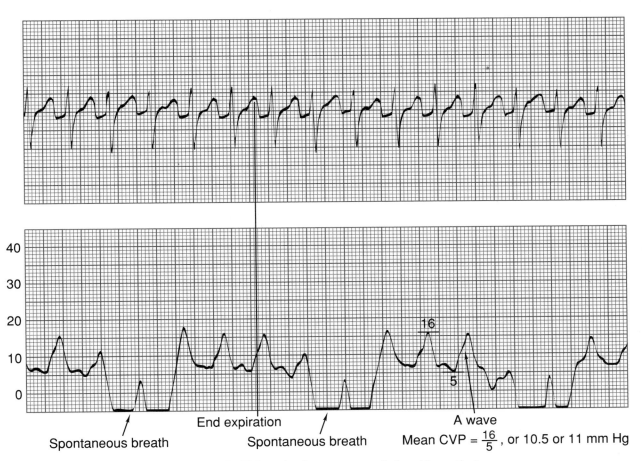

Waveform 6–3. CVP tracing in a spontaneously breathing patient.

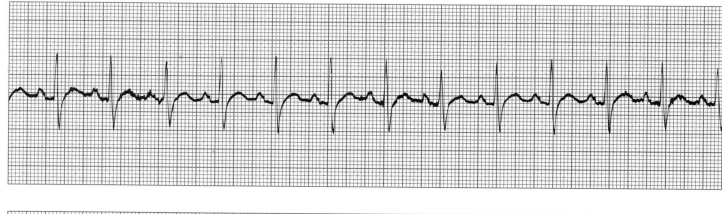

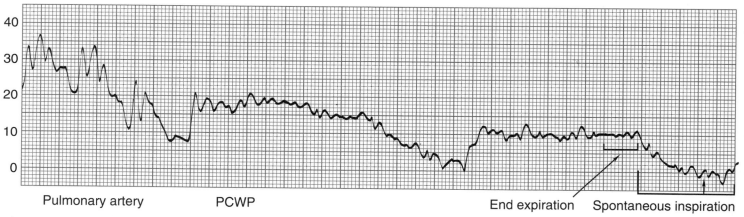

Pulmonary artery   PCWP   End expiration   Spontaneous inspiration

Mean PCWP = 10 mm Hg

Waveform 6–4. PCWP tracing in a spontaneously breathing patient.

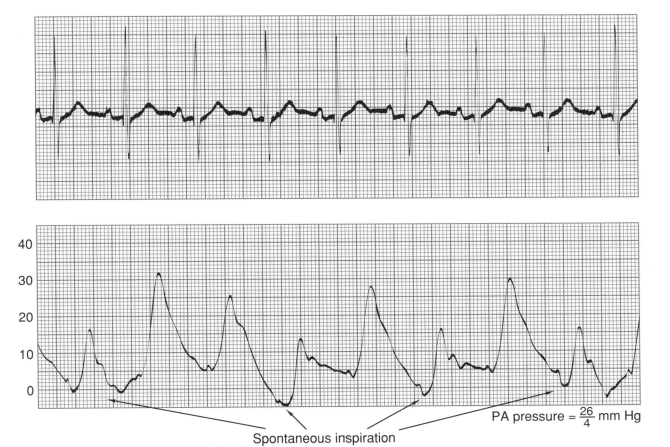

Waveform 6–5. Pulmonary artery waveform in a spontaneously breathing patient.

produces the most distortion is a spontaneously generated breath. Even when the patient is on mechanical ventilation, a spontaneously triggered respiration can produce substantial distortion in the waveform. Mechanical ventilation tends to produce less effect on the waveform because the positive pressure breath from the ventilator is introduced to the airways, not directly to the pleural space. Pressure changes during mechanical ventilation must reach the intrapleural space through the pulmonary tissue. Any air or mass between the airway and the pleural space will tend to absorb the ventilator-induced pressure. In healthy people, with compliant lungs, the pressure is fairly easily conducted across the lungs owing to minimal consolidation or lung water accumulation. However, in patients with poor lung compliance, the pressures are not readily transmitted across the lungs owing to consolidation or large amounts of air trapping. Waveforms clearly illustrate the implication of poor compliance on hemodynamic readings. Mechanical ventilator breaths, for example, tend to produce less artifact than will spontaneously generated breaths. The following sections will help illustrate this point.

SPONTANEOUS BREATHING

In a patient with spontaneous breathing, the waveform will decrease when compared with normal values (Waveform 6–6). In order to identify the correct location at which to read the waveform, note the point just prior to the inspiratory induced artifact. One must be careful to read the pressure wave that is free of inspiratory artifact, which means reading the wave prior to the inspiratory dip. Waveforms 6–7 and 6–8 illustrate the correct method of reading spontaneously generated breaths.

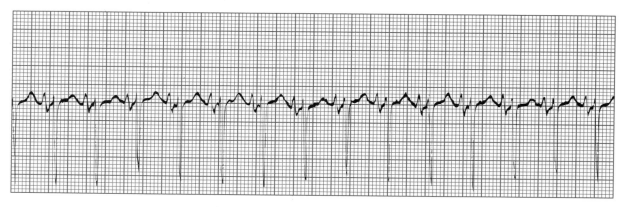

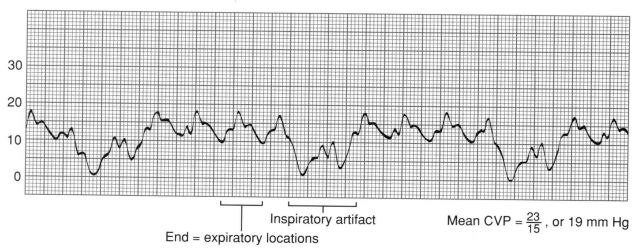

Inspiratory artifact

End = expiratory locations

Mean CVP = $\frac{23}{15}$, or 19 mm Hg

Waveform 6–6. CVP tracing with inspiratory artifact.

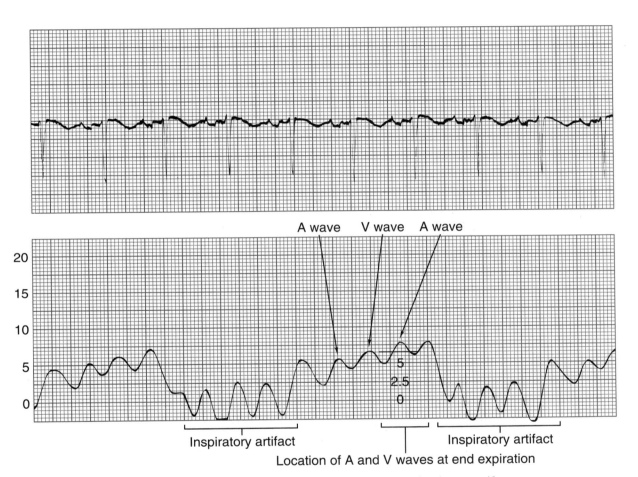

Waveform 6–7. Reading CVP waveforms with spontaneous inspiratory artifact.

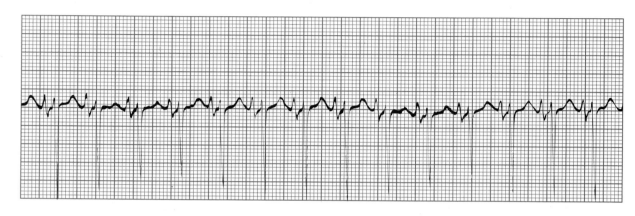

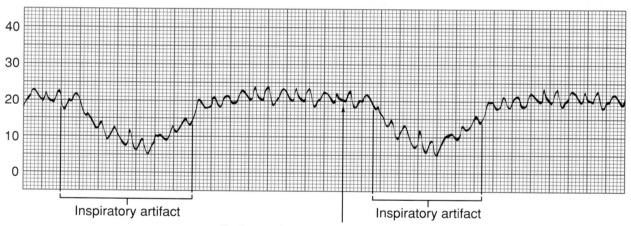

Inspiratory artifact

End = expiratory points for reading values

Inspiratory artifact

Mean PCWP = 20 mm Hg

Waveform 6–8. Reading PCWP waveforms with spontaneous inspiratory artifact.

Because inspiration is typically shorter than expiration, inspiratory artifact can be identified by noting which part of the waveform is larger. Waveform 6–9 illustrates a normal inspiratory/expiratory (I:E) ratio pattern of 1:2 (1-second inspiration/2-second expiration).

Typically, the largest waveform component is expiration. Two potential exceptions to this rule exist. In inverse I:E ratio ventilation, expiration becomes shorter than inspiration. The rule is now reversed. The relationship of transmural pressure to readings taken on patients with inverse I:E ratio ventilation is not well researched. A good possibility exists that these readings are also artificially high, owing to the limited time to reach end expiration.

The second exception is the patient who is breathing rapidly, greater than 30 breaths per minute (bpm). Inspiratory and expiratory time become nearly equal (Waveform 6–10) in patients with respiratory rates near 30 bpm. At this point, the patient's breathing will produce such distortions that the waveform may not be able to be correctly interpreted.[48] During rapid respiration, there may not be any point where zero gas flow exists. Without a point for zero gas flow, intrapleural pressure will always be different than the assumed normal value of near −3 mm Hg. As a rule, the intrapleural pressure is higher than expected because of the active expiration. The result is artificially elevated hemodynamic waveforms.

Clinicians may use several techniques to try to obtain more accurate readings. The simplest method would be to have the patient hold his or her breath after a normal expiration.[49] If the patient can perform this request for even a few seconds, a stable baseline can be noted (Waveform 6–11). Be careful that the patient does not bear down during breath holding, which will cause

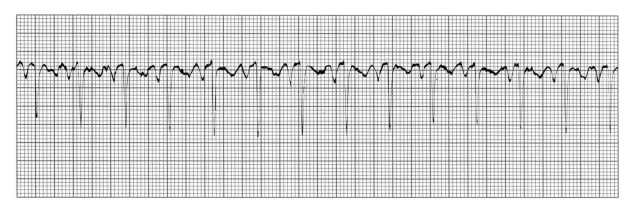

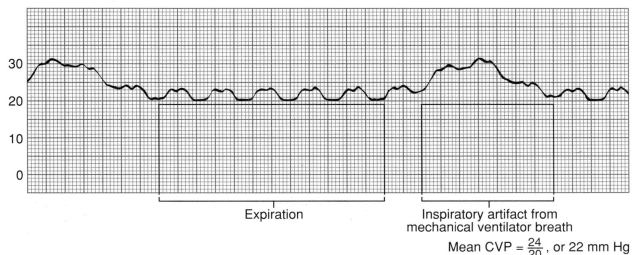

Expiration   Inspiratory artifact from
                mechanical ventilator breath

Mean CVP = $\frac{24}{20}$, or 22 mm Hg

Waveform 6–9. Normal inspiratory/expiratory ratio effect on waveform appearance.

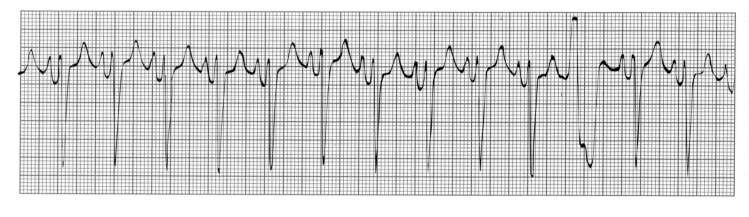

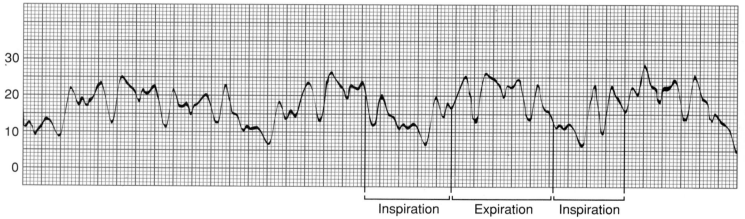

Waveform 6–10. Inspiratory/expiratory ratio effect on waveform appearance with rapid breathing.

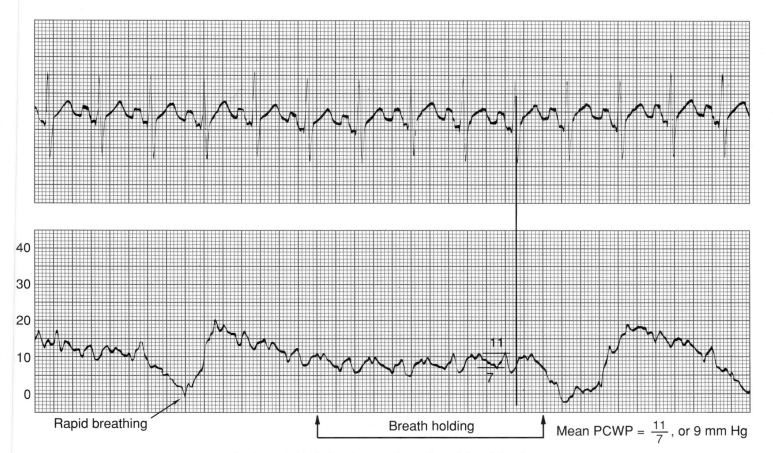

Rapid breathing

Breath holding

Mean PCWP = $\frac{11}{7}$, or 9 mm Hg

Waveform 6–11. Stabilizing waveforms through breath holding.

pressures to increase (Waveform 6–12). Similar to the waveform change that occurs with bearing down during exhalation is the waveform observed in the patient with forced exhalations, which may occur with obstructive airway disease. Waveform 6–13 illustrates the effect of forced exhalation on the waveform.

Unfortunately, many patients are breathing quickly because they are short of breath, and are unable to hold their breath even for a few seconds. If this occurs, a second method to stabilize the baseline would be to have the patient take several breaths quickly. If the patient is on a ventilator, give several breaths with the manual inspiration control or with a manual resuscitator (Ambu bag), which should reduce the arterial P_{CO_2} a few millimeters. If the Pa_{CO_2} is reduced, the drive to breathe will temporarily be reduced. Again, the goal is to stabilize the baseline for just a few seconds.

Should neither of these methods work, administering a short-acting muscle paralyzing agent will remove respiratory effort. Succinylcholine is an example of such an agent. Obviously, such a method could only be used in an intubated patient. In addition, make sure the patient is aware of the temporary loss of muscle control. The use of sedation simultaneously with the paralyzing agent is necessary to ensure patient comfort.

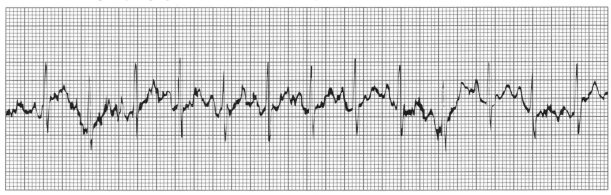

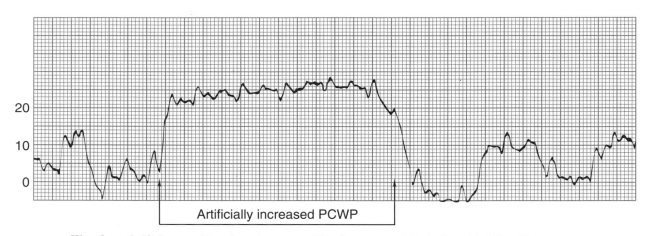

Waveform 6–12. Increased intrathoracic pressure (Valsalva manuever) during breath holding. The pressure values are artificially elevated during this event.

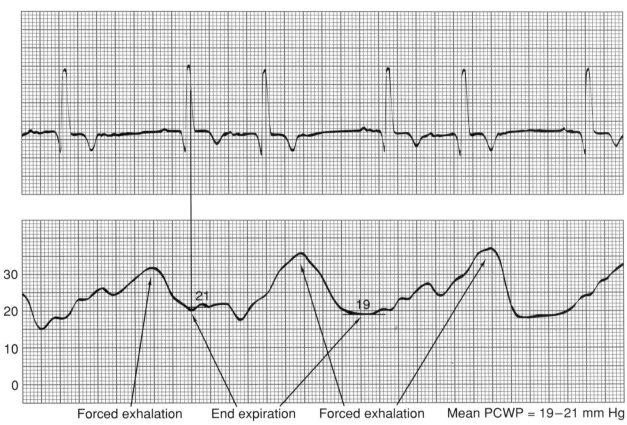

Forced exhalation   End expiration   Forced exhalation   Mean PCWP = 19–21 mm Hg

Waveform 6–13. Forced exhalation producing elevation in pressures. Read waveform after forced exhalation.

ASSISTED MANDATORY VENTILATION (ASSIST/CONTROL)

When a patient is on assisted mandatory ventilation (AMV), the location of waveform interpretation depends on whether the patient is triggering the ventilator or must rely on the ventilator to perform all respiration.

In the patient who is not triggering the ventilator, the only waveform distortion will be that produced by the ventilator positive pressure breath (Fig. 6–4). The ventilator artifact may or may not be pronounced, depending on the patient's pulmonary compliance. As a rule, the positive pressure will produce a slight upward deflection of the baseline (Waveforms 6–14 and 6–15).

If the patient is triggering the ventilator, the spontaneously generated breath will produce a dip in the waveform. This dip may be followed by positive pressure artifact from the ventilator (Fig. 6–5). The key to reading this type of artifact is identification of the inspiratory dip artifact and reading the wave before this dip (Waveforms 6–16 and 6–17). The inspiratory dip and the subsequent rise in the waveform are influenced by intrapleural pressures and should be avoided. Location of end expiration, just prior to the inspiratory deflection or dip, is necessary to obtain accurate values.

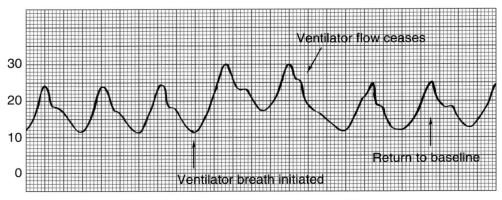

Figure 6–4. Ventilator-induced respiratory artifact in hemodynamic waves.

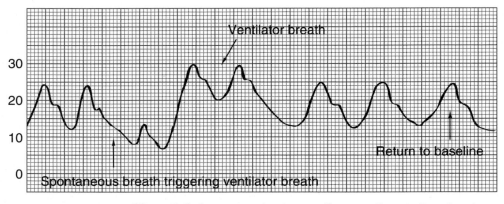

Figure 6–5. Spontaneous inspiratory effort preceding ventilator breath.

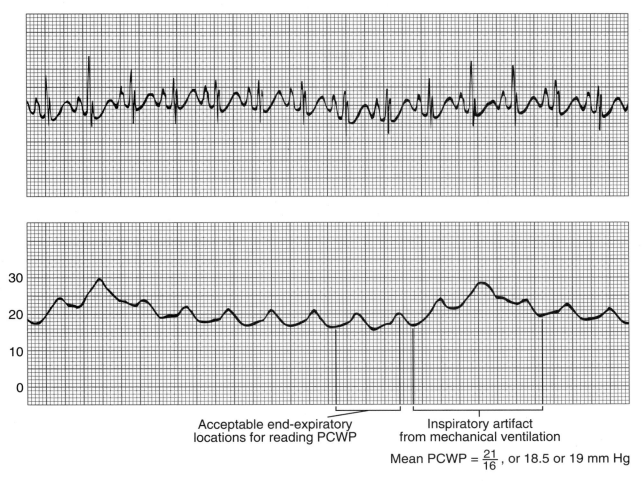

Acceptable end-expiratory
locations for reading PCWP

Inspiratory artifact
from mechanical ventilation

Mean PCWP = $\frac{21}{16}$, or 18.5 or 19 mm Hg

Waveform 6–14. Identifying end expiration in the patient receiving mechanical ventilation.

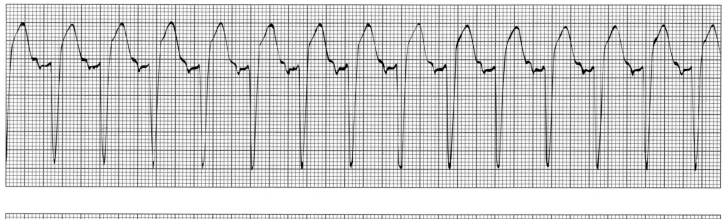

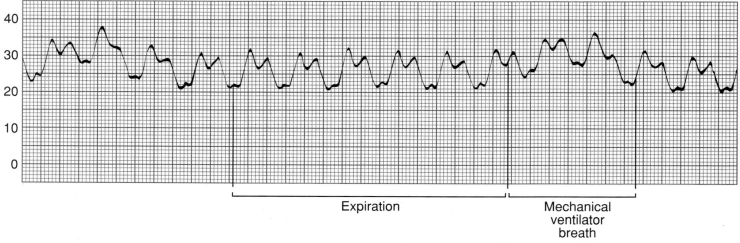

Expiration

Mechanical
ventilator
breath

$$\text{PA pressure} = \frac{31}{21} \text{ mm Hg}$$

Waveform 6–15. Effect of mechanical ventilation on waveform appearance.

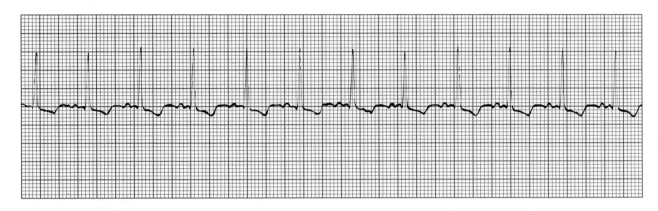

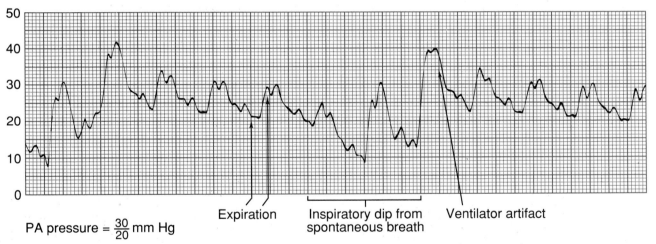

Expiration   Inspiratory dip from   Ventilator artifact
                  spontaneous breath

PA pressure = $\frac{30}{20}$ mm Hg

Waveform 6–16. Effect of mechanical ventilation triggered by a spontaneous breath on waveform appearance.

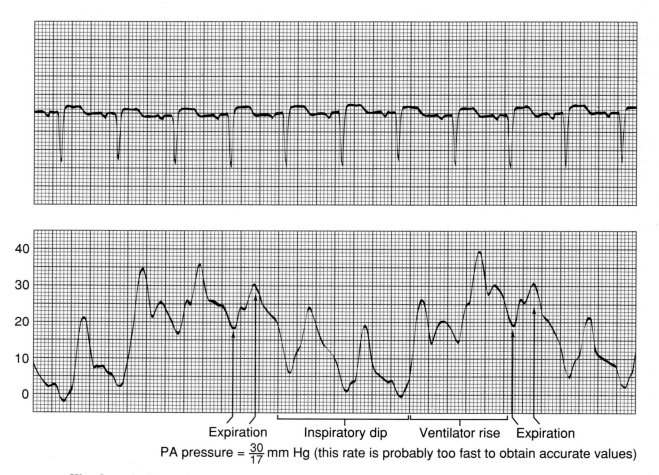

Expiration   Inspiratory dip   Ventilator rise   Expiration

PA pressure = $\frac{30}{17}$ mm Hg (this rate is probably too fast to obtain accurate values)

Waveform 6–17. Effect of mechanical ventilation triggered by rapid spontaneous breaths on waveform appearance.

INTERMITTENT MANDATORY VENTILATION

In the patient receiving intermittent mandatory ventilation (IMV), both spontaneous and positive pressure artifacts are possible. In this mode, however, the artifacts may be independent of each other. For example, in AMV, an inspiratory artifact would be immediately followed by positive pressure artifact. In IMV, spontaneous breathing is independent of mechanically delivered breaths. If the patient is not breathing spontaneously, then reading the waves is identical to reading the waves of the patient on AMV who is not breathing faster than the set rate. However, when the patient is spontaneously breathing, note inspiratory dips and avoid reading the artifact caused by these decreases in pressure. Positive pressure artifacts, if present, are noted by the slight upward deflection. Avoid these inflated readings. Waveform 6–18 illustrates the types of waveform variations in the IMV mode of ventilation. Figure 6–6 illustrates how to read hemodynamics in all the presented modes of ventilation.

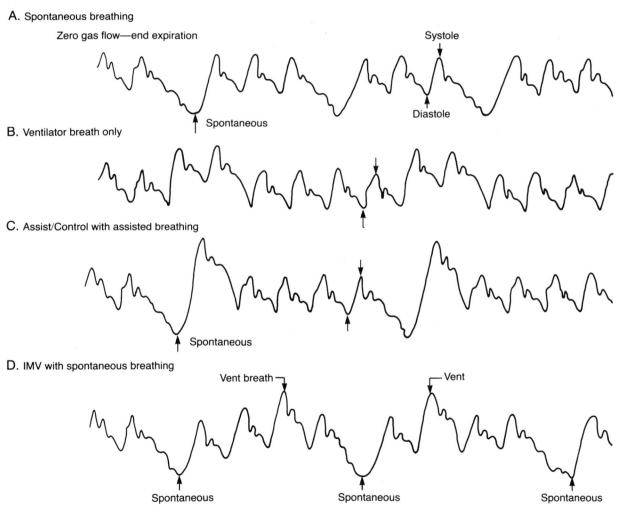

Figure 6–6. Identification of end expiration in different respiratory cycles.

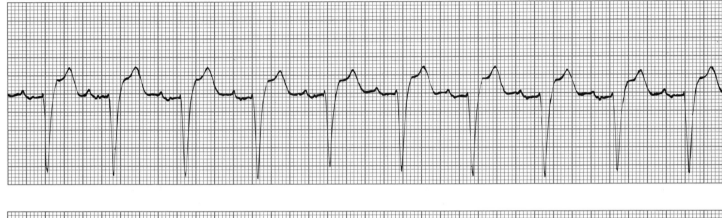

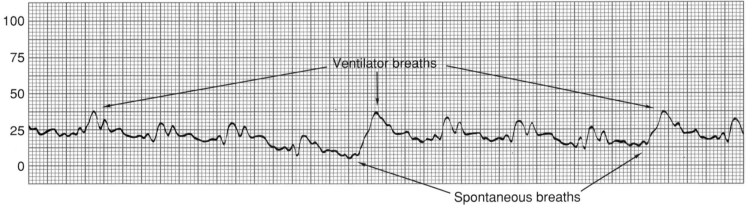

Waveform 6–18. IMV mode of ventilation and the effect on a PA waveform.

AIRWAY PRESSURE MONITORING TO IDENTIFY END EXPIRATION

The use of airway pressure monitoring to identify specific points in the respiratory cycle has great potential to aid in obtaining more accurate waveform analysis.[50] Airway pressure monitoring is relatively simple, requiring only a transducer and amplifier connection to the ventilator tubing near the endotracheal tube (Fig. 6–7).

Airway pressure monitoring allows easy identification of end expiration through monitoring changes in the patient airway pressures. Although pleural pressures are not measured, changes in the airway pressure that may affect hemodynamic values are clearly measured. As the patient inspires, the airway pressure records a decrease in pressure. If inspiration is generated from a ventilator, airway pressures rise. Exhalation is marked by a fall in airway pressures. As the patient exhales, end expiration is the point of zero gas flow, accompanied by zero pressure (Fig. 6–8).

Inspiratory artifacts, both patient- and ventilator-generated, are easily identified. Spontaneous breaths generate subatmospheric pressures (or pressures below positive end-expiratory pressure [PEEP]/continuous positive airway pressure [CPAP] levels); ventilator breaths produce positive pressure distortion. Waveforms 6–19 and 6–20 provide examples of spontaneous and ventilator-induced changes in airway pressures. Once inspiratory artifact can be identified, reading end expiration is simplified. Waveforms 6–21 and 6–22 provide examples of reading end expiration with the aid of airway pressure monitoring.

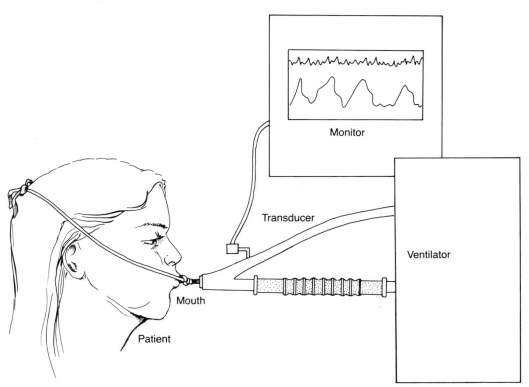

Figure 6–7. Airway pressure transducer mounting in ventilator circuit.

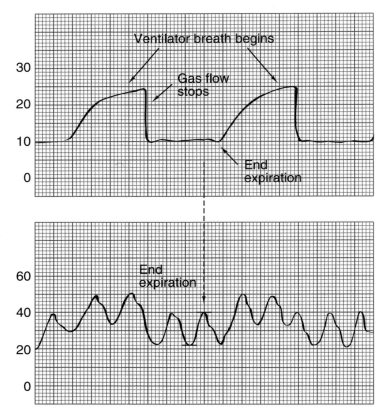

Figure 6–8. Simultaneous use of airway pressures and hemodynamic waveforms to identify end expiration.

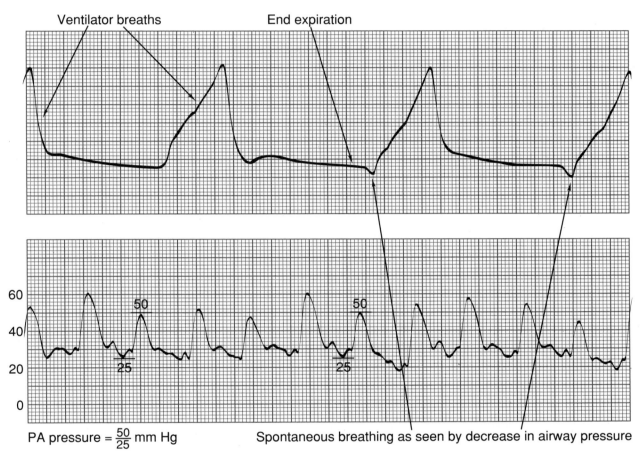

Ventilator breaths

End expiration

60

50

40

25

20

0

50

25

50

25

PA pressure = $\frac{50}{25}$ mm Hg

Spontaneous breathing as seen by decrease in airway pressure

Waveform 6–19. Spontaneous and ventilator-induced changes in airway pressure.

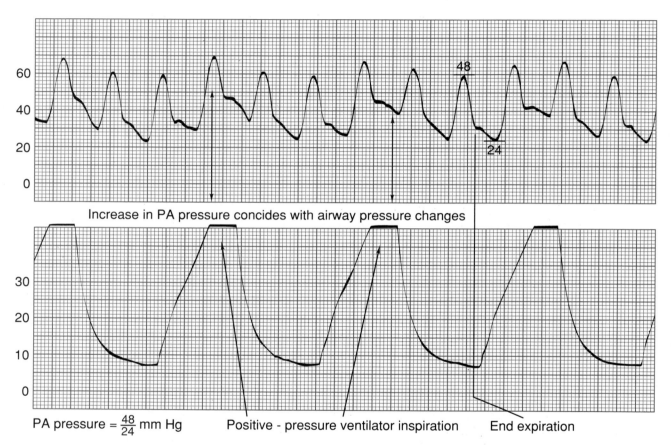

Increase in PA pressure concides with airway pressure changes

PA pressure = $\frac{48}{24}$ mm Hg   Positive - pressure ventilator inspiration   End expiration

Waveform 6–20. Ventilator-induced changes in airway pressure.

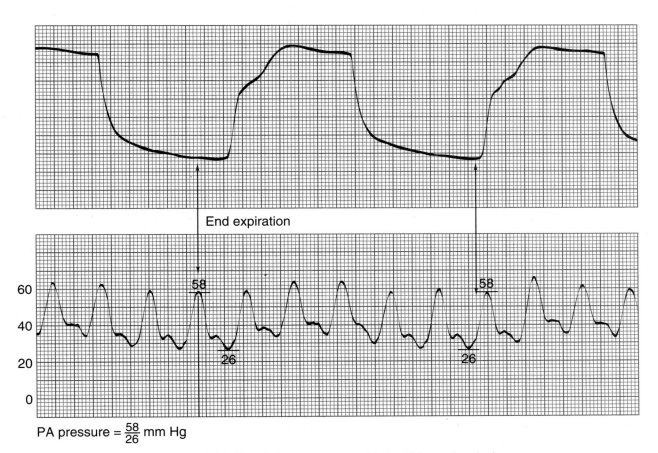

PA pressure = $\frac{58}{26}$ mm Hg

Waveform 6–21. Use of airway pressure to aid identifying end expiration.

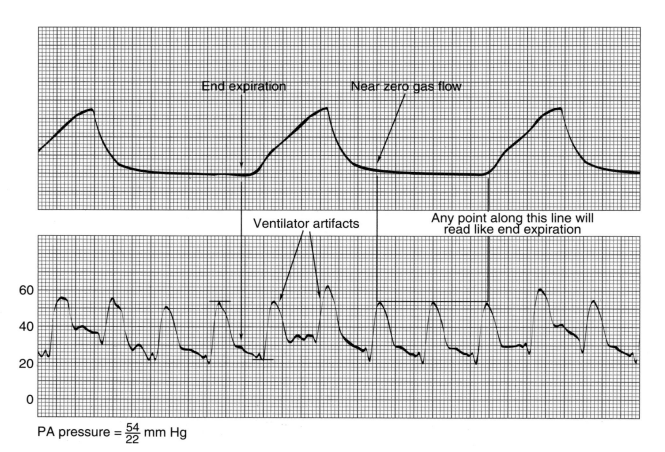

PA pressure = $\frac{54}{22}$ mm Hg

Waveform 6–22. Airway pressure and end expiration.

CONCEPT OF AUTO-PEEP

In a mechanically ventilated patient with rapid respirations, the inability to completely exhale before starting another inspiration may trap pressure inside the lungs. The air or pressure trapping is referred to as an auto-PEEP effect.[51] The increased pressure from the auto-PEEP can cause reductions in the cardiac output and increase the incidence of barotrauma to the lungs. All readings will potentially be altered (usually elevated) from the auto-PEEP.

In a patient breathing rapidly, the presence of auto-PEEP can be verified relatively easily. If the ventilator in use does not have an expiratory pause feature, the procedure must be manual. With the manual technique, the first step is to locate the exhalation valve on the ventilator. Second, after a ventilator-delivered inspiration and immediately before the next ventilator breath, temporarily obstruct the expiratory tubing. Third, after blocking the expiratory line, note the pressure on the pressure manometer.[52] If auto-PEEP is present, the pressure will not return to zero (or the preset desired PEEP level).

If airway pressure monitoring is available, use of the airway pressure waveform simplifies measurement of auto-PEEP. Measurement of auto-PEEP is readily identified by obtaining an airway pressure reading during the auto-PEEP measurement. If auto-PEEP is present, the airway pressure reading will readily be evident (Waveform 6–23).

If auto-PEEP is present, ventilator adjustments such as increasing inspiratory flow rates, reducing the respiratory rate or tidal volume, or sedating the patient may be necessary to prevent the hemodynamic problems associated with auto-PEEP. Identification of auto-PEEP is important due to the inability of normal ventilator monitoring to detect the trapped pressures. Any patient with high ventilatory demands should have auto-PEEP checked on a routine basis, e.g., every 2 hours or when the respiratory rate increases.

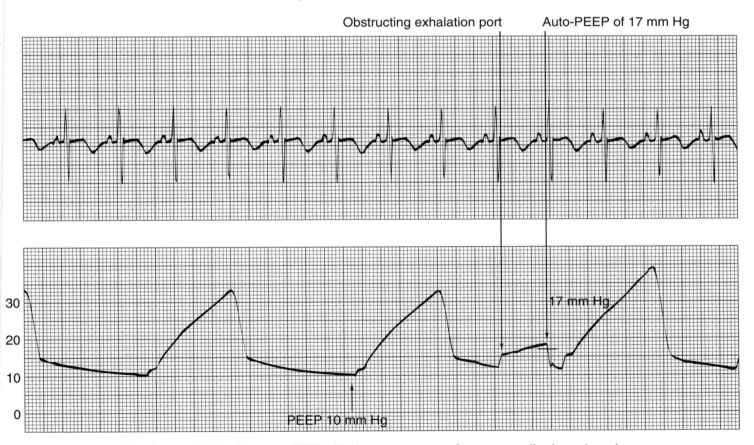

Waveform 6–23. Identifying auto-PEEP with airway pressure waveforms temporarily obstructing exhalation value.

Remember that obstruction of the expiratory tubing during measurement for auto-PEEP is performed in a matter of seconds or less. Do not block the expiratory tubing for any more than the second or two necessary to note the auto-PEEP effect. If the exhalation port is obstructed while the next ventilator breath is delivered, the resultant breath will produce higher airway pressures. The higher airway pressures could potentially cause barotrauma to develop.

SUMMARY

Differentiating appropriate end-expiratory points to read the waveforms is important for obtaining consistent values. Even the most recent monitoring systems have difficulty in consistently identifying the optimal location to read the pressure tracing with respiratory artifact.[51] Inasmuch as the monitoring systems cannot be consistently trusted for accurate values, the clinician is responsible for reading the waveform correctly.

PRACTICE WAVEFORMS

Practice Waveforms 6–1 through 6–9 review the major waveform distortions noted with respiratory artifact. Try to interpret the waveforms to assess your skill with waveform interpretation.

PRACTICE WAVEFORM 6–1. In this pulmonary artery tracing with spontaneous inspiratory artifact, where would you read the waveform?

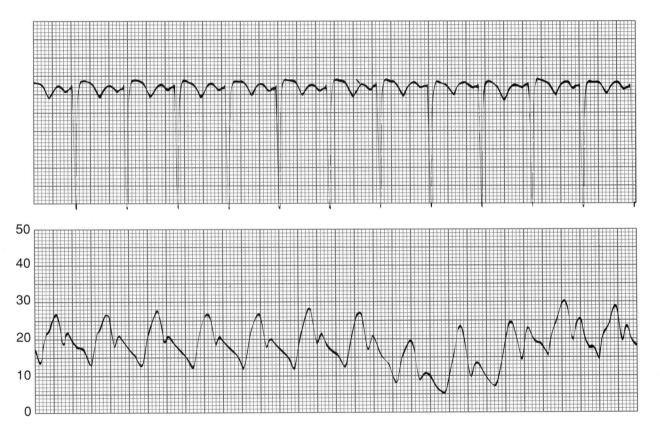

PRACTICE WAVEFORM 6–1. *Analysis:* End-expiratory values are located as marked, immediately prior to the negative deflections produced by the inspiratory effort.

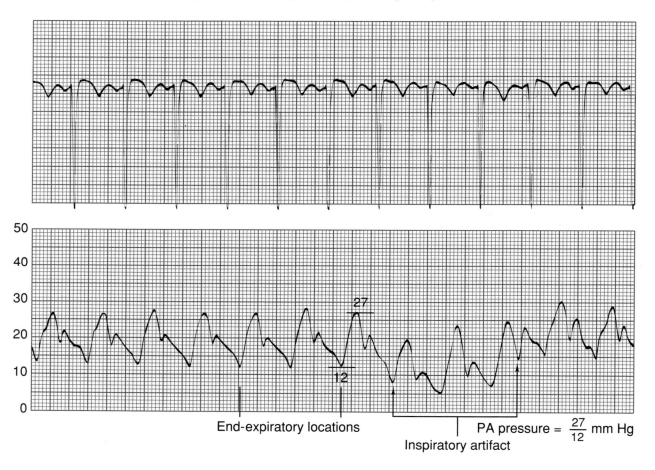

End-expiratory locations

Inspiratory artifact

PA pressure = $\frac{27}{12}$ mm Hg

PRACTICE WAVEFORM 6–2. Spontaneously breathing patient with rapid respiratory rate. Where would you read this waveform?

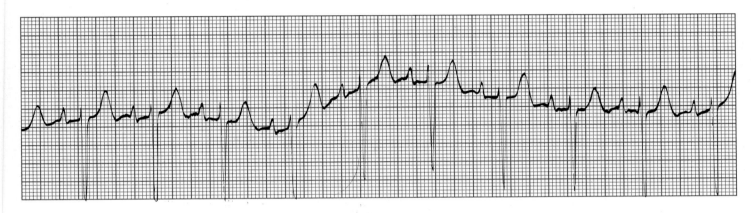

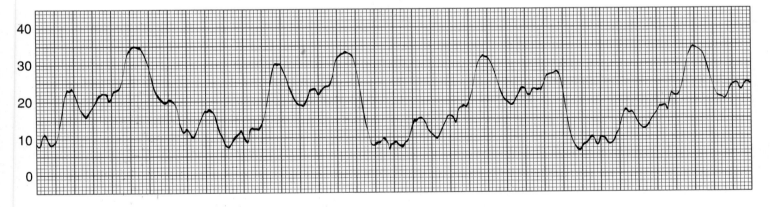

PRACTICE WAVEFORM 6–2. *Analysis:* End expiration is identified as marked. In this fast respiratory rate, no clear end-expiratory value is present, although potential sites are noted.

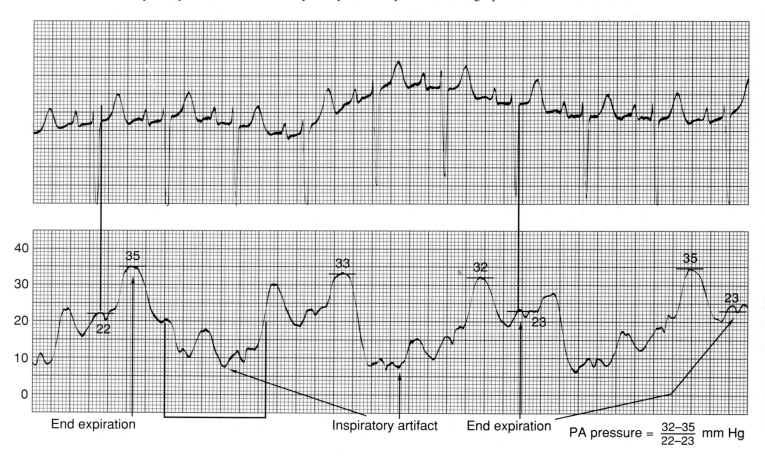

End expiration   Inspiratory artifact   End expiration   PA pressure = $\dfrac{32-35}{22-23}$ mm Hg

PRACTICE WAVEFORM 6–3. In this patient on assist/control ventilation with spontaneous inspiratory efforts, where would you read the waveform?

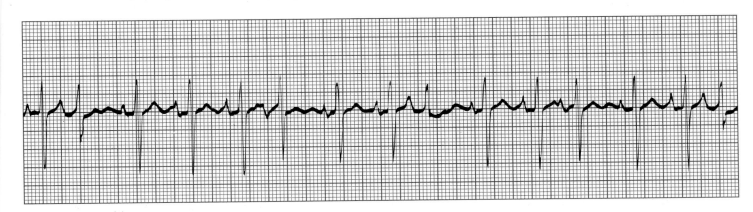

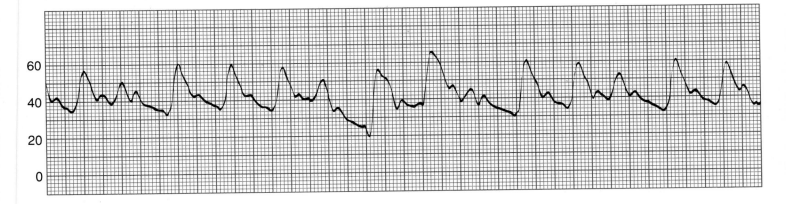

PRACTICE WAVEFORM 6–3. *Analysis:* Inspiratory artifact and end-expiration values are marked.

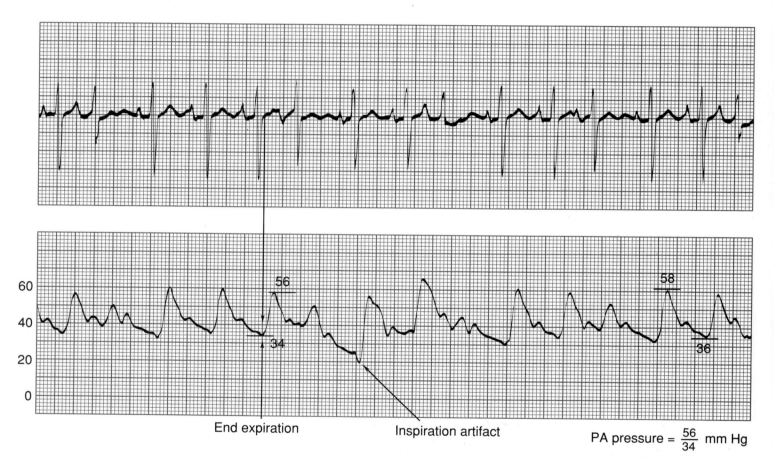

End expiration   Inspiration artifact   PA pressure = $\dfrac{56}{34}$ mm Hg

PRACTICE WAVEFORM 6–4. Assist/control ventilation in a patient without spontaneous inspiratory artifact. Where would you read this pulmonary artery waveform?

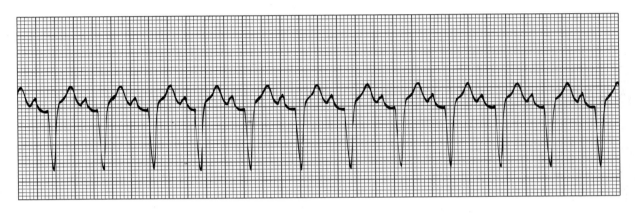

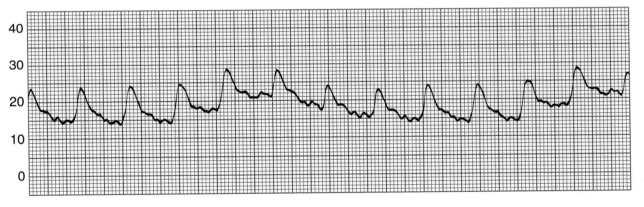

PRACTICE WAVEFORM 6–4. *Analysis:* Inspiratory artifact and end-expiration values are marked.

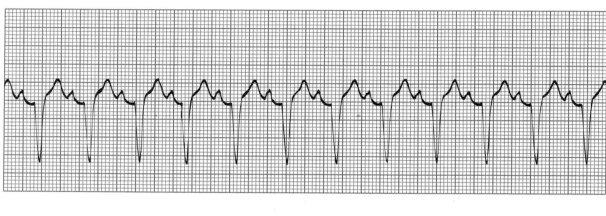

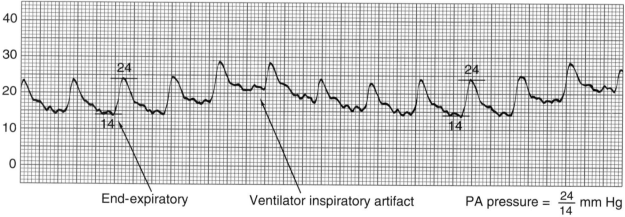

End-expiratory   Ventilator inspiratory artifact   PA pressure = $\frac{24}{14}$ mm Hg

PRACTICE WAVEFORM 6–5. In this CVP tracing in a patient receiving IMV mode of ventilation, rate of 10 with a total rate of 20, where is the tracing read?

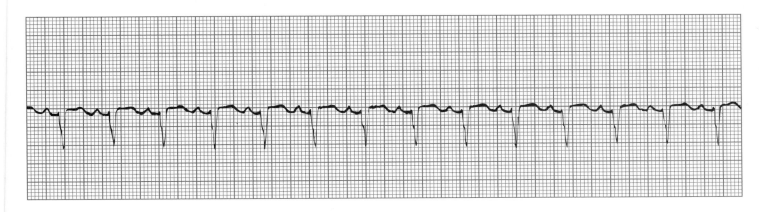

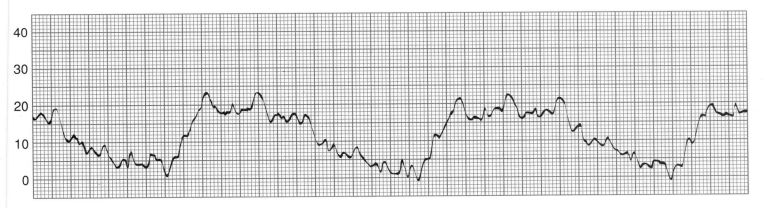

PRACTICE WAVEFORM 6–5. *Analysis:* Note end expiration is at the peak plateau, not the lower levels. The lower levels are a reflection of the distortion of spontaneous inspiratory efforts on the waveform. No overt ventilator effect is present.

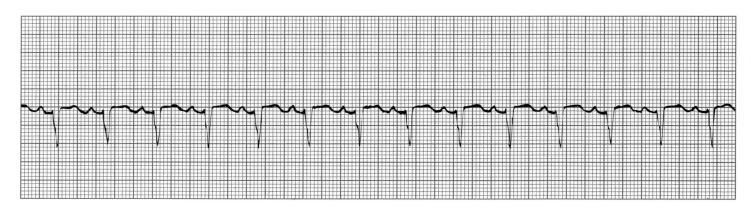

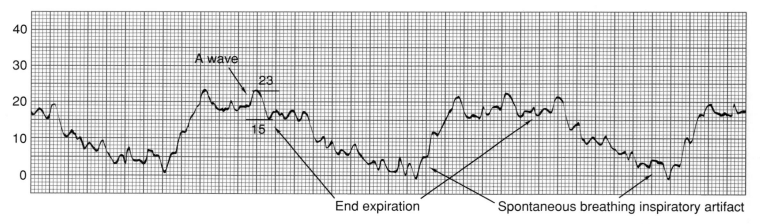

A wave

23

15

End expiration

Spontaneous breathing inspiratory artifact

Mean CVP = $\frac{23}{15}$, or 18 mm Hg

PRACTICE WAVEFORM 6–6. Pulmonary artery waveform in a spontaneous breathing patient. No mechanical ventilation is present. Where would you read this pulmonary artery waveform?

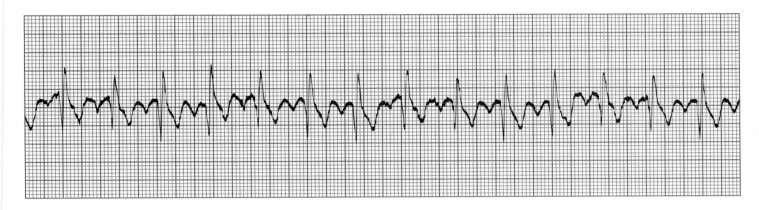

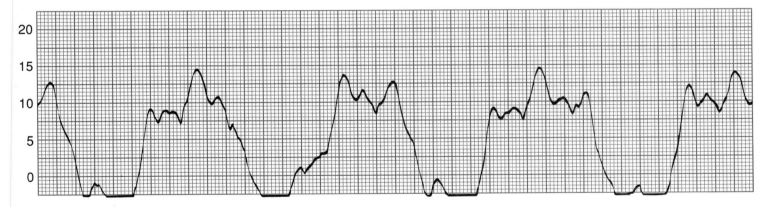

PRACTICE WAVEFORM 6–6. *Analysis:* Inspiratory artifact and end-expiration values are marked. Note the marked changes in waveform values due to the inspiratory effort and the small scale.

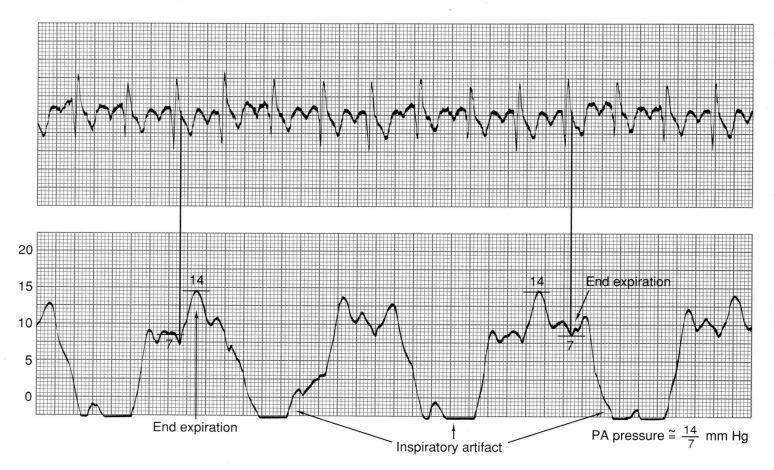

PRACTICE WAVEFORM 6–7. This dual waveform illustrates both a radial artery waveform and a pulmonary artery wave. Considering this patient is not on mechanical ventilation, where would each of these waveforms be read?

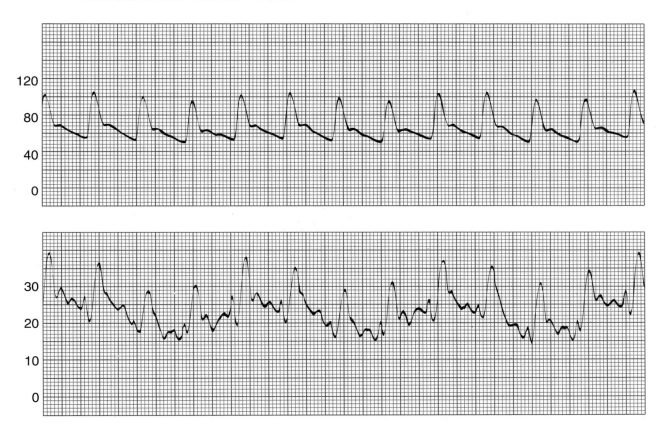

PRACTICE WAVEFORM 6–7. *Analysis:* The pulmonary artery wave is read at end expiration, as marked. The radial artery wave must be summed because the changes in waveform appearance with the radial wave are real, not artifact.

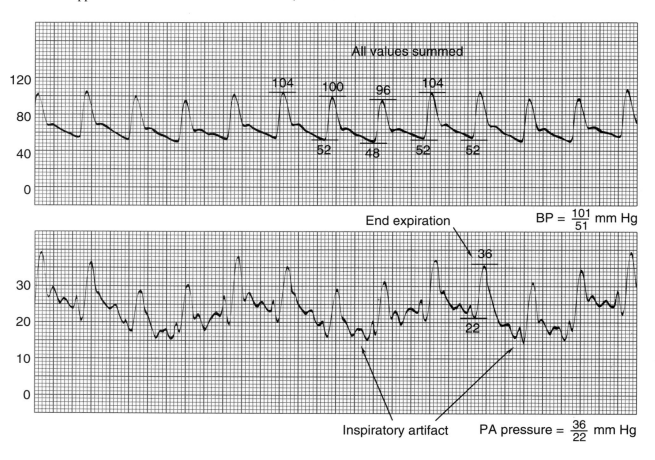

All values summed

104 100 96 104

52 48 52 52

$$BP = \frac{101}{51} \text{ mm Hg}$$

End expiration

36

22

Inspiratory artifact $PA \text{ pressure} = \frac{36}{22} \text{ mm Hg}$

PRACTICE WAVEFORM 6–8. This CVP tracing is from a patient receiving assist/control ventilation without spontaneous breathing. Where would you read this CVP waveform?

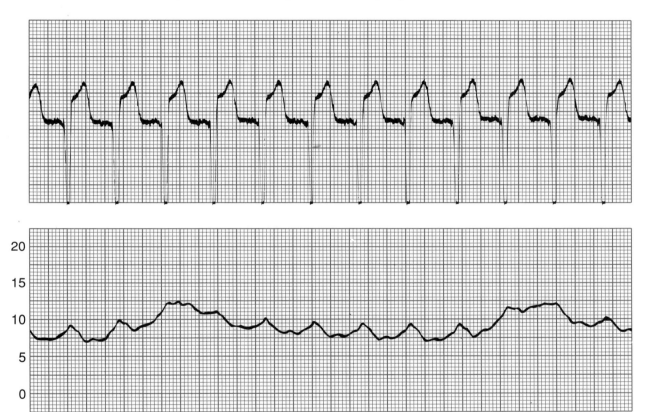

PRACTICE WAVEFORM 6–8. *Analysis:* Read end expiration in front of the ventilatory artifact (end expiration).

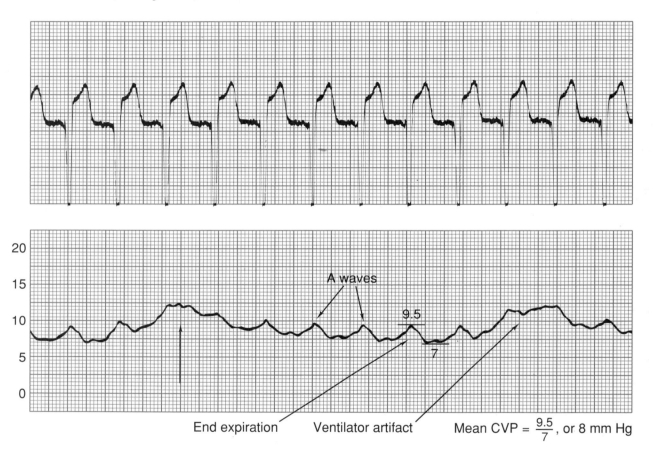

PRACTICE WAVEFORM 6–9. CVP tracing in a patient with spontaneous breathing. Where would you read this CVP waveform?

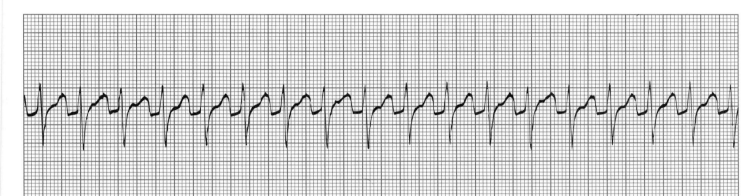

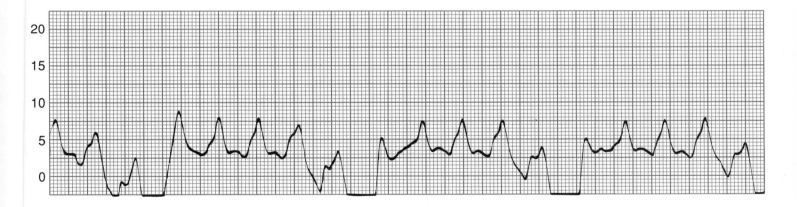

PRACTICE WAVEFORM 6–9. *Analysis:* Inspiratory artifact and end-expiration values are marked.

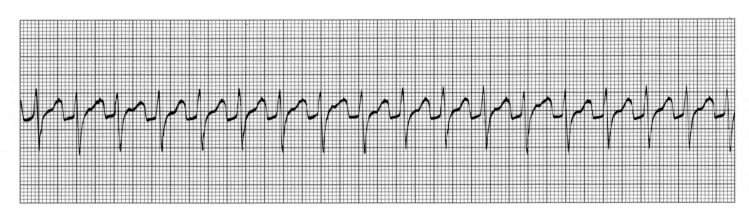

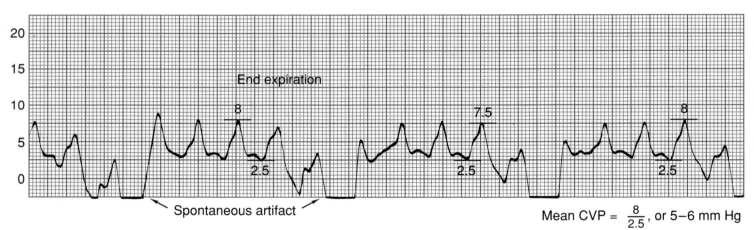

End expiration

Spontaneous artifact

Mean CVP = $\frac{8}{2.5}$, or 5–6 mm Hg

7 Technical Considerations in Obtaining Hemodynamic Waveform Values

Technical issues regarding hemodynamic monitoring are frequently confusing to clinicians. In this chapter, we present concepts relating to technical issues commonly encountered by critical care nurses. These concepts are presented in such a way as to address technical issues without becoming too complex or confusing. Understanding the technical issues involving hemodynamic monitoring, including troubleshooting, is crucial to obtaining accurate values. The goal of this chapter is to present key technical issues clearly and in a manner nurses find practical.

INTRODUCTION TO TECHNICAL ISSUES IN HEMODYNAMIC MONITORING

Hemodynamic monitoring depends on obtaining waveforms as they occur in the blood vessel. Several aspects regarding the technical features of reproducing the waveform can interfere with obtaining accurate waveform values. The nurse must be aware of these factors in order to avoid obtaining inaccurate values. Major factors influencing hemodynamic monitoring include: (1) the components of the tubing-catheter system; and (2) transducer/amplifier function (zeroing and calibration). A thorough understanding of these features ensures that the clinician can obtain accurate hemodynamic waveform values.

Potential technical problems in waveform reproduction will also be explored in this chapter, including catheter-induced artifact, verifying a pulmonary capillary wedge position, accuracy of peripheral arterial catheters, troubleshooting monitoring equipment, and the appropriate use of bedside monitor display information.

INTRODUCTION TO WAVEFORM MEASUREMENT

Obtaining accurate waveform values depends greatly on proper functioning of the fluid-filled tubing system feeding the waveform from its source (the blood vessel) to the monitoring system. Although the specific technical functioning of the mechanical components in waveform reproduction (transducers and pressure amplifier systems) is beyond the scope of this text, the nurse should understand a few key concepts in order to interpret waveforms accurately.

Three components of the system are important to the nurse in regard to their impact on accurate waveform reproduction: (1) zero balancing of the transducer/amplifier system; (2) calibration of the transducer/amplifier system; and (3) adequate frequency response and damping coefficient of the catheter tubing system.

Understanding these three aspects, however, requires a basic understanding of physics and electronic principles—information typically not in most health care academic curriculums, at least to the extent that may be helpful in understanding waveform reproduction. Most nurses, therefore, are unfamiliar with basic principles of waveform reproduction. Although much more in-depth information is available on the scientific background necessary to understand the technical nature of hemodynamic monitoring, the focus of this chapter will be practical rather than theoretical. The reader is referred to several very good references for more complete information on these technical aspects of hemodynamic monitoring.[53,54,55]

For waveforms to be reproduced on the amplifier display panel, the typical invasive monitoring system must have the following components: (1) A fluid-filled catheter tubing system; (2) a transducer capable of reproducing accurate pressures; and (3) an amplifier that will integrate with the transducer and catheter tubing system to faithfully reproduce the transducer values to the display (Fig. 7–1). Each of these components needs to be briefly explained in order to provide an understanding of their importance and potential effect on waveform interpretation.

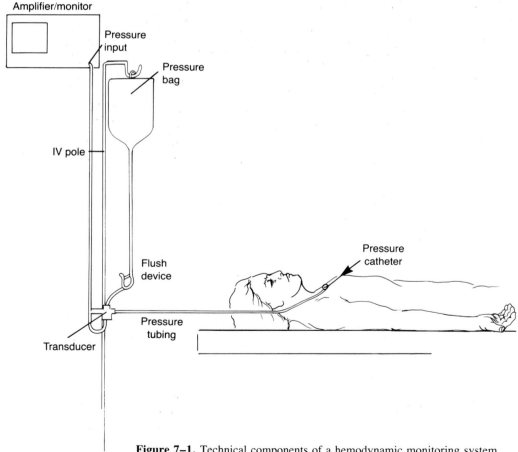

Figure 7–1. Technical components of a hemodynamic monitoring system.

THE CATHETER TUBING COMPONENT

The first component of the catheter tubing system is the catheter, which is introduced directly into the blood vessel. Located immediately after the catheter is the tubing or tubing set, which transfers the pressure back to the transducer. The tubing set may also include various stopcocks or drug infusion ports. For practical purposes, the catheter and tubing are considered as one unit, and we will, for the sake of clarity, refer to the catheter and tubing set simply as the tubing set.

The first consideration to be noted regarding the tubing set is that the tubing must be filled with fluid for the waveform to be reproduced. Fluid is the transport mechanism that delivers the vascular pressures to the transducer. Fluid is essentially noncompressible, allowing the pressure waveform to be transmitted across relatively long distances.

Not all substances are good transmitters of the pressure waveform. An air bubble in the tubing, for example, is compressible and will distort the waveform. The presence of air in the system will interfere with the tubing set's ability to accurately deliver correct information to the transducer. Therefore, care must be taken to avoid the presence of air in the system.

Air is only one of many factors that may distort the waveform. Any factor that affects the impulse transmission can change the waveform's appearance. One factor is a change in the density of the fluid within the tubing set. If blood is present in the tubing set, the blood may absorb more of the waveform than normal saline.

Another factor is the tubing itself. If the tubing distends during the waveform pulsation, the waveform can be dissipated as the tubing expands. Compliant tubing tends to absorb energy from the fluid and then return it to the system a very short time later. The result is an inaccurate representation of the measured waveform. In order to avoid this problem, tubing manufactured for pressure monitoring is made to be highly noncompliant. The more rigid (noncompliant) the tubing, the better it will function. Noncompliant tubing is readily identified on touch, as it feels very rigid in comparison with normal tubing.

Another factor that may alter the waveform is the length of tubing. The longer the tubing, the more likely the waveform will not be faithfully reproduced. As a general guideline, keeping the tubing as short as possible will help obtain more accurate waveforms.

An important point to remember is that problems in the tubing set are the only clinical aspects of the measurement system that will actually change the waveform *appearance*. Problems with zero balancing and calibration may change the overall values, but will not change the appearance of the waveform. Thus, if the waveform's appearance changes, something is wrong with the tubing set.

Assessing the Adequacy of the Tubing Catheter Set

Measurement of Frequency Response and Damping Coefficients

Frequency response (FR) and *damping coefficient* (DC) are terms used during assessment of the tubing catheter system. Abnormalities in FR or DC can produce errors in the systolic and diastolic values of the blood pressure. A basic understanding of these terms allows us to appreciate how they may influence waveform reproduction and blood pressure values.

Frequency response and damping coefficient measure the overall system's ability to accurately reproduce a signal. One analogy of this concept is that of a home stereo system. Typically accepted values for high-quality equipment are a frequency response of 20 Hertz (Hz) to 20,000 Hz (1 Hz = 1 cycle/second). Although there are some components of music that are outside of this range, they are not important to reproduce because the human ear cannot distinguish them. Hemodynamic monitoring is very similar. The accepted FR for clinical diagnostic waveform reproduction is 1/2 Hz to 40 Hz. Although there are some components of the waveforms that are outside of this range, they are not necessary for typical intensive care monitoring needs. Most current hemodynamic monitoring equipment (tubing sets, transducer, and amplifiers) has the necessary FR characteristics, although these characteristics should be carefully investigated before purchasing equipment. For the purpose of this text, we shall assume the equipment meets the desired requirements.

    A tubing set can reproduce waveforms accurately if the system has adequate FR and DC.[56] The FR refers to the system's ability to reproduce all of the waveform components being generated. Arterial waveforms generate multiple components, and the inability to reproduce any of the components can affect the waveform's ultimate appearance (Fig. 7–2).

Example A

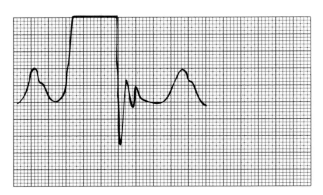

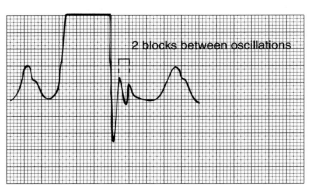

$$\frac{25}{2} = 12.5 \text{ Hz}$$

Example B

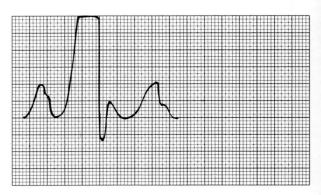

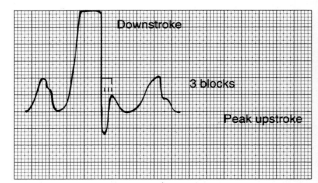

1. Perform square wave test.
2. Note the number of blocks between oscillations.
3. Divide number of blocks into paper speed (usually set at 25 mm) This number gives the frequency response.

If no oscillations are noted, measure the number of blocks between the downstroke of the square wave and the peak of the upstroke.

$$\frac{25}{3} = 8.3 \text{ Hz}$$

Figure 7–2. Method for measuring frequency response of the tubing catheter system. Note that measuring frequency response often yields an approximation rather than an exact value.

The DC can be thought of as the ability to reproduce the changes in the actual waveform. A good example to illustrate the damping principle is the shock absorbers on your car. If their ''damping coefficient'' is too low (i.e., shocks are no good), any bump in the road will cause your car to continue to bounce up and down, even after the bump is gone. If the ''damping coefficient'' is too high (i.e., extra stiff shocks), a bump in the road could cause the tires to come off the road momentarily.

Interaction Between Frequency Response and Damping Coefficient

If the FR of the system is too low, the waveform cannot be reproduced accurately even if the system has a good DC. Also, large variations in DC will produce errors, even if the system has a good FR. If the system has a reduced FR, such as would occur with air in the line, the system cannot be relied upon to accurately reproduce the waveforms. Mechanisms that distort waveforms, such as air or changes in the viscosity of fluid, act by changing the FR or DC, or both.

All hemodynamic waveforms contain many different frequency components. A technique used to analyze these components is called Fourier analysis. This analysis breaks down a waveform into individual components, each with a single frequency. Waveforms that change rapidly have more high frequency components than those that change more slowly. To illustrate this, consider the typical arterial waveform. Portions of the waveform change more rapidly than others. The dicrotic notch and the point at which the aortic valve opened represent the most rapidly changing portions of the arterial waveform. These portions also have higher frequency components than the other portions of the waveform. If the system has too low of an FR, the system may accurately reproduce the majority of the waveform, but smooth over the dicrotic notch and aortic valve opening point.

Using the same waveform for an example, a system with a very low DC (underdamped), would tend to ''ring'' and exaggerate the dicrotic notch (Waveform 7–1). A high DC (overdamped) would smooth out the waveform, creating an effect similar to that caused by a low frequency response.

Fortunately, the nurse does not need to have an in-depth understanding of physics in order to determine if a system has an adequate FR and DC. Several authors have reported a simple method to estimate the adequacy of the tubing set through an application of the square wave test.[57,58] The square wave test is simple to perform, relatively easy to read, and provides the nurse with a practical method to determine the adequacy of the tubing set.

The square wave test is performed by activating the fast flush device on the pressure tubing. Although some fast flush systems may perform the square wave test better than others, most commercial fast flush systems can be used to perform square wave tests. When the fast flush device is activated, the transducer is exposed to the pressure in the flush solution bag (typically 300 mm Hg). The result is a rapid rise in pressure that exceeds the display capacity, resulting in a squaring off of the pressure wave or the waveform going off scale (Fig. 7–3). Upon release of the flush device, the pressure wave should rapidly return to the baseline. A few oscillations of the waveform will be noted below and above the baseline. The distance between these oscillations can be measured to reflect the frequency response. Frequency response can be estimated by recording the waveform on paper, noting the distance between oscillations, and then dividing the distance into the paper speed. For example, if the distance between oscillations is 2 mm and the paper speed is normal at 25 mm per second, then the FR is calculated to be $25/2 = 12.5$ Hz. Adequate FR must be higher than 8.1 Hz.[59]

The height of the oscillations can be used to determine the adequacy of the DC. If the damping coefficient is abnormal, the difference in height between oscillations varies. Generally,

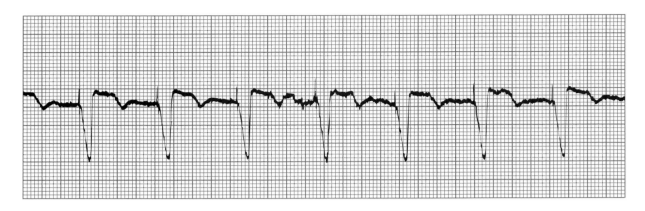

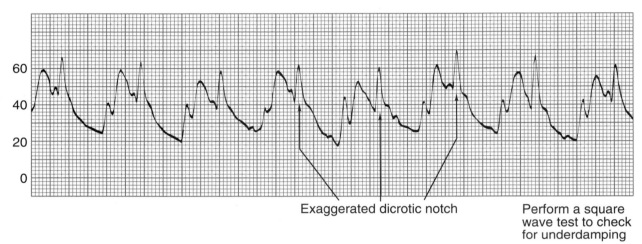

Exaggerated dicrotic notch

Perform a square
wave test to check
for underdamping

Waveform 7–1. Exaggerated dicrotic notch in an underdamped pulmonary artery tracing.

the greater the height of the oscillations, the lower the DC (underdamping). Loss of oscillation or of small deflections reflects high DCs (overdamping). The DC is the more difficult of the two to measure because it requires a conversion scale. Figures 7–4 and 7–5 provide examples of typical square wave tests and the measurement of FR and DC.

If the tubing set is unable to reproduce a waveform accurately, the square wave test will detect the problem in either FR or DC. If the FR is low, the system is slow to respond and upon the release of the fast flush device, the square wave pattern widens between oscillations (Waveform 7–2).

It is important to remember that the higher the FR of the system, the less impact an abnormal DC will have on producing errors within the system. Because of the relatively low frequency characteristics of blood pressure waveforms in general, if the FR is significantly higher than is normally required, then relatively large errors in the DC can be tolerated before any notable effect is generated in the waveform.

The interaction between FR and DC should produce an optimally damped waveform (Waveform 7–3). If a problem exists with either FR or DC, two basic types of errors, overdamping and underdamping, can occur. Overdamping will diminish the systolic and may slightly elevate the diastolic values. Underdamping will potentially increase the systolic and may decrease the diastolic values. An overdamped tracing is illustrated in Waveform 7–4, and an underdamped tracing is presented in Waveform 7–5.

1. Activate fast flush device.
2. Hold flush device open for less than 1 second.
3. Quickly release flush device.
4. Note square wave pattern on monitor or strip recorder.

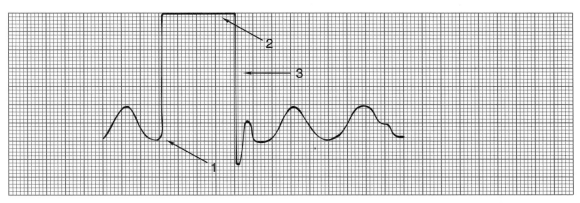

Squaring off occurs as transducer is exposed to 300 mm Hg pressure in continuous flush pressure bag.

Rapid downstroke as flush device is released.

Square wave pattern is now ready to be analyzed for frequency response and damping coefficient.

Figure 7–3. Performing the square wave test.

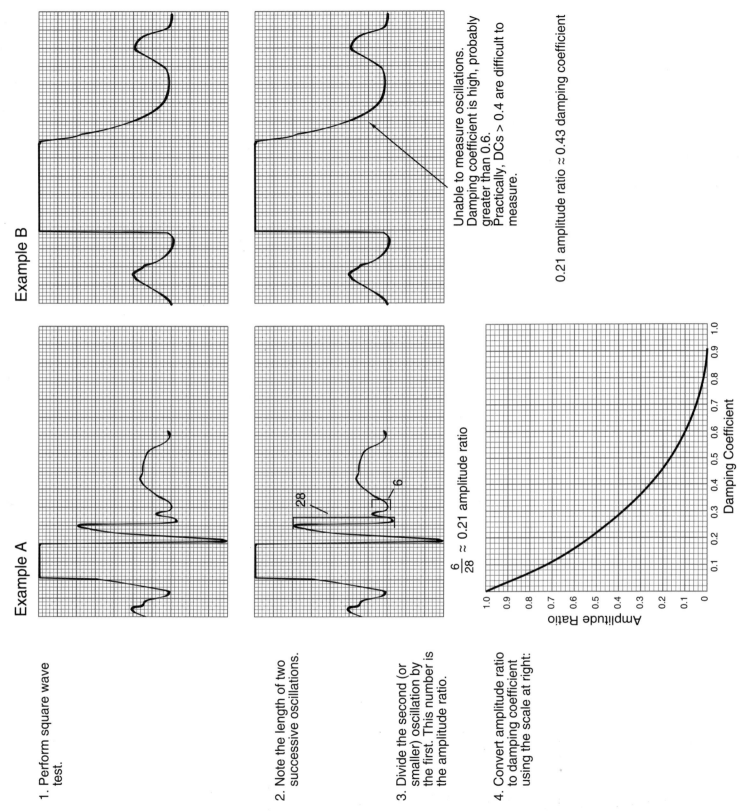

Figure 7–4. Method of measuring the damping coefficient of the tubing catheter system. Measuring the DC frequently yields an estimate rather than an exact value.

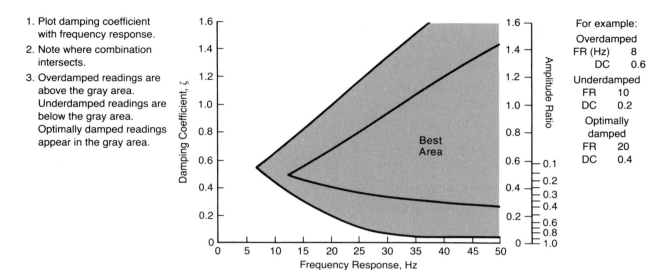

1. Plot damping coefficient with frequency response.
2. Note where combination intersects.
3. Overdamped readings are above the gray area. Underdamped readings are below the gray area. Optimally damped readings appear in the gray area.

For example:
Overdamped
FR (Hz)   8
DC   0.6
Underdamped
FR   10
DC   0.2
Optimally damped
FR   20
DC   0.4

Figure 7–5. Use of frequency response and damping coefficients to determine if the tubing catheter system is generating accurate pressure values. Note that waveforms can have different dynamic response requirements. Attempt to keep the combination of DC and FR well within the acceptable range to avoid potential variations in waveform requirements.

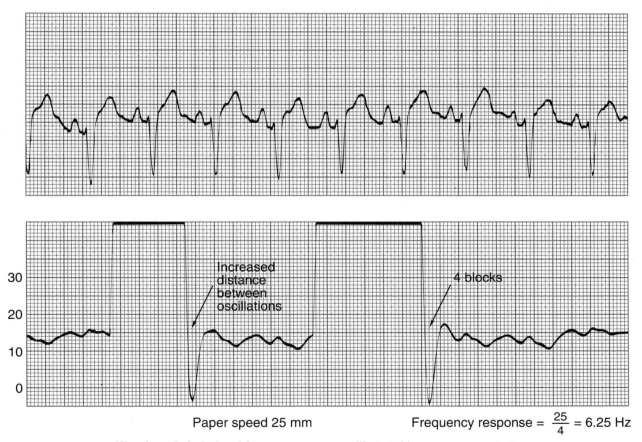

Increased distance between oscillations

4 blocks

Paper speed 25 mm   Frequency response = $\dfrac{25}{4}$ = 6.25 Hz

Waveform 7–2. Reduced frequency response as illustrated by a square wave test.

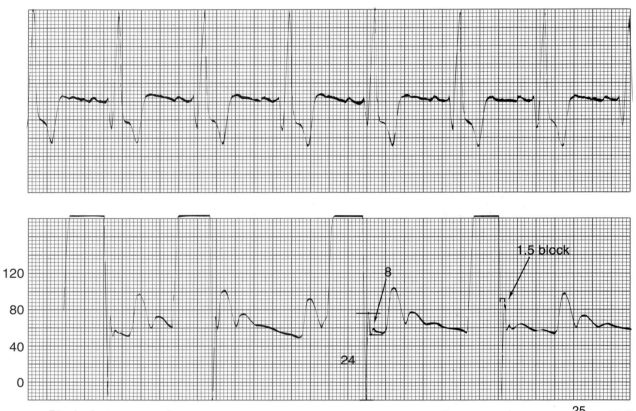

Blocks between peaks

Frequency response: $\frac{25}{1.5}$ = 16.6

Damping coefficient: $\frac{8}{24}$ = 0.33 amplitude ratio = 0.37 damping coefficient

Waveform 7–3. Optimally damped waveform as illustrated by a square wave test.

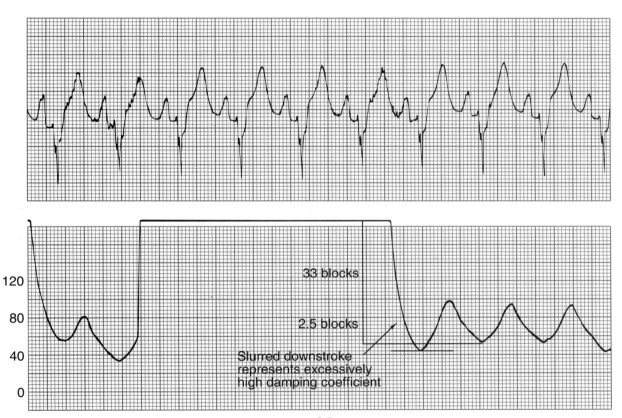

Probable damping coefficient: $\frac{2.5}{33}$ = 0.8 amplitude ratio = 7.6 damping coefficient

Waveform 7–4. Overdamped waveform as illustrated by a square wave test. Lack of oscillations following release of fast flush device indicates excessively low frequency response.

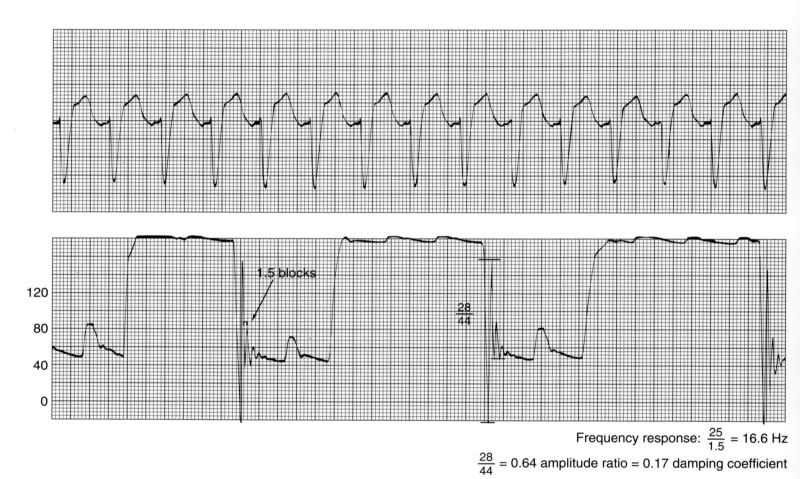

Frequency response: $\dfrac{25}{1.5}$ = 16.6 Hz

$\dfrac{28}{44}$ = 0.64 amplitude ratio = 0.17 damping coefficient

Waveform 7–5. Underdamped waveform as illustrated by a square wave test.

Overdamping is difficult to measure exactly under clinical circumstances. The slurring on the downstroke of the square wave test is an indication of a high DC. Actual measurement of the DC can be difficult because oscillations may be completely absent. Refer to Figure 7–5 for help in reading square wave tests without oscillations.

Nursing Implications

Keeping the FR as high as possible will diminish the effect of overdamping and underdamping. Factors that alter FR include air or blood in the tubing and loose connections. If the square wave test indicates an overdamped or underdamped system, reporting of only the mean pressures is more accurate. Mean pressures are less likely to be affected by over- and underdamped systems.

The square wave test can also be used to identify if the line is obstructed (such as with a kink in the line or with a blood clot). When the line is obstructed, an overdamped waveform will appear during the square wave test.

Overdamping and underdamping are of real concern only in arterial waveforms, inasmuch as venous waveforms are normally reported as mean values. Subsequently, the square wave test is most important when reading arterial or pulmonary artery (PA) waves. Central venous pressure (CVP) and pulmonary capillary wedge pressure (PCWP) readings are less affected by overdamping or underdamping due also to the magnitude of the signal involved and the characteristics of the waveform itself. It is still important, however, to be aware of any aspect that will affect the accuracy of the analysis. Square wave tests should be initiated before each reading to ensure no changes have occurred that may have affected the quality of the waveform.

THE TRANSDUCER/AMPLIFIER SYSTEM

Leveling and Zero Balancing

Although performing the square wave test is important, an even more important aspect of obtaining accurate waveform readings is the leveling and zero balancing of the transducer/ amplifier system. Errors in leveling and zero balancing can produce the largest errors of any aspect in hemodynamic monitoring.[60]

The principle of zero balancing is relatively simple. The transducer system must first be given a zero point in order to establish a reference level for all measured signals. An analogy can be made with a weight scale. A weight scale must be set to read 0 before any weight is applied.

The reference point for the monitoring system is atmospheric pressure, which is assumed to be 0. While this is technically not true, for the purpose of monitoring it is acceptable. A brief explanation of the transducer and amplifier system may be helpful at this point.

A transducer is a device that allows conversion of energy from one form to another. In the case of a blood pressure transducer, it takes the pressure generated by the contraction of the heart and converts it into an electrical signal. The conversion takes place through the displacement in the transducer of a diaphragm. The change in diaphragm in the transducer alters the electrical flow characteristics in the transducer. The electrical flow change is then inputted into the amplifier (monitor), displayed as a waveform, and analyzed to determine specific values.

Transducers are made in a wide variety of configurations. In the past, the vast majority of the reusable transducers were made using a simple strain gauge. New transducers and all of the disposable transducers that are common in most critical care settings today use a semiconductor-based system to convert the signal. Because the transducer is continuously connected to the system and a pressure is constantly applied, the process of zeroing the system must be completed when the system is first being assembled. This process should take place after the tubing set has been assembled and the transducer is attached to the monitor. Many different transducers and pressure monitoring systems exist. The following steps, however, will apply to all models.

The transducer system must be opened to air in order to read atmospheric pressure. This is usually best accomplished at a stopcock. Most institutions use the stopcock on the transducer to zero the transducer system, but any stopcock in the tubing set that is open to air could be used.

Proper leveling techniques must also be observed when zeroing the system. The stopcock should be open at the point where the end of the catheter is located (this process is referred to as leveling). Many institutions have the first person performing the zeroing procedure mark the catheter location for reference and have all subsequent readings based on this marking.

Confusion frequently arises regarding the correct point to use for reference. For intercardiac pressures, the location used for leveling is usually the fourth intercostal space at the midaxillary line (MAL) or about 5–6 cm under the sternal angle (angle of Louis). This location has been identified by a variety of investigators.[61,62] Peripheral arterial lines are not leveled to the MAL unless the end of the catheter is in this plane. One must frequently estimate the end catheter position for arterial lines and, once this is identified, everyone should use the same location as the reference point.

The goal of any pressure monitoring is to read the pressure existing in the cannulated blood vessel. Referencing must take place at this blood vessel location. This point continues to be misunderstood by many clinicians. Figures 7–6, 7–7, 7–8, and 7–9 demonstrate four methods for zeroing and leveling the transducer. All of these methods are acceptable for exposing the transducer to atmospheric pressure and zeroing the system.

The midaxillary line is used because it has been determined by radiologic studies that the CVP line is near this location.[63] When PA catheters were first introduced, this location was continued although evidence suggests that the MAL may not be the most accurate reference location.[64] The reasons arterial lines should be referenced at their source can be illustrated by a simple example. Assume that an arterial line is in the patient's pedal artery and the person is standing. Where would the correct point be for the transducer to be zeroed? If it were zeroed at the MAL, the reading would be substantially reduced due to the failure to account for the pressure column from the foot of the patient to the heart. Clinically this point is illustrated in Figure 7–10.

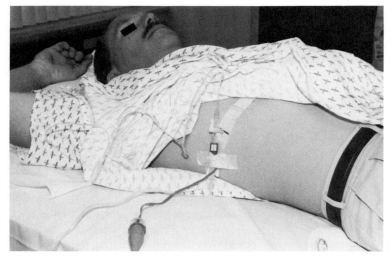

Figure 7–6. Transducer taped to midaxillary line.

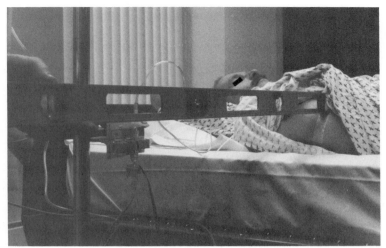

Figure 7–7. Midaxillary line aligned with stopcock via carpenter's level.

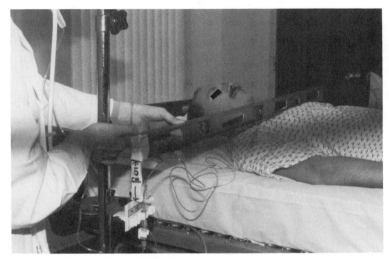

Figure 7–8. Five centimeters below the sternal angle.

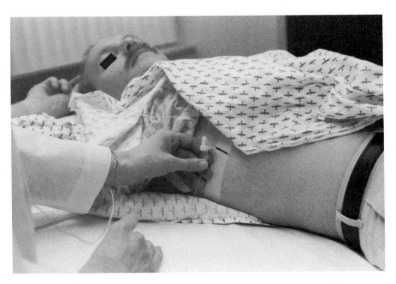

Figure 7–9. Stopcock held to midaxillary line.

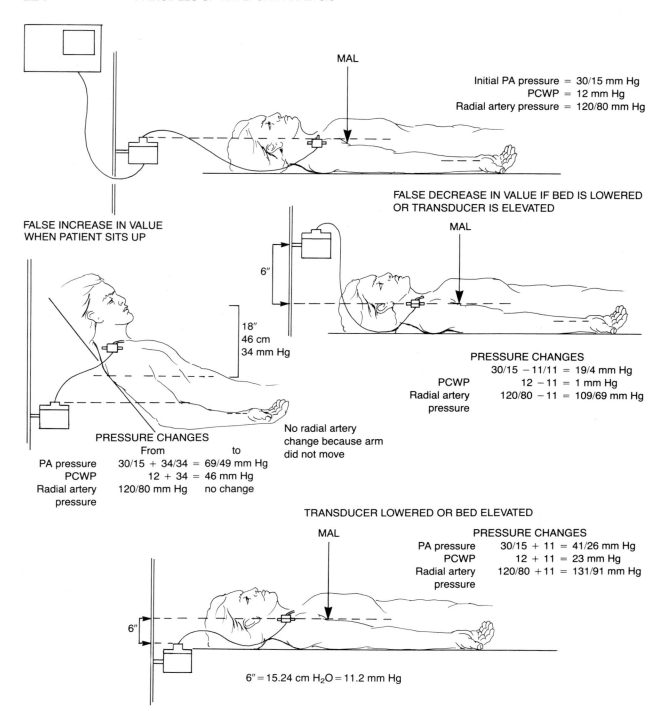

MAL

Initial PA pressure = 30/15 mm Hg
PCWP = 12 mm Hg
Radial artery pressure = 120/80 mm Hg

FALSE DECREASE IN VALUE IF BED IS LOWERED
OR TRANSDUCER IS ELEVATED

MAL

6"

FALSE INCREASE IN VALUE
WHEN PATIENT SITS UP

18"
46 cm
34 mm Hg

PRESSURE CHANGES
30/15 − 11/11 = 19/4 mm Hg
PCWP   12 − 11 = 1 mm Hg
Radial artery   120/80 − 11 = 109/69 mm Hg
pressure

No radial artery
change because arm
did not move

PRESSURE CHANGES
From   to
PA pressure   30/15 + 34/34 = 69/49 mm Hg
PCWP   12 + 34 = 46 mm Hg
Radial artery   120/80 mm Hg   no change
pressure

TRANSDUCER LOWERED OR BED ELEVATED

MAL

PRESSURE CHANGES
PA pressure   30/15 + 11 = 41/26 mm Hg
PCWP   12 + 11 = 23 mm Hg
Radial artery   120/80 + 11 = 131/91 mm Hg
pressure

6"

6" = 15.24 cm H_2O = 11.2 mm Hg

Figure 7–10. Effect of position changes on hemodynamic values.

This point can also be demonstrated with a patient who has both a PA line and peripheral catheter. Zero the system and obtain the first readings with the person flat. Then, without repeating the zeroing process, have the person sit up to a 45° angle. Notice how the PA and CVP readings increase, but the arterial values stay about the same. If one were to rezero all lines at the MAL, the PA readings would return to pre–position change values, but the arterial pressures would decrease. This example illustrates that the location of zero balancing should be the end of the catheter.

Once the transducer is open to air, zeroing the system occurs by activating the zero function on the monitor. This may be as simple as depressing an autozero button. Most of the current monitoring systems have a single button zeroing function while older systems require several steps. When the zero function is activated, the amplifier reads the current input from the transducer as zero and remembers this point as the reference value. Any subsequent pressure applied to the transducer is now indicated and referenced to this zero point.

The patient does not need to remain flat in bed when the readings are obtained.[65,66] Several studies have indicated patients can be at an approximately 45° angle (or less) and still have similar readings to when they were lying flat. It is especially important to avoid placing an orthopneic patient in a flat position because exacerbation of the orthopnea without improvement in the accuracy of the waveform values would be the likely result.

The effect of movement on the zero/level point can be clinically significant. Once the leveling has been accomplished, the patient and transducer must remain in the same position. If movement is necessary, then releveling needs to be repeated in the new position. For example, if the transducer is lowered or the patient's position raised, all readings will increase due to the increased effect of hydrostatic pressure on the transducer. The increase is directly proportional to the amount of change. An increase in patient position of only 2 inches amounts to approximately a 4 mm Hg change in indicated pressure. The 4 mm Hg change is computed by the following process: Begin with 1 inch = 2.54 cm H_2O, so 2 inches = 2 × 2.54 = 5.08 cm H_2O. Because the amplifier displays in mm Hg, convert this change in height from centimeters of water to millimeters of mercury by dividing the 5.08 by 1.36. This is 3.74, or about 4 mm Hg. If the patient had a PCWP of 14 and the patient's position was raised 2 inches, the indicated pressure would now read 18. Remember, no change in the actual patient PCWP has occurred; only the indicated numbers have changed. The change will occur in both directions, i.e., if the patient is lowered or the transducer raised, the indicated values will decrease. Because of the critical nature of the zero balancing process and its ability to cause drastic errors in the results, it is recommended that zero balancing be repeated frequently, i.e., prior to each reading. With increased accuracy from disposable transducers and new monitoring systems, rezeroing may not need to be performed before each reading. The appropriate frequency of zeroing may be as low as every day or every other day. However, the ideal frequency of zeroing will not be clear until further research has been completed in this area.

The only exception to frequent zeroing is if the transducer is patient mounted. When patient mounted, the transducer will not lose the relationship to the end of the catheter (as long as movement is in the same plane, i.e., not turning to the side). For patient-mounted transducers, zeroing could be reduced to once a shift or potentially even longer.

Calibration

Once the zeroing process is complete, the calibration process is used to ensure indicated values are correct by checking that the system correctly reads a known pressure. With the advent of disposable transducers, this step has diminished in importance. The disposable transducers now typically have an accuracy rate of 1–2%.[67] Coupled with the amplifier accuracy, which is also typically 1–2%, the maximum error of properly functioning equipment is about 4%. Because disposable transducers are precalibrated prior to gas sterilization and shipping, calibration is usually very good and further calibration of the system need not be completed. However, in order to verify transducer accuracy, calibration should be performed at least once, upon initial assembly of the tubing set.

The procedure for calibration can be done with a sphygmomanometer or with a sterile water column. Inasmuch as most intensive care units are converting to disposable transducers, the water column method is preferable due to the sterility and safety features.[68] Although the water column method primarily measures static and not dynamic responses, for clinical purposes this method of measuring calibration is acceptable.

To perform calibration with the water column, one must have a length of sterile tubing with a known height, e.g., IV extension tubing. From the known height of the extension tubing, one can compute the weight it will generate. For example, if the height of the column of water is 30 inches, this can be converted to mm Hg by first converting inches to centimeters of water; $30'' \times 2.54 = 76.2$ cm H_2O. Now convert to mm Hg by dividing 76.2 by 1.36, which gives 56 mm Hg. When this weight is applied to the transducer, the monitor should read 56 mm Hg. If it does not, the amplifier can be adjusted to offset any difference. Because amplifier adjustment is company specific, you should consult your individual manual for the exact steps. Figures 7–11 and 7–12 illustrate one method of checking calibration.

Keep in mind one relevant point when obtaining the height of the extension tube.[69] Measurement is focused on the total height of the water column within the tubing, stopcock, and transducer. If a transducer is used that is manifold mounted, then when the extension tube is inserted, height may be lost. The actual height of the tubing should be measured from where it plugs into the transducer (Fig. 7–12).

The procedure for calibration is as follows:

1. Zero the transducer system.
2. Attach a known length of sterile tubing.
3. Fill the tubing with water by activating the flush device (a pressure bag should be in place or if not, hold the tubing below the height of the solution bag until it fills).
4. The monitor should now read the weight displaced by the fluid column (pressure).
5. If the monitor does not read the correct value, adjust the amplifier using the monitor manufacturer's defined calibration procedure until the desired reading is obtained (termed the *calibration factor*).

Be cautious if the amplifier cannot readily correct for a discrepancy in readings. If the initial value is greater than 10% in error, the amplifier/monitor may need to be checked or replaced. The amplifier/monitor is usually checked first because no cost is associated with this step (most current monitors have a self-test mode that is quite easy to initiate). If checking the amplifier/monitor does not correct the problem, replace the transducer and again begin the zero and calibration procedure. If the transducer value cannot correctly read the pressure at this point, the clinical engineering department should be notified and the entire unit may need replacement.

Accuracy

The transducer/amplifier system, if properly zeroed and leveled, calibrated, and with acceptable frequency response and damping coefficients, will produce waveform values within 4% of the actual value. The waveforms produced should be accurate enough to be accepted for clinical decision making. A few exceptions to this rule may be present, primarily in peripheral arterial lines. In the presence of peripheral vasoconstriction, blood pressure values may not be accurately displayed from the arterial line.[70,71] Vasoconstriction-induced errors are common in the immediate postoperative phase. Generally, the peripheral arterial pressure, such as with radial lines, underestimates the central blood pressure.

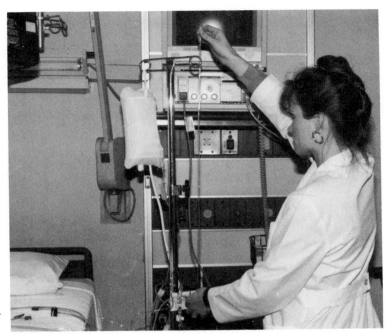

Figure 7–11. Method of performing sterile calibration of the transducer with water column.

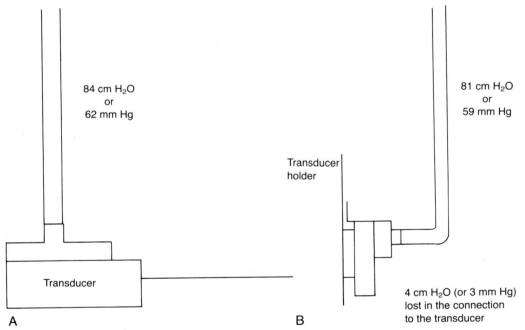

Figure 7–12. Effect of changing the height of the water column reference on calibration values. Tubing must be held to full height (no slack in the tubing) during both methods.

As a rule, the transducer/amplifier system will display a blood pressure value more accurately than a sphygmomanometer (cuff) method. If the sphygmomanometer method generates a blood pressure higher than the arterial pressure line, some problem must exist in the arterial line. Checking the arterial line for problems is necessary. To check the accuracy of hemodynamic monitoring, simple application of the previously discussed principles is necessary. The following section on troubleshooting potential problems summarizes the method to determine if the transducer/amplifier system is displaying accurate values.

TROUBLESHOOTING PRESSURE MONITORS

In order to avoid errors in hemodynamics, nurses should take the following steps:

1. Zero and level the transducer to the end of the catheter before each reading.
2. Check the square wave test before each reading.
   a. If underdamped, insert a damping device and adjust until the square wave test is optimally damped.
   b. If overdamped, check for obstructions in the line or the presence of air or blood in the tubing set or for excessive tubing.
3. Calibration should be performed when the transducer is initially set up and when it is changed.

These steps will eliminate most errors in hemodynamic monitoring.

SPECIFIC PROBLEMS IN MONITORING

1. *Arterial line pressure is higher than sphygmomanometer value:*
   This is normal under most circumstances. It may be abnormal when the line is underdamped.
2. *Arterial line pressure is lower than sphygmomanometer value:*
   This is abnormal in most circumstances. Check for an overdamped waveform.
3. *No value is displayed on the monitor:*
   Make sure the amplifier is on and stopcocks are open to the patient. Perform a calibration check to see if the transducer/amplifier can read a pressure. If no pressure is displayed during a calibration check, replace the amplifier if possible (replace the amplifier module). If the new module does not read a pressure, replace the transducer. It will be unusual for these methods not to work; however, if neither of these methods results in a pressure being displayed, consult your clinical engineering department.

ARTIFACTS IN THE PRESSURE WAVEFORM

Several types of artifact exist in hemodynamic waveforms. The artifact can be from excessive catheter movement or underdamped waveforms. Applying a few basic principles can help eliminate many of the artifacts that occur.

One of the more helpful principles is application of the electrocardiogram (ECG) components to the waveform. For example, arterial systolic values are associated with near end-QRS locations. Peak values that occur later than the T wave may represent artifact (Waveform 7–6).

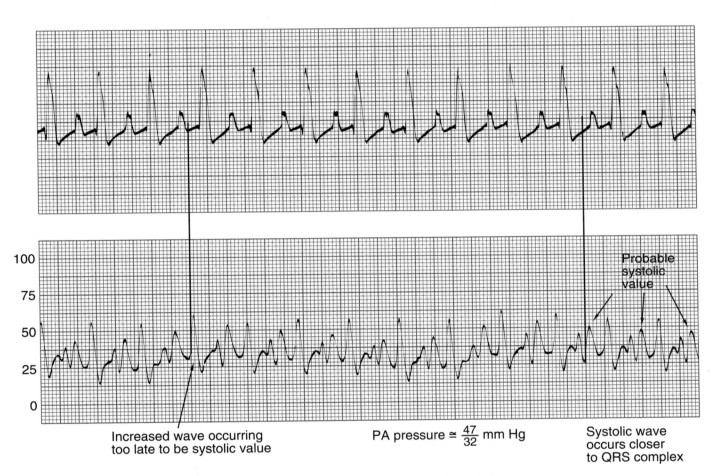

Increased wave occurring
too late to be systolic value

PA pressure $\simeq \dfrac{47}{32}$ mm Hg

Systolic wave
occurs closer
to QRS complex

Probable
systolic
value

Waveform 7–6. Artifact identified through ECG correlation.

Waveforms tend to be smooth and without marked, sharp changes. When waveforms have sharp fluctuations in appearance, suspect that artifact may be present. For example, in underdamped waveforms, certain aspects of the wave may be exaggerated. In Waveform 7–7, note how the presystolic wave is markedly enlarged. The waveform is not smooth but has sharp fluctuations from the normal diastolic runoff. This waveform is most likely artifact and the real diastolic value is higher than would appear.

When arterial waveforms have more than the normal number of waves, i.e., a triphasic pattern, either excessive catheter movement is present, the line is underdamped, or the catheter is near a valve (Waveforms 7–8 and 7–9). A square wave test will help to demonstrate which problem exists.

Several solutions can be attempted to reduce the degree of artifact:

1. A damping device can be placed in the line to increase the damping coefficient.[72]
2. In a pulmonary artery line, the balloon can be inflated slightly to see if the inflated balloon would reduce the degree of catheter movement. Be careful when inflating the balloon to avoid overinflation, which can be seen when the waveform begins to rise sharply beyond physiologic values. The sharp pressure increase is due to the balloon obstructing the end of the catheter and the catheter now reading the pressure in the pressure bag (Waveform 7–10).
3. Either advancing or pulling back on the catheter can place the catheter in a less turbulent blood flow area.

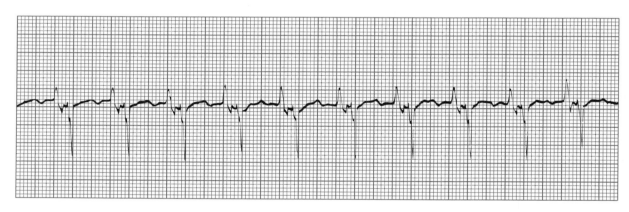

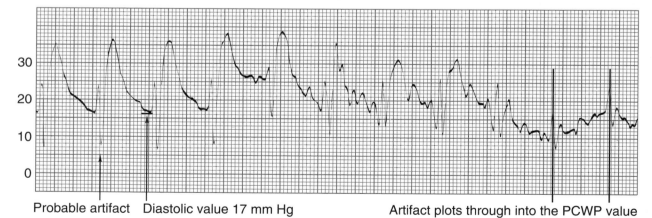

Probable artifact   Diastolic value 17 mm Hg   Artifact plots through into the PCWP value

Waveform 7–7. Presystolic artifact in pulmonary artery waveform.

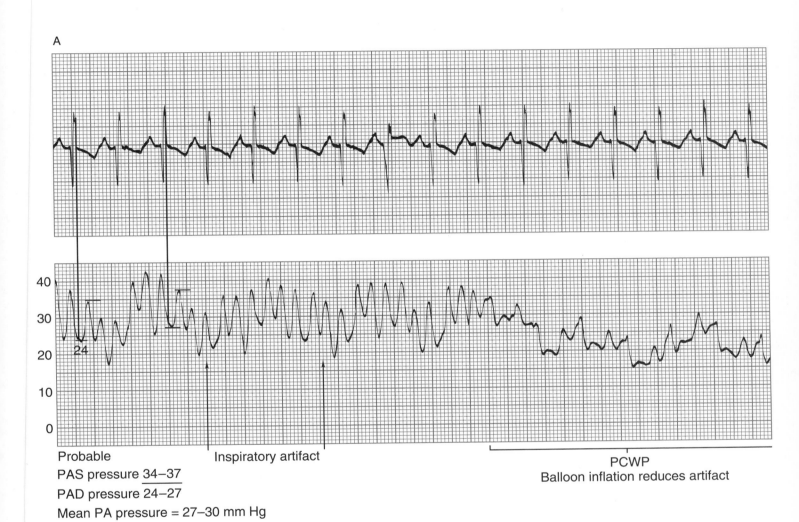

A

Probable
PAS pressure 34–37
PAD pressure 24–27
Mean PA pressure = 27–30 mm Hg

Inspiratory artifact

PCWP
Balloon inflation reduces artifact

Waveform 7–8. *A*, Multiphased pulmonary artery tracing due to artifact. Excessive artifact requires that only mean values be reported.

B

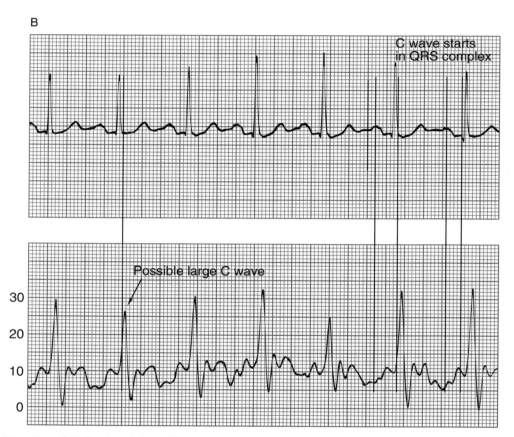

Waveform 7–8 *Continued. B,* Artifact from catheter location near the tricuspid valve. Exaggerated wave could be a large C wave if the catheter was near the tricuspid valve. The artifact disappeared when the catheter was pulled back a few centimeters.

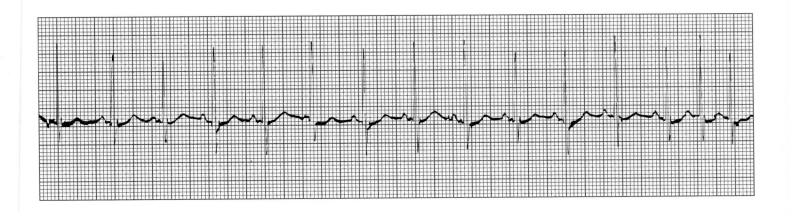

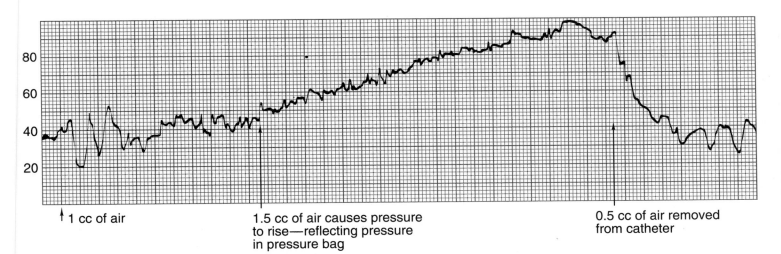

↑ 1 cc of air   1.5 cc of air causes pressure   0.5 cc of air removed
                       to rise—reflecting pressure   from catheter
                       in pressure bag

Waveform 7–9. Overinflation of pulmonary artery balloon produces an ''overwedged'' tracing.

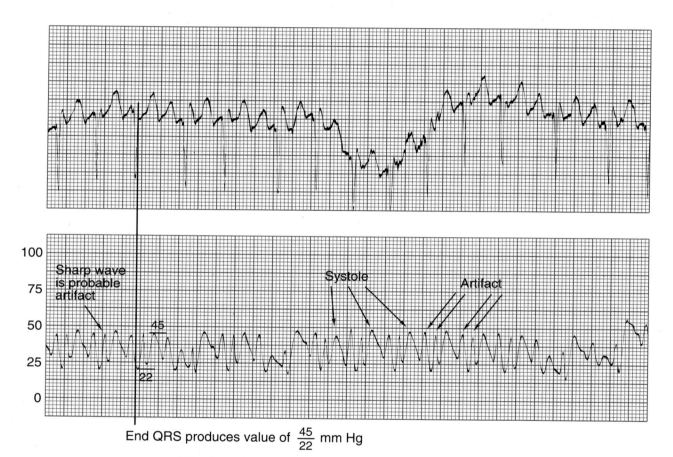

End QRS produces value of $\frac{45}{22}$ mm Hg

Waveform 7–10. Use of the ECG to read pressure waveform.

SUMMARY

Obtaining hemodynamic readings with accuracy (Table 7–1) depends on understanding essential components of the hemodynamic monitoring equipment. The key components of accurate waveform replication include zeroing, leveling, and calibration of the transducer/amplifier system, and assessing the frequency response and damping coefficients of the tubing catheter system. Zeroing and leveling are the most crucial actions to perform when obtaining hemodynamic values because of the degree of error that can occur in these areas. Assessing the frequency response and damping coefficients through a square wave test is the next most important action when obtaining readings. Calibration is less important and is only necessary to perform upon initial assembly of the transducer system.

Waveform values are only as accurate as the nurse's understanding of the components of the hemodynamic technical system. Simple errors in pressure value interpretation can be avoided if nurses incorporate routine checks of the technical features of hemodynamic monitoring into their practice.

Table 7–1. PROCEDURES FOR OBTAINING HEMODYNAMIC READINGS

Before Each Reading	When Setting Up or Changing Transducers
1. Check for proper leveling.	1. Check for leveling.
2. Zero the transducer/amplifier.	2. Zero the transducer/amplifier.
3. Perform square wave test.	3. Calibrate the transducer/amplifier.

Definitions

Leveling: Establishment of a reference point between the end of the catheter and the zero point of the transducer.
  Method—Place an open stopcock port in the same plane (level) as the end of the catheter being used to obtain values. Leveling should be done whenever the patient or transducer moves from the position where zeroing was performed.

Zeroing: Electrically balancing the transducer/amplifier to read no (zero) pressure.
  Method—Open a stopcock vent port to air and activate (push) the zero function key on the amplifier (monitor). Zeroing should be perfromed at least once a day. Many institutions prefer to zero before each reading, although zero drift is less common with disposable transducers.

Calibration: Verification that the transducer/amplifier system can read a known pressure accurately.
  Method—Open a stopcock to air, zero the transducer/amplifier, and insert a tubing with a known height and weight. Check to see that the monitor displays the same pressure as the weight of the tubing. Calibration needs to be performed when the transducer is initially set up or changed (every 48 hours.)

Square Wave Test: Assessment of the ability of the tubing catheter system to accurately reproduce a wave and pressure.
  Method—Activate the fast flush device for about 1 second and note the monitor or strip recorder for the square wave pattern. Square wave tests should be done any time the line is entered or manipulated, including before each reading.

PRACTICE WAVEFORMS

Practice Waveforms 7–1 through 7–11 provide examples of waveforms with technical components for your practice analysis. Interpreting these waveforms will give you an opportunity to apply principles presented in this chapter.

PRACTICE WAVEFORM 7–1. In this radial artery tracing, is the tracing optimally damped?

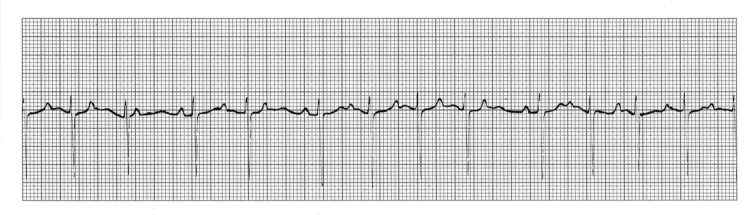

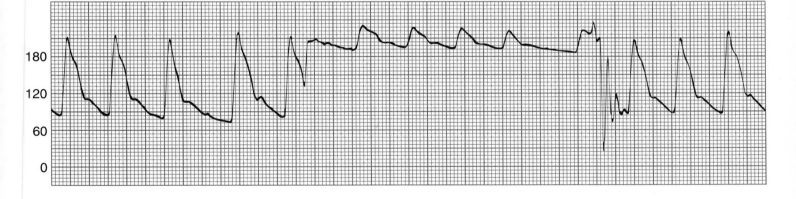

PRACTICE WAVEFORM 7–1. *Analysis:* The tracing indicates a low DC (0.21) with a barely acceptable FR (10 Hz). The tracing is underdamped (see Fig. 7–5) based on these values. Also note that the square wave test does not produce a flat line at the top of the scale but shows a pressure wave. This is due to the pressure bag containing less than 300 mm Hg. Inflate the bag to proper pressures when this occurs.

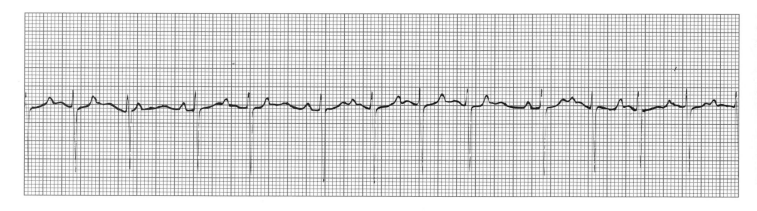

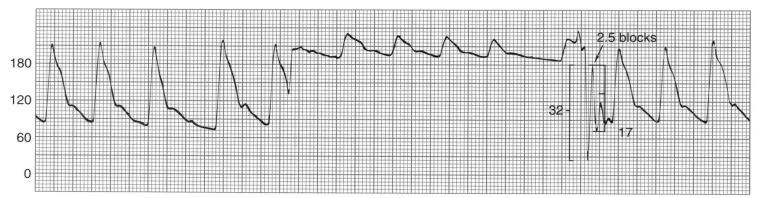

Frequency response $\dfrac{25}{2.5} = 10$ Hz

$\dfrac{17}{32} = 0.53$ amplitude ratio = 0.21 damping coefficient

PRACTICE WAVEFORM 7–2. In this femoral artery waveform, is the tracing optimally damped?

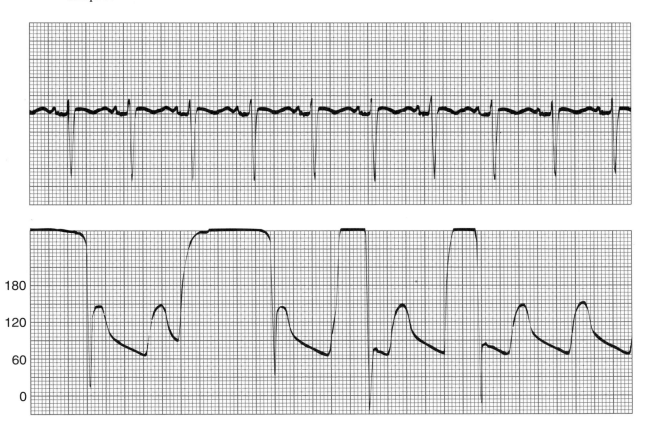

PRACTICE WAVEFORM 7–2. *Analysis:* Yes, based on a good FR (25 Hz). The DC is low but is offset by the high FR.

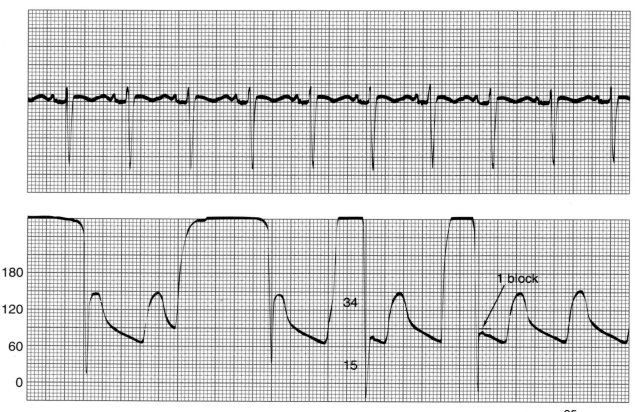

Frequency response: $\frac{25}{1}$ = 25 Hz

Damping coefficient: $\frac{15}{34}$ = 0.44 amplitude ratio = 0.22 damping coefficient

PRACTICE WAVEFORM 7–3. In this PA waveform, is the tracing optimally damped?

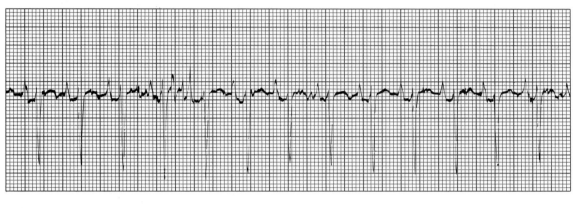

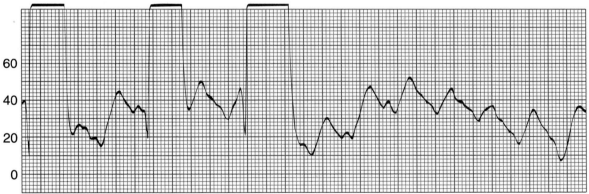

PRACTICE WAVEFORM 7–3. *Analysis:* No. The lack of clear oscillations following release of the fast flush device indicates a low FR. In addition, the slurring on the downstroke of the square wave indicates a high DC. The tracing is overdamped.

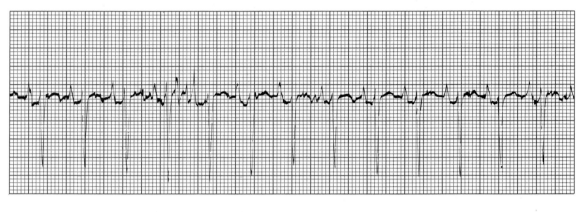

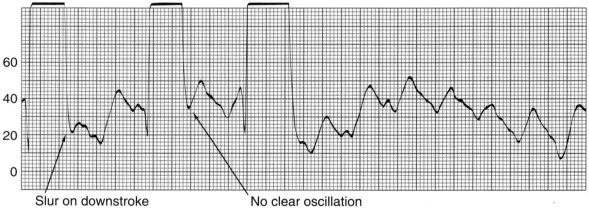

Slur on downstroke   No clear oscillation

PRACTICE WAVEFORM 7–4. In this CVP tracing, no clear A and V waves exist, although a sharp oscillation is noted after the QRS complex. What is the cause of this oscillation?

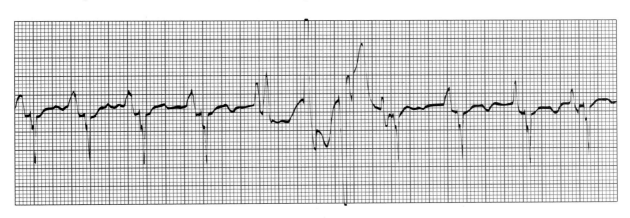

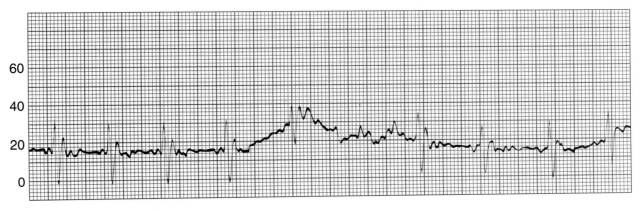

PRACTICE WAVEFORM 7–5. *Analysis:* An unclear PA waveform is present in this tracing, indicating probable artifact. Diastole can be located by finding the end-QRS complex and drawing a line to the pressure wave. Systole is more difficult to identify owing to the multiphased upstrokes on the PA waveform. Systole appears to be about 55 mm Hg, although because of the artifact, it might be better simply to report mean values.

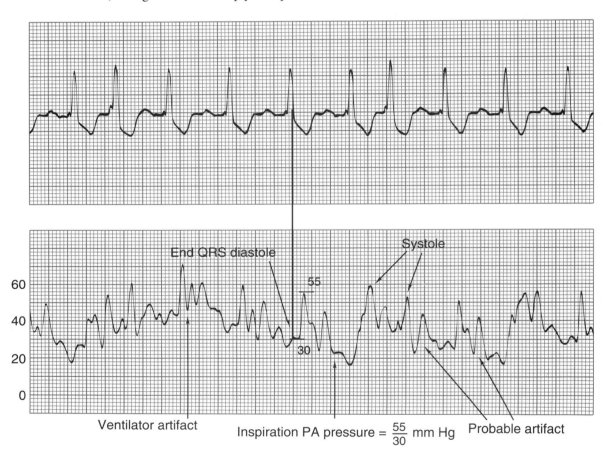

PRACTICE WAVEFORM 7–6. In this PA waveform, is the tracing optimally damped?

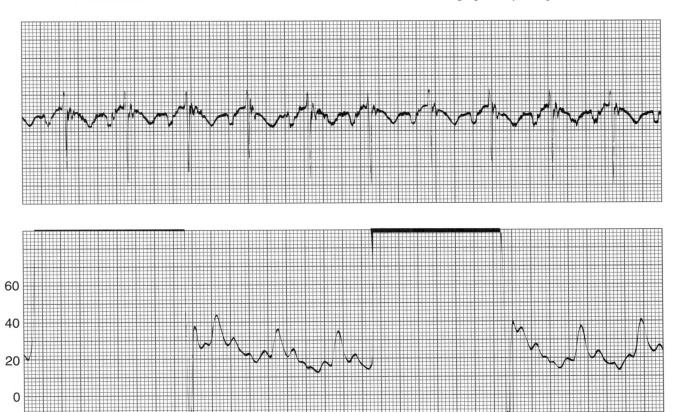

PRACTICE WAVEFORM 7–6. *Analysis:* The FR is slightly low (10 Hz) but a good DC is present (0.43). This combination results in a slightly underdamped waveform (see Fig. 7–5). In addition, the scale did not quite allow for maximal wave deflection on the downstroke of the square test, potentially generating a lower than reported DC.

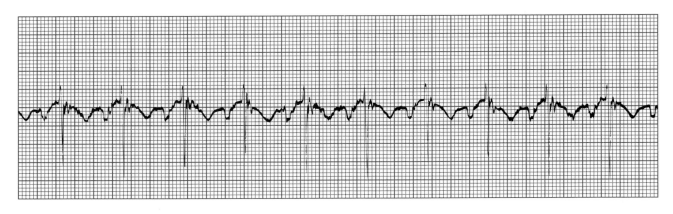

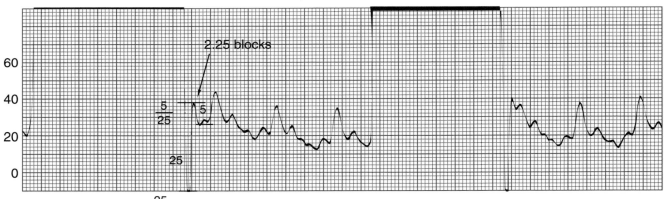

Frequency response: $\dfrac{25}{2.5} = 10$ Hz

Damping coefficient: $\dfrac{5}{25} = 0.2$ amplitude ratio = 0.43 damping coefficient

PRACTICE WAVEFORM 7–7. In this PA waveform, is the tracing optimally damped?

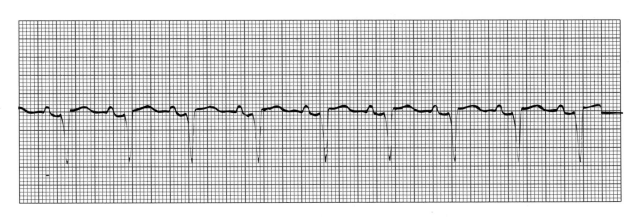

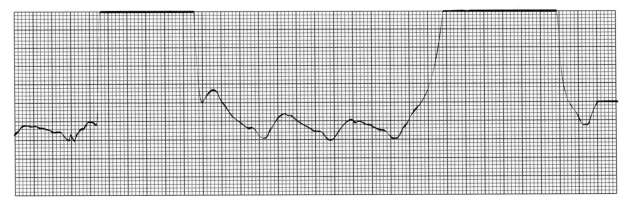

PRACTICE WAVEFORM 7–7. *Analysis:* The lack of oscillations and the slurring on the downstroke of the square wave test indicate both low FR and high DC. The tracing is over-damped.

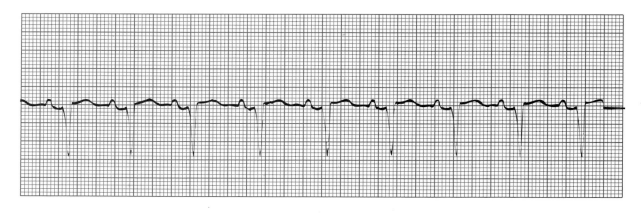

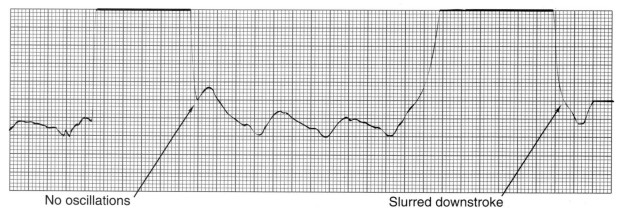

No oscillations   Slurred downstroke

PRACTICE WAVEFORM 7–8. Where is this PA waveform read? The patient is on assist/control ventilation, with a rate of 10, but triggering the ventilator at a rate of 20 breaths per minute.

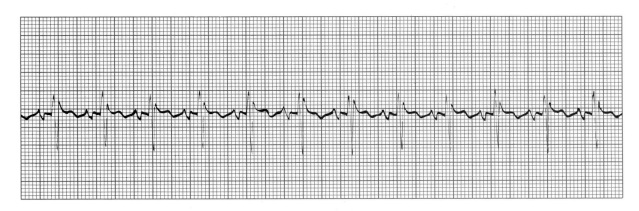

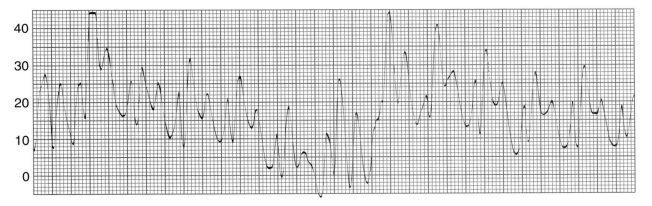

PRACTICE WAVEFORM 7–8. *Analysis:* After locating end expiration, find diastole by using the end of the QRS complex. Note the multiphased PA waveform, indicating artifact or an underdamped tracing. Avoid the presystolic artifact and read the systolic value near 27. Perform a square wave test and determine if a damping device would be useful in this case.

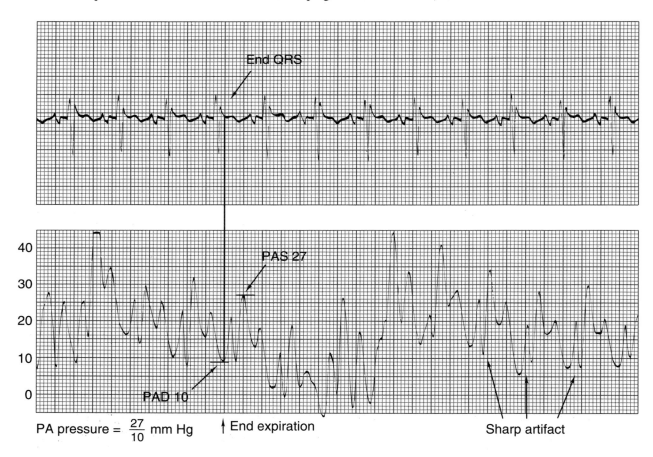

PA pressure = $\frac{27}{10}$ mm Hg   ↑ End expiration

PRACTICE WAVEFORM 7–9. Is this radial arterial waveform optimally damped?

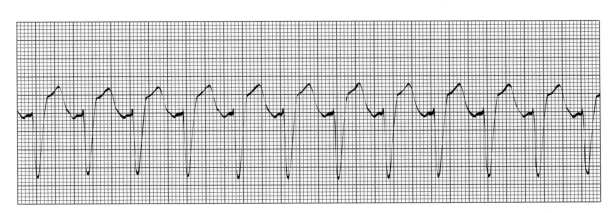

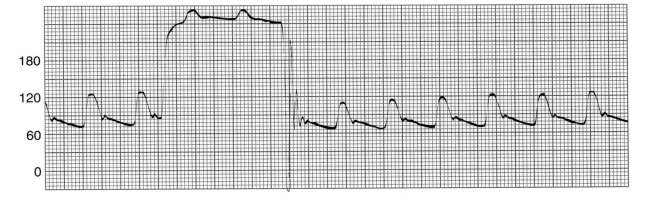

PRACTICE WAVEFORM 7–9. *Analysis:* No, the tracing is underdamped as indicated by a low DC (0.18). The FR is adequate (16.6 Hz) but not high enough to offset the low DC.

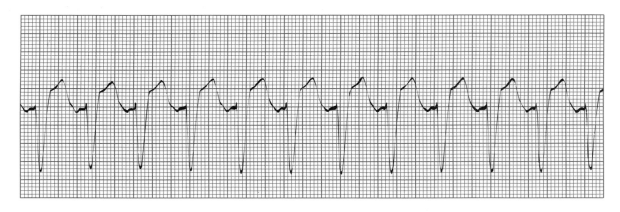

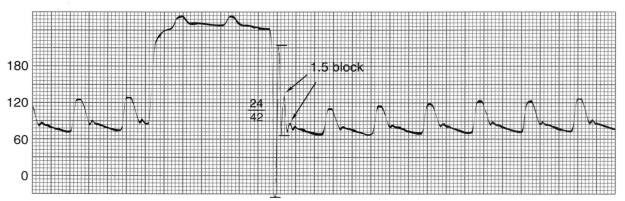

Systolic values may be amplified

Damping coefficient: $\frac{24}{42}$ = 0.57 amplitude ratio = 0.18 damping coefficient

Frequency response: $\frac{25}{1.5}$ = 16.6 Hz

PRACTICE WAVEFORM 7–10. In this femoral artery waveform, is the tracing optimally damped?

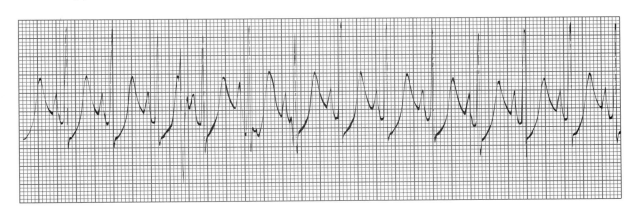

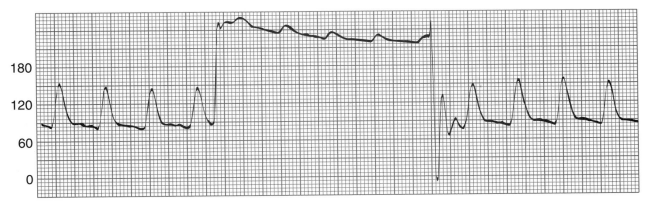

PRACTICE WAVEFORM 7–10. *Analysis:* No, the tracing is underdamped due to a low DC (0.21) and FR (7 Hz).

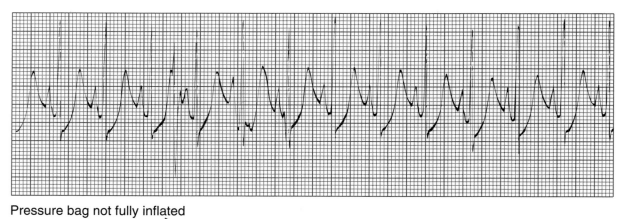

Pressure bag not fully inflated

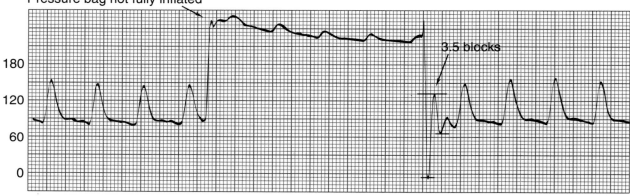

3.5 blocks

Frequency response: $\frac{25}{3.5}$ = 7.1 Hz

Damping coefficient: $\frac{11}{23}$ = 0.49 amplitude ratio = 0.21 damping coefficient

PRACTICE WAVEFORM 7–11. In this femoral artery waveform, is the tracing optimally damped?

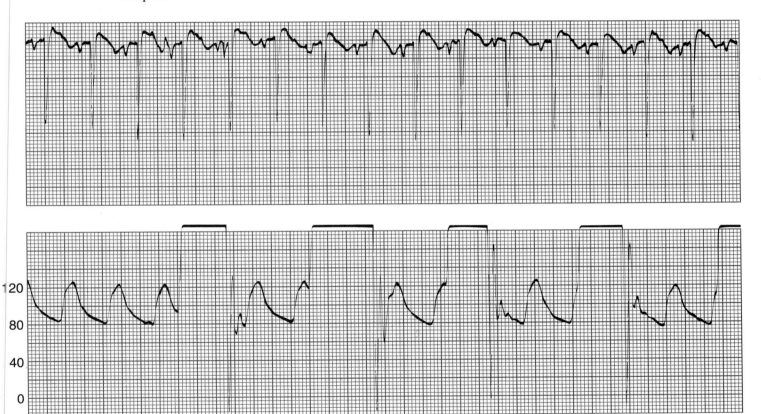

PRACTICE WAVEFORM 7–11. *Analysis:* No, the DC is low (0.22) and the FR (14.3 Hz) is not high enough to offset the low coefficient.

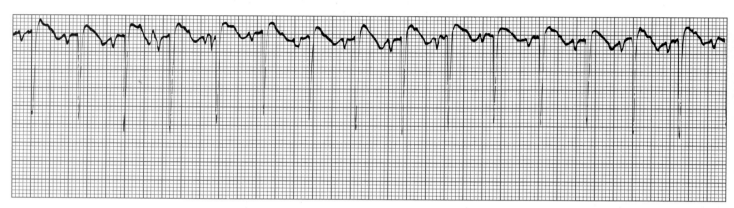

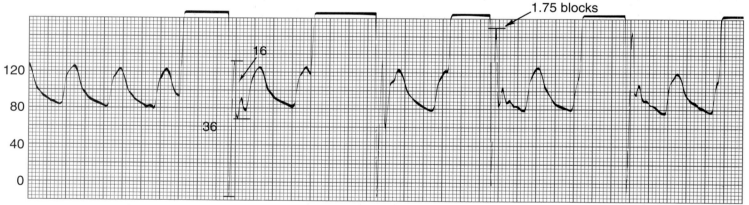

Underdamped arterial waveform

Frequency response: $\frac{25}{1.75}$ = 14.3 Hz

Damping coefficient: $\frac{16}{36}$ = 0.44 amplitude ratio = 0.22 damping coefficient

III PRACTICE IN WAVEFORM ANALYSIS

8 Practice Waveform Analysis

In this chapter, we present waveforms that cover all situations discussed in the text. The waveforms are not presented with any information other than identification of the respiratory pattern and from which monitoring port the wave was obtained. This chapter serves as a method for you to assess your ability to interpret waveforms without help from clinical scenarios. In so doing, your ability to apply waveform interpretation principles will be developed. Answers to Practice Waveforms are presented on the back of each page. Good luck with your interpretations.

PRACTICE WAVEFORM 8–1. In this waveform obtained from the distal port, the patient was receiving IMV ventilation without spontaneous breathing. What is the tracing and the value associated with the waveform?

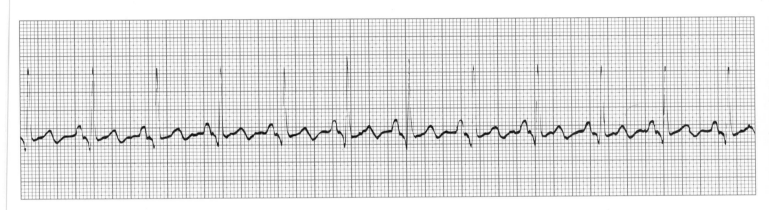

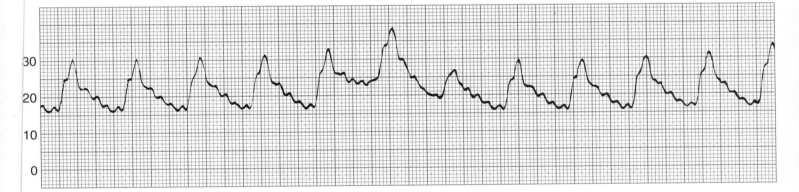

PRACTICE WAVEFORM 8–1. *Analysis:* Pulmonary artery pressure = 32/17 mm Hg. Note waveform between 4th and 5th and 11th and 12th ECG complexes for examples of where to read the tracing.

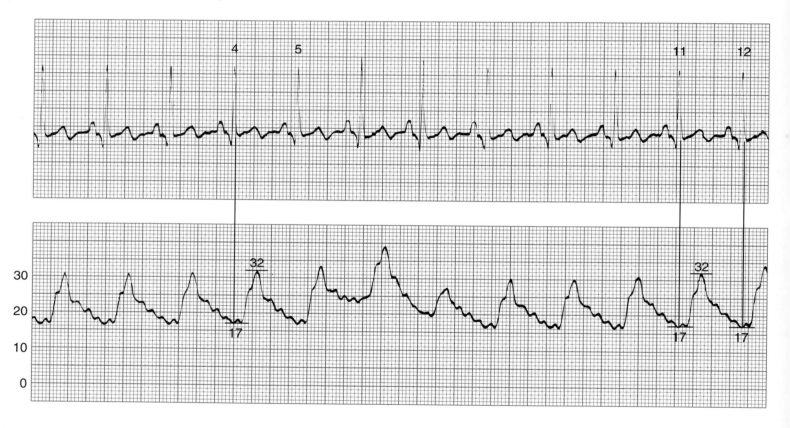

PRACTICE WAVEFORM 8–2. In this waveform obtained from the distal port, the patient was receiving mechanical ventilation via the assist/control mode. No spontaneous ventilation was present. What is the tracing and the value associated with the waveform?

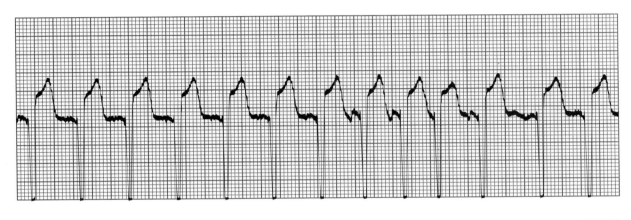

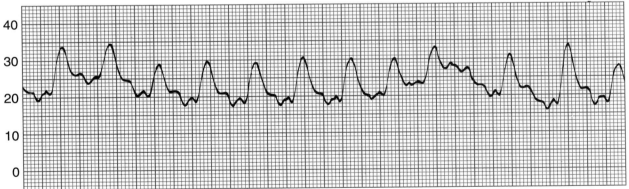

PRACTICE WAVEFORM 8–2. *Analysis:* Pulmonary artery pressure = 30/18 mm Hg. Note waveforms between the 7th and 8th ECG complexes for an example of where to read the waveforms before each mechanical ventilator breath.

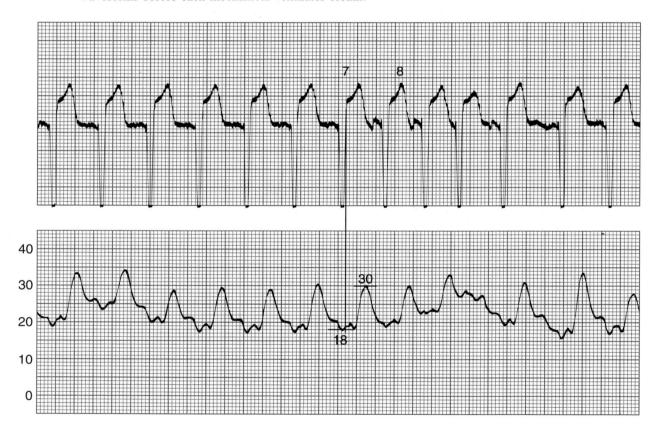

PRACTICE WAVEFORM 8–3. In this waveform obtained from the distal port, the patient was on assist/control ventilation with no spontaneous breathing. What is the tracing and the value associated with the waveform?

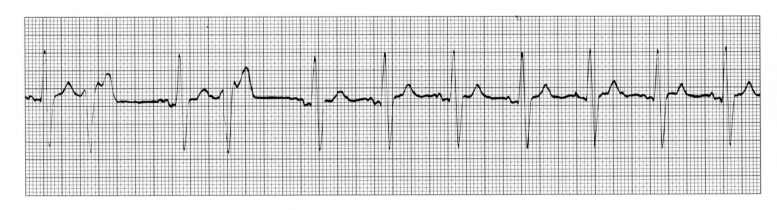

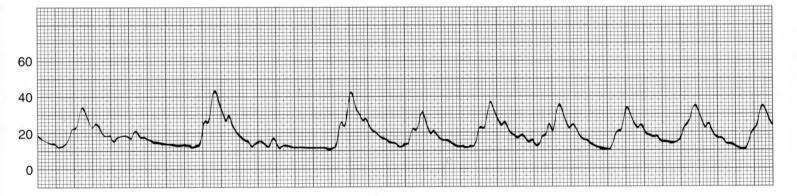

PRACTICE WAVEFORM 8–3. *Analysis:* Pulmonary artery pressure = 35/14 mm Hg. Waveforms between the 8th and 9th and between the 10th and 11th ECG complexes illustrate where to read the waveform.

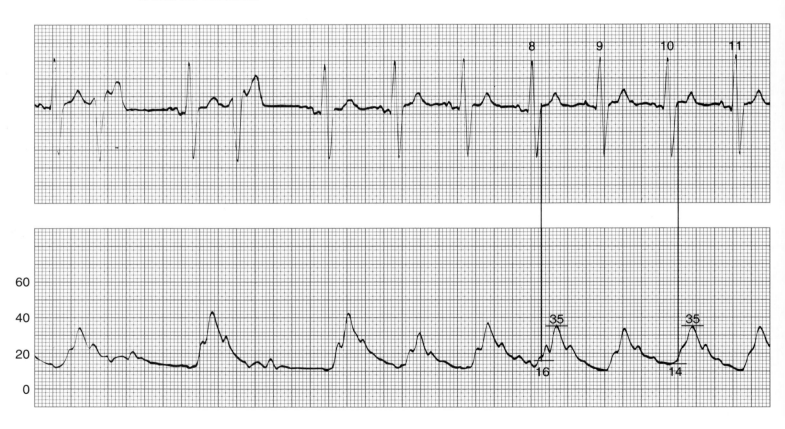

PRACTICE WAVEFORM 8–4. In this waveform obtained from the distal port, the patient was on assist/control ventilation with no spontaneous breathing. What is the tracing and the value associated with the waveform?

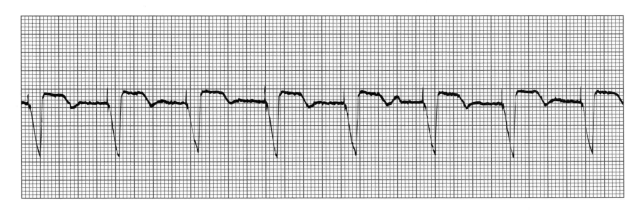

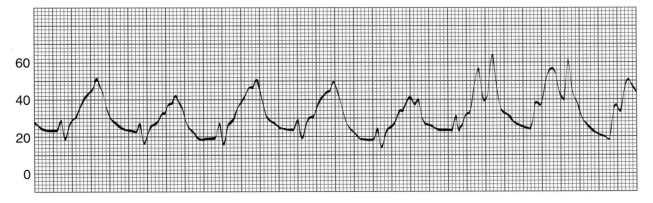

PRACTICE WAVEFORM 8–4. *Analysis:* Waveform is a pulmonary capillary wedge tracing changing to a pulmonary arterial waveform. The PCWP waveform has a giant V wave. The PCWP value is approximately 23 mm Hg, as seen beneath the 1st and 2nd QRS complexes. The PA tracing has artifact as illustrated by a high sharp wave after the T wave. This wave is probably not a physiologic wave and should not be used as the peak systolic pressure. The PA pressure is likely about 56/23 mm Hg, illustrated beneath the 7th and 8th QRS complexes.

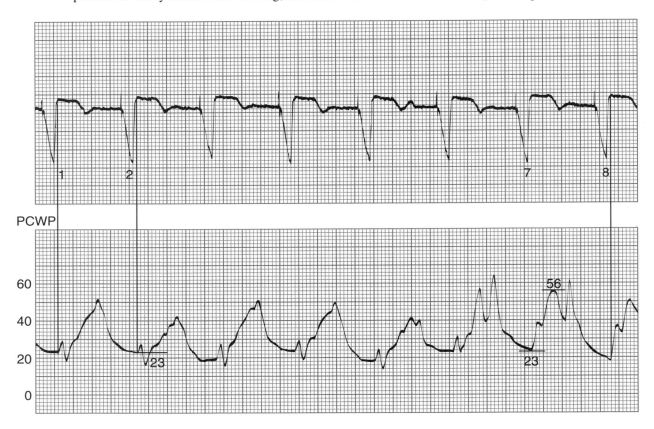

PRACTICE WAVEFORM 8–5. In this waveform obtained from the proximal port, the patient was breathing spontaneously. What is the tracing and the value associated with the waveform?

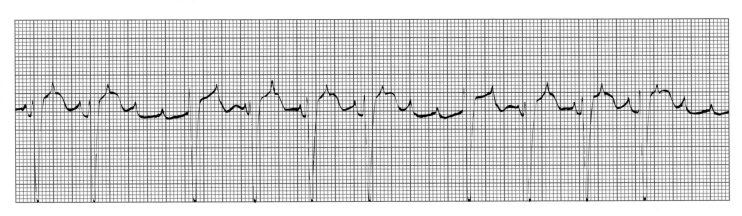

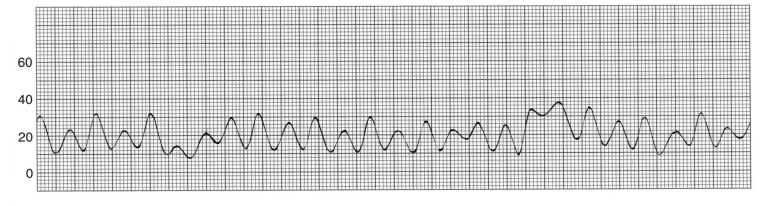

PRACTICE WAVEFORM 8–5. *Analysis:* This is a CVP waveform with multiple A waves due to the atrial flutter rhythm. CVP is read near the end of the QRS under these circumstances in order to try to approximate end-diastolic ventricular pressures. Value would be about 19 mm Hg, as illustrated beneath the 2nd, 4th, and 5th ECG complexes.

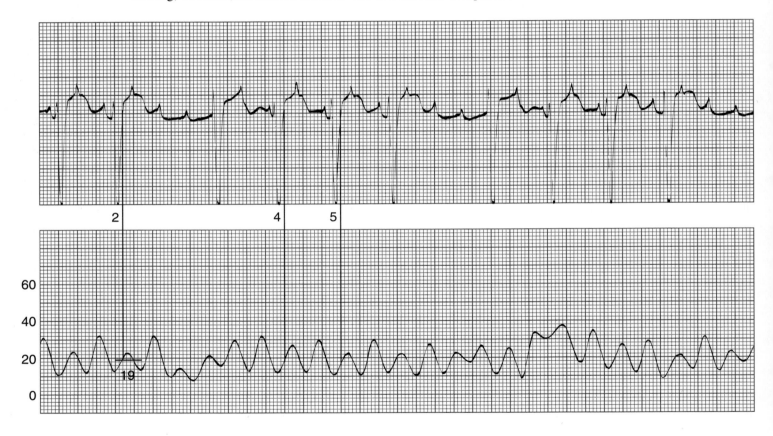

PRACTICE WAVEFORM 8–6. In this waveform obtained from the proximal port, the patient was receiving mechanical ventilation, IMV mode, with spontaneous breathing efforts. What is the tracing and the value associated with the waveform?

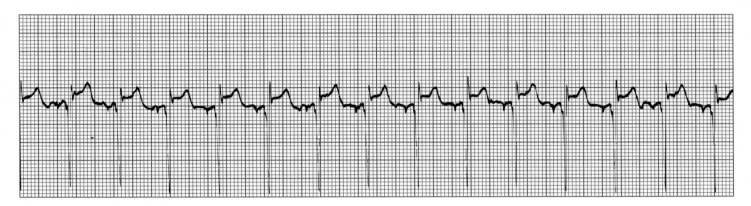

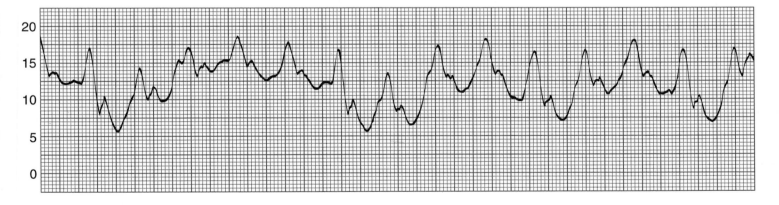

PRACTICE WAVEFORM 8–6. *Analysis:* This is a CVP waveform with clear A and C waves but no clear V wave. Spontaneous breathing efforts and mechanical ventilator breaths are marked. CVP value would be approximately 14 mm Hg, as illustrated beneath the 9th–10th and 13th–14th ECG complexes.

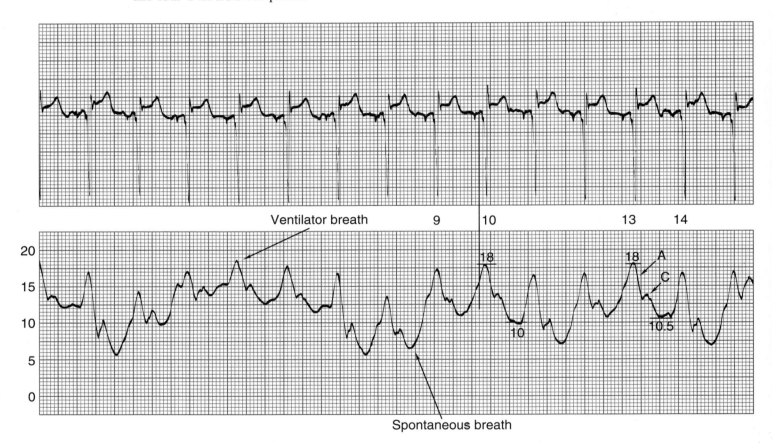

PRACTICE WAVEFORM 8–7. In this waveform obtained from the proximal port, the patient was on assist/control ventilation. What is the tracing and the value associated with the waveform?

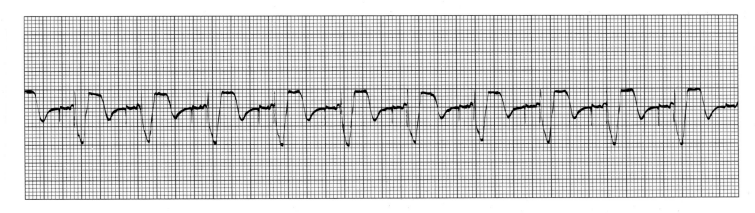

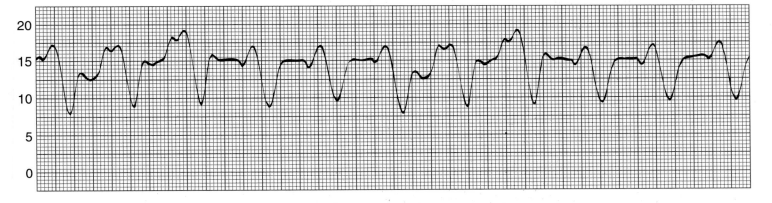

PRACTICE WAVEFORM 8–7. *Analysis:* This is a CVP waveform with an ECG rhythm demonstrating an A-V sequential pacemaker. No clear A waves are visible, although a large V wave is present. In the absence of A waves, read at the end of the QRS complex. Value of the CVP is about 15 mm Hg. Locations to read the waveform are marked.

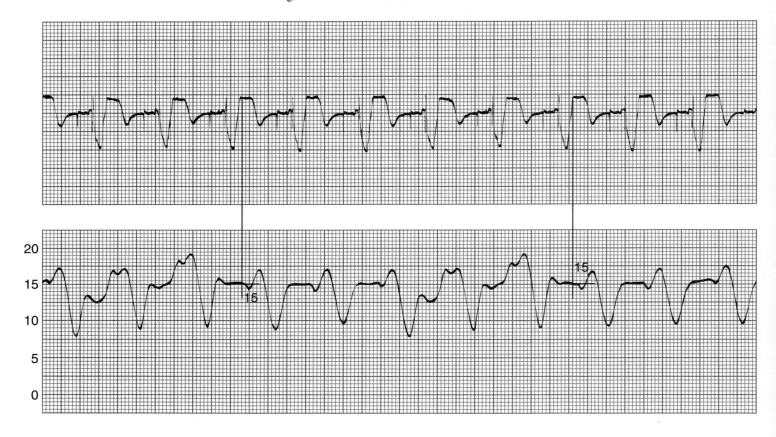

PRACTICE WAVEFORM 8–8. In this waveform obtained from the distal port, the patient was breathing spontaneously. What is the tracing and the value associated with the waveform?

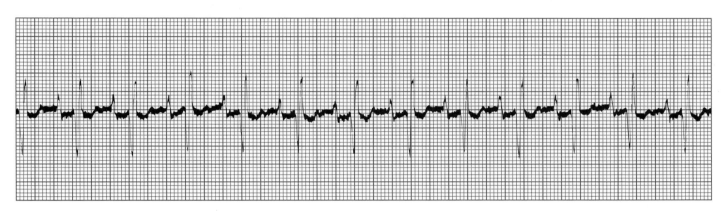

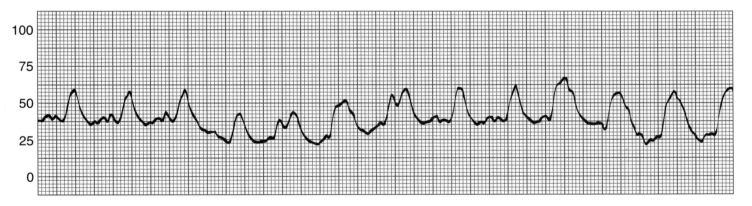

PRACTICE WAVEFORM 8–8. *Analysis:* This is a PCWP waveform changing into a PA waveform. Note the large V wave in the T–P interval during the PCWP tracing. Read the A wave beneath the QRS complex to obtain a PCWP value of about 38 mm Hg. Avoid the spontaneous breathing efforts marked during the tracing. Also note the transition between the PCWP and PA waveforms between the 11th and 12th QRS complexes.

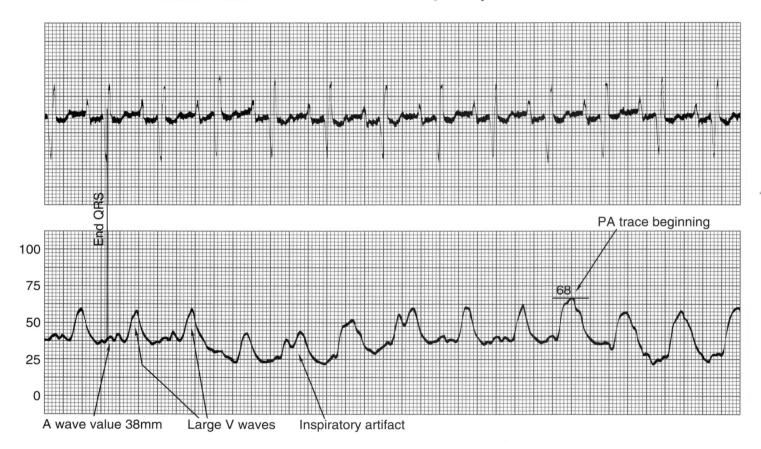

PRACTICE WAVEFORM 8–9. In this waveform obtained from the distal port, the patient was on assist/control ventilation with no spontaneous breathing. What is the tracing and the value associated with the waveform?

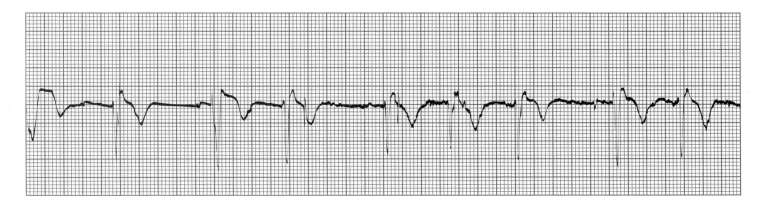

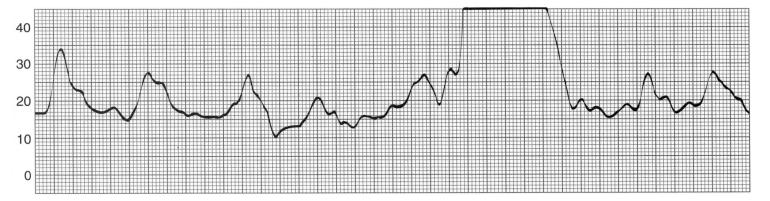

PRACTICE WAVEFORM 8–9. *Analysis:* The waveform is a PA tracing. The square wave test indicates an overdamped tracing, potentially decreasing systolic and elevating diastolic values. The ECG rhythm shows occasional ventricular pacing, causing inconsistent arterial values. The fluctuation in arterial values represents not artifact but actual physiologic variations. The pressure should be read by averaging all waves or taking a representative waveform. An approximate PA value is marked near 27/18 mm Hg. Keep in mind the PAS pressure may be slightly lower and the PAD pressure slightly higher due to the overdamping.

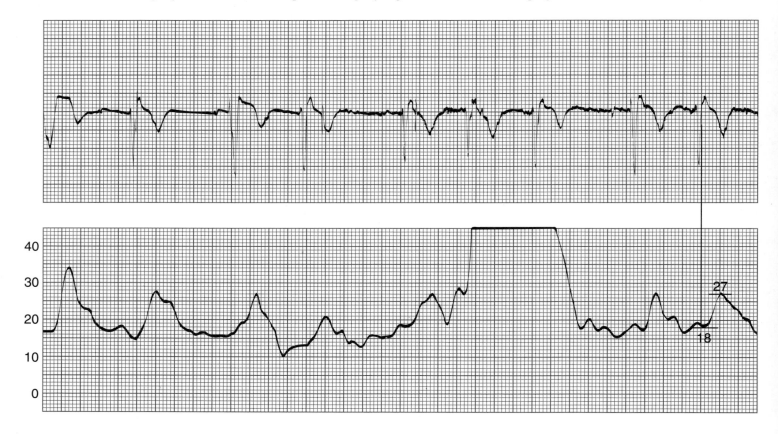

PRACTICE WAVEFORM 8–10. In this waveform obtained from the proximal port, the patient was breathing spontaneously. What is the tracing and the value associated with the waveform?

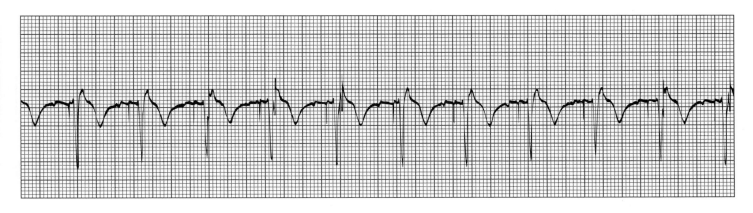

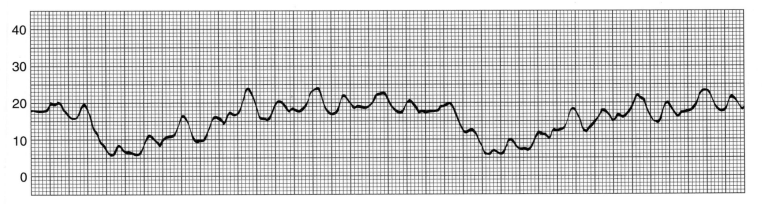

PRACTICE WAVEFORM 8–10. *Analysis:* This is a CVP waveform with clear A and V waves. Avoid inspiratory artifact as marked. CVP value is about 19 mm Hg.

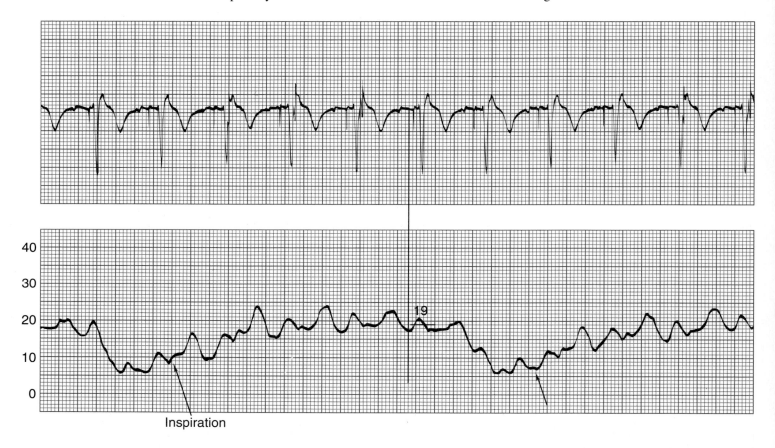

Inspiration

PRACTICE WAVEFORM 8–11. In this waveform obtained from the distal port, the patient was on assist/control ventilation plus spontaneously initiating each breath. What is the tracing and the value associated with the waveform?

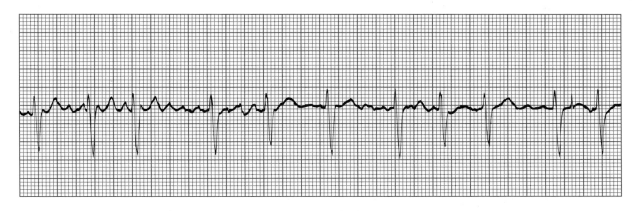

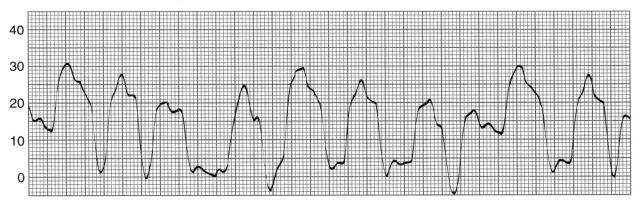

PRACTICE WAVEFORM 8–11. *Analysis:* This is a ventricular waveform as reflected in the rapid diastolic drop and terminal rise. The PA catheter is not advanced far enough and has fallen back into the right ventricle. The ventricular value is about 20–26/3 mm Hg, depending on the diastolic filling time. The catheter needs to be advanced or replaced. Remember that if a right ventricular value is present, the end-diastolic ventricular value should be used instead of the CVP value.

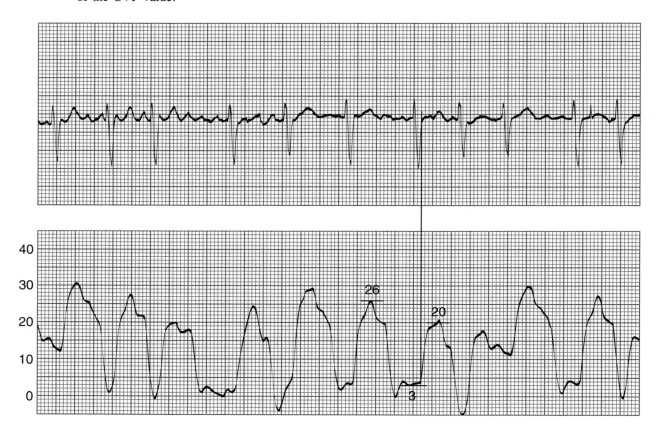

PRACTICE WAVEFORM 8–12. In this waveform obtained from the distal port, the patient was breathing spontaneously. What is the tracing and the value associated with the waveform?

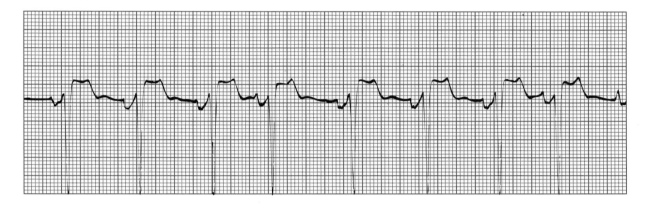

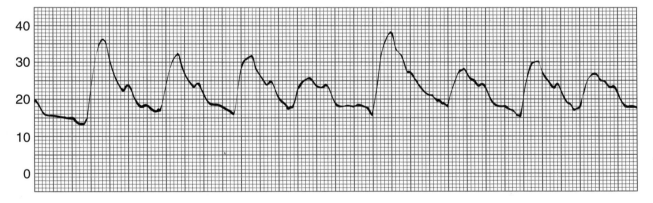

PRACTICE WAVEFORM 8–12. *Analysis:* This is a PA waveform in an ECG rhythm of frequent atrial premature contractions. The variations in pressures are physiologic, not artifactual. Note that each increased PA pressure waveform follows a long diastolic filling phase. Approximate PA pressure is 32/16 mm Hg, although this pressure does not include the occasional increased pressures.

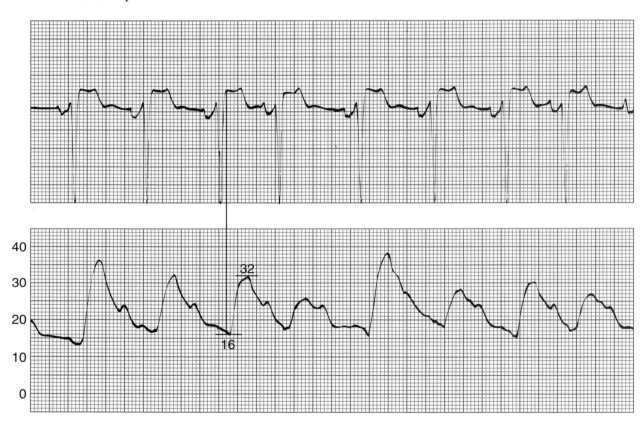

PRACTICE WAVEFORM 8–13. In this waveform obtained from the distal port of a PA catheter, the patient was on assist/control ventilation with no spontaneous breathing. What is the tracing and the value associated with the waveform?

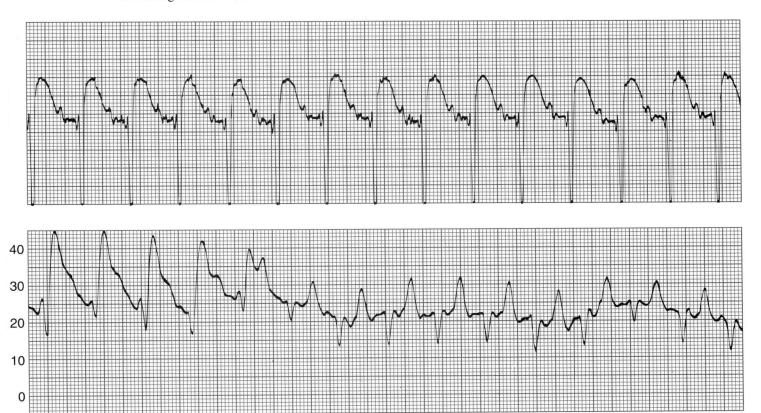

PRACTICE WAVEFORM 8–13. *Analysis:* This is a PA tracing changing to a PCWP wave. This tracing is interesting due to the presence of artifact producing false low values. Notice the sharp decreases in pressures in both the PA and PCWP waveforms. These decreases are inconsistent with normal waveforms. Read this waveform at end diastole for both the PCWP and PAD pressure. The PA value would be about 42/23 mm Hg, with a PCWP of about 22 mm Hg.

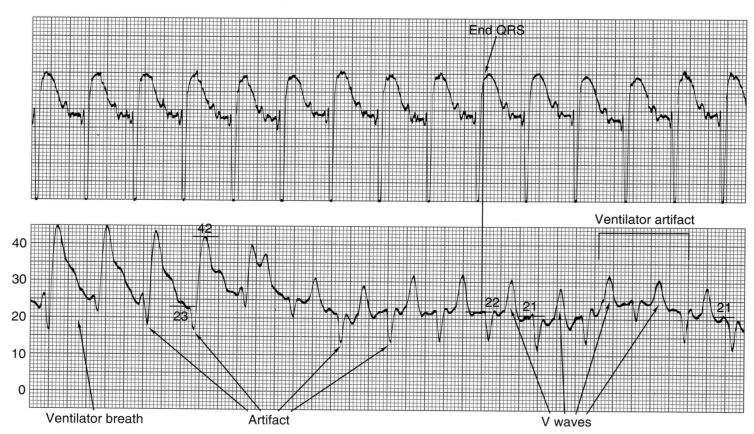

No clear A wave is present   Probable mean PCWP = 21–22 mm Hg

PRACTICE WAVEFORM 8–14. In this waveform obtained from the proximal port, the patient was breathing spontaneously. What is the tracing and the value associated with the waveform?

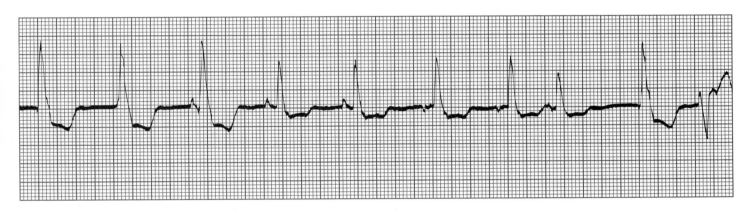

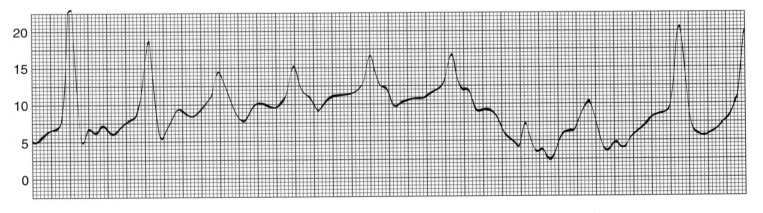

PRACTICE WAVEFORM 8–14. *Analysis:* This is a CVP waveform with occasional giant A waves when the P wave is lost in the QRS complex. Normal A waves occur when atrioventricular synchrony occurs in the middle of the rhythm strip. Approximate value is 12 mm Hg. Note that when the giant A waves occur, an approximate value can still be obtained if the end-QRS value is read.

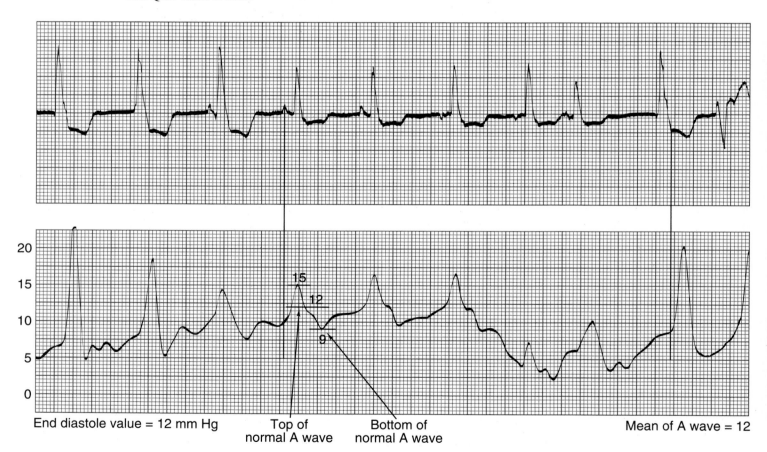

End diastole value = 12 mm Hg   Top of normal A wave   Bottom of normal A wave   Mean of A wave = 12

PRACTICE WAVEFORM 8–15. In this waveform obtained from the proximal port, the patient was breathing spontaneously. What is the tracing and the value associated with the waveform?

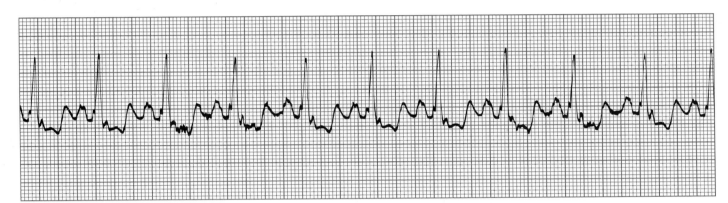

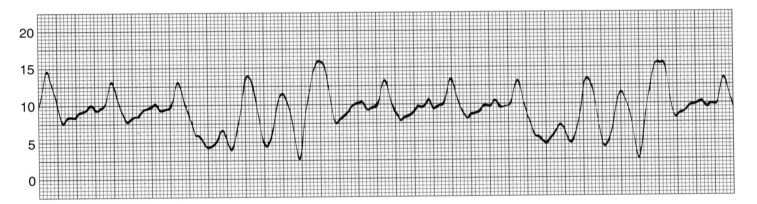

PRACTICE WAVEFORM 8–15. *Analysis:* This is a CVP waveform with a clear A wave and small V wave. Note the exaggerated A and V waves with each spontaneous breath. CVP value is approximately 11 mm Hg.

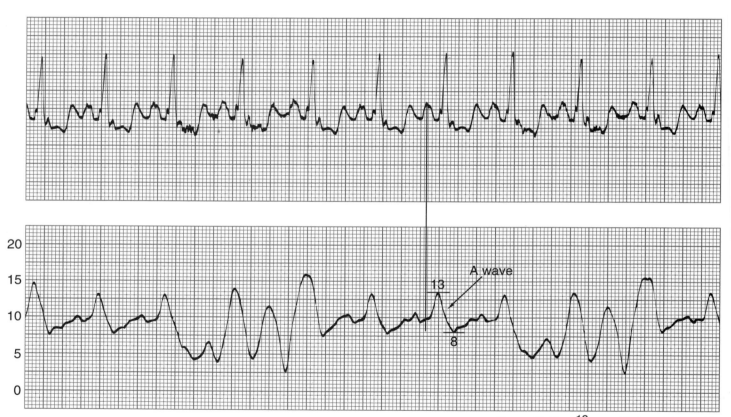

Mean CVP = $\frac{13}{8} \approx$ or 10.5 or 11 mm Hg

PRACTICE WAVEFORM 8–16. In this waveform obtained from the distal port, the patient was on assist/control ventilation plus spontaneous initiation of each breath. What is the tracing and the value associated with the waveform?

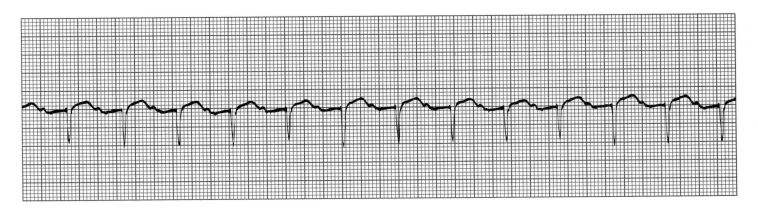

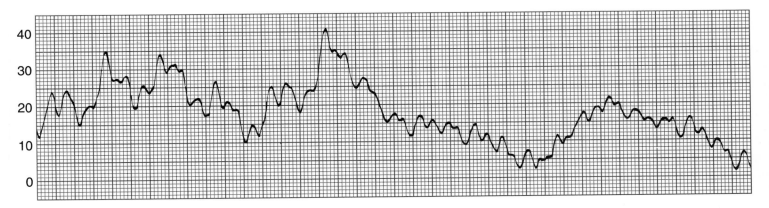

PRACTICE WAVEFORM 8–16. *Analysis:* This is a PA waveform changing to a PCWP waveform. The rapid respiratory pattern makes reading end expiration difficult. Reading the PA and PCWP just prior to inspiratory dips increases the likelihood of accurate values. PA value is about 34/20 mm Hg, and the PCWP is about 13 mm Hg.

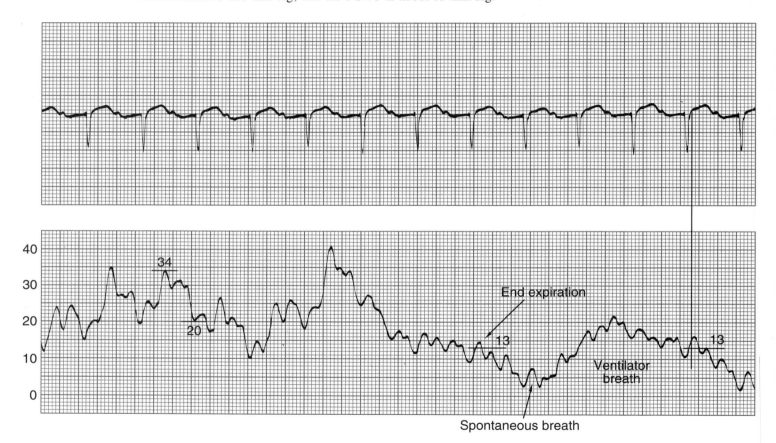

PRACTICE WAVEFORM 8–17. In this waveform obtained from the distal port, the patient was breathing spontaneously. What is the tracing and the value associated with the waveform?

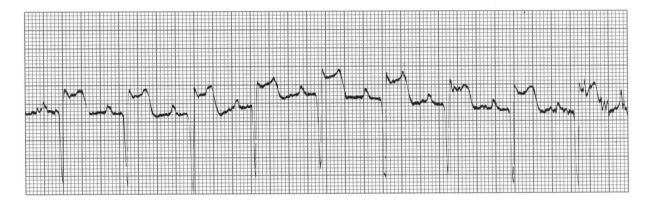

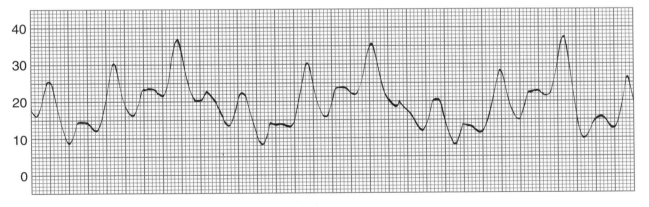

PRACTICE WAVEFORM 8–17. *Analysis:* This is a PCWP waveform with clear A and V waves. The V wave is larger than the A wave, as can be seen by the V waves' appearance late in the T–P interval. Respiratory artifact is also present. PCWP value is about 22 mm Hg.

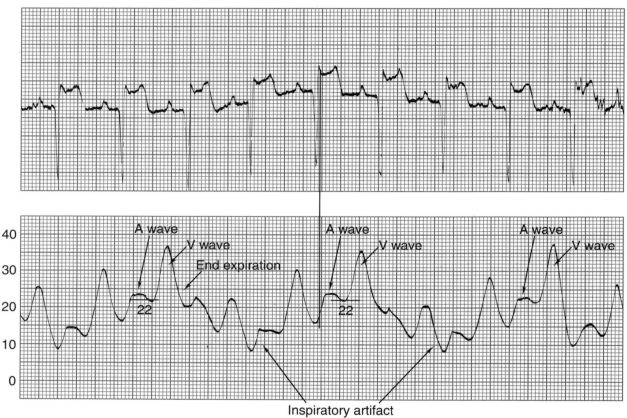

PRACTICE WAVEFORM 8–18. In this waveform obtained from a radial artery line, the patient was on assist/control ventilation without spontaneous breathing. What is the tracing and the value associated with the waveform?

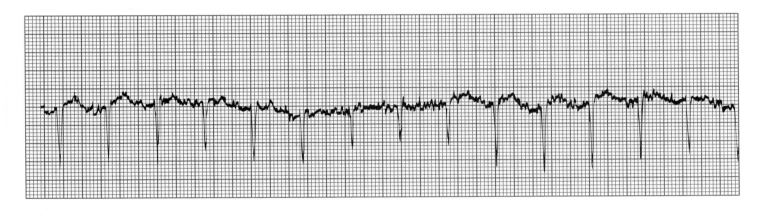

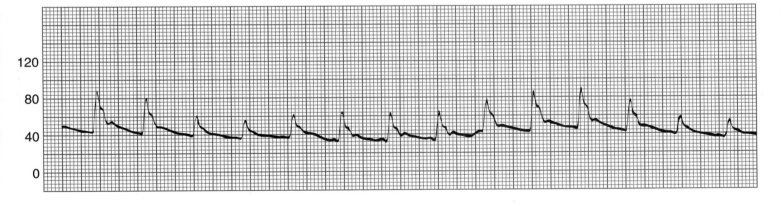

PRACTICE WAVEFORM 8–18. *Analysis:* Radial artery waveform changing with each ventilator breath. The waveforms are actual physiologic values and not artifact. Systolic values fluctuate between 56 and 92 mm Hg, with diastolic values changing between 32 and 44 mm Hg. The average systolic value over one respiratory cycle (10 QRS complexes) is 71 mm Hg, and the average diastolic value is 37. In this type of situation, average the waveforms over a representative respiratory cycle and compare these values to the monitor values. This method will let you know if the waveform values on the monitor are to be trusted.

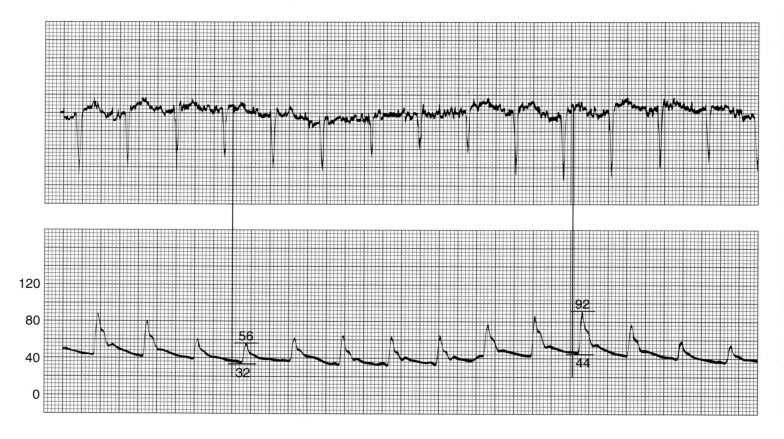

PRACTICE WAVEFORM 8–19. In this waveform obtained from the proximal port, the patient was on spontaneous ventilation. What is the tracing and the value associated with the waveform?

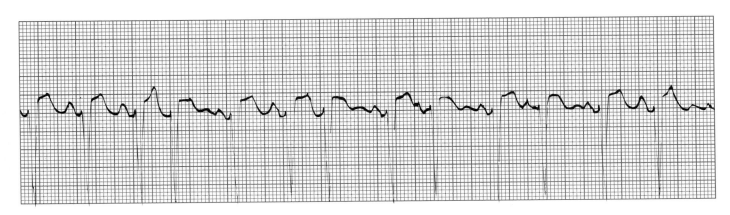

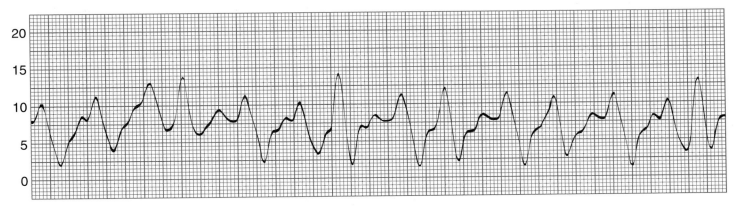

PRACTICE WAVEFORM 8–19. *Analysis:* This is a CVP waveform with large A waves and diminished V waves owing to the tachycardia. Note larger A waves with each ectopic beat (beneath each P–R interval). Also note the clear V wave when a longer diastolic filling time is present. CVP value is about 6–7 mm Hg.

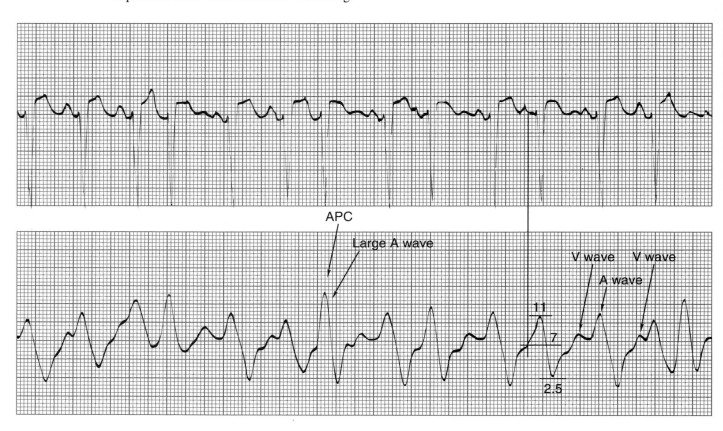

PRACTICE WAVEFORM 8–20. In this waveform obtained from the proximal port, the patient was on IMV ventilation with spontaneous breathing. What is the tracing and the value associated with the waveform?

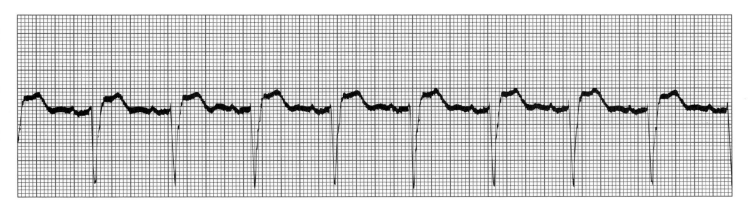

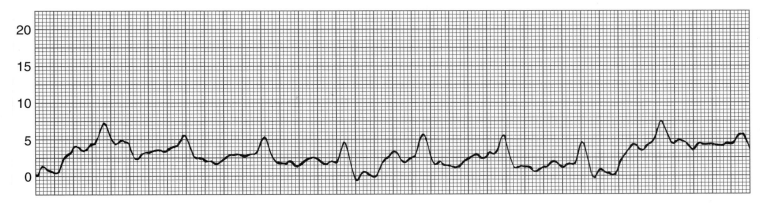

PRACTICE WAVEFORM 8–20. *Analysis:* This is a CVP waveform with multiple respiratory artifact patterns. Interpretation requires avoiding spontaneous breaths as well as the ventilator breaths. Average CVP value is about 4 mm Hg.

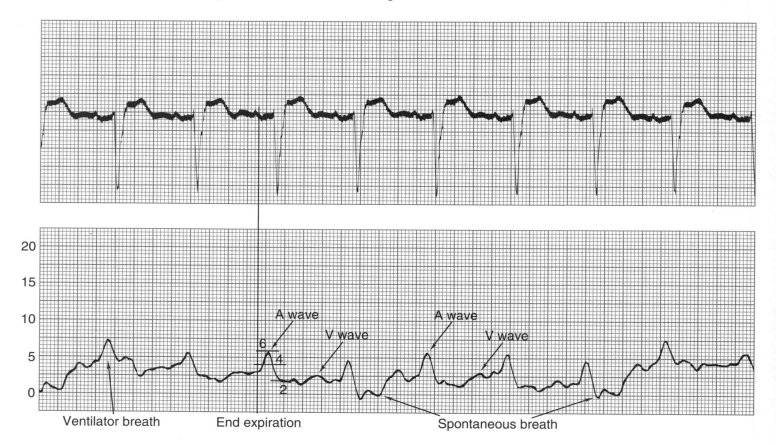

PRACTICE WAVEFORM 8–21. In this waveform obtained from the proximal port, the patient was on assist/control ventilation plus intermittent spontaneous initiation of ventilator breaths. What is the tracing and the value associated with the waveform?

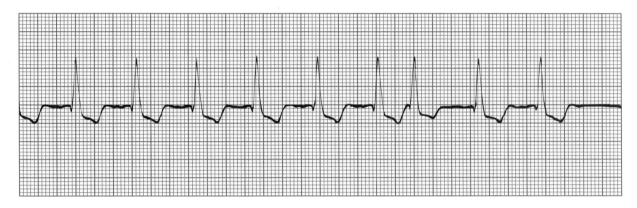

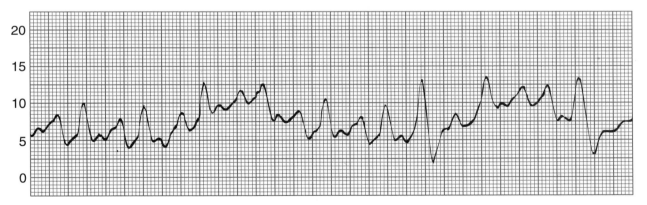

PRACTICE WAVEFORM 8–21. *Analysis:* This is a CVP waveform with frequent respiratory artifact, large A waves with atrial premature contractions (APCs) and clear normal A and V waves. To obtain a CVP reading, avoid the spontaneous and ventilator breath artifacts as well as the large A waves associated with APCs. CVP value is about 7–8 mm Hg.

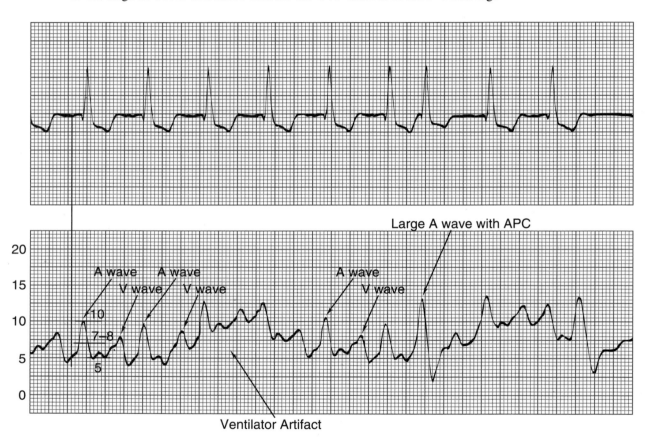

PRACTICE WAVEFORM 8–22. On this waveform, try to interpret the wave without knowing which port was used to obtain the wave. The patient was breathing spontaneously and was in respiratory distress. What is the tracing and the value associated with the waveform?

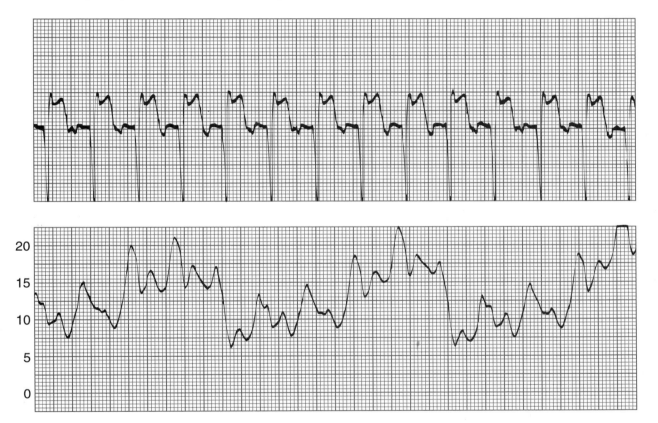

PRACTICE WAVEFORM 8–22. *Analysis:* This is a CVP waveform, as distinguished by the large wave occurring before the QRS complex, ruling out a PA and a PCWP wave. The respiratory rate is so fast as to make it questionable whether an accurate value will be obtained, even with end-expiratory readings. The nurse should attempt to have the patient hold his or her breath after a normal exhalation for a few seconds, if possible. From this tracing, the value is about 18–19 mm Hg. Keep in mind that the actual value may be lower because expiratory effort may maintain positive airway pressure during exhalation.

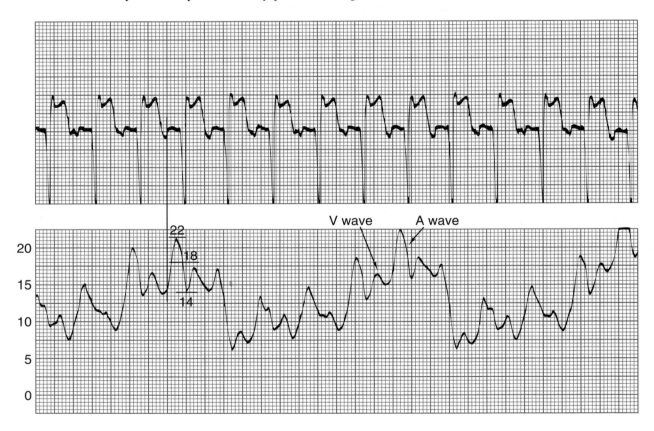

PRACTICE WAVEFORM 8–23. In this waveform obtained from the proximal port, the patient was on assist/control ventilation plus intermittent spontaneous initiation of ventilator breaths. What is the tracing and the value associated with the waveform?

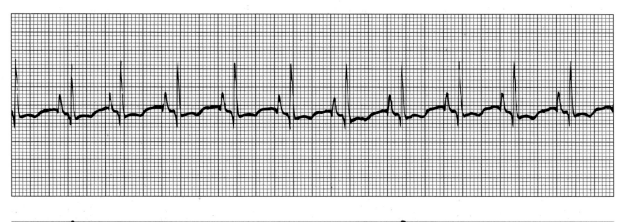

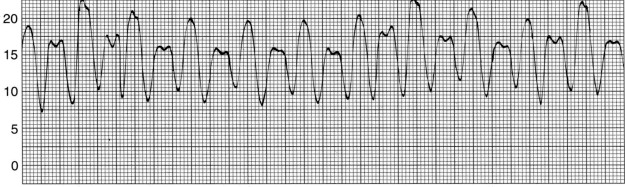

PRACTICE WAVEFORM 8–23. *Analysis:* This is a CVP tracing with large A and V waves. Note that the A wave is slightly larger by aligning the A wave with the P–R interval. The CVP value obtained before ventilator breaths is about 14 mm Hg.

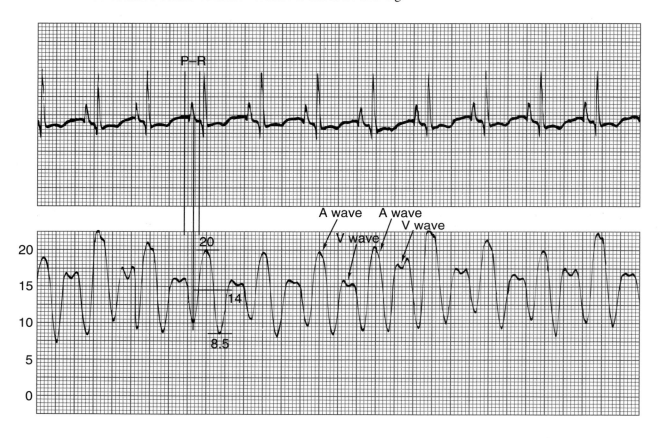

PRACTICE WAVEFORM 8–24. In this waveform obtained from the distal port, the patient demonstrated inverse ratio ventilation. What is the tracing and the value associated with the waveform?

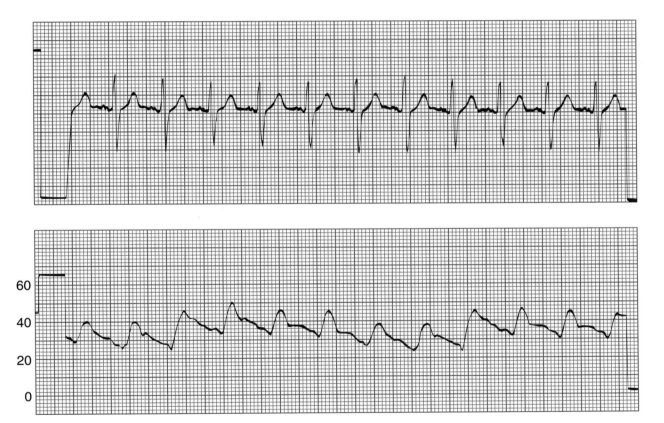

PRACTICE WAVEFORM 8–24. *Analysis:* This is a PA waveform. In inverse ratio ventilation, the values are obtained at the brief expiratory phase. Positive pressure artifact is present during most of the ventilatory cycle. Note end-expiratory value of about 38/24 mm Hg.

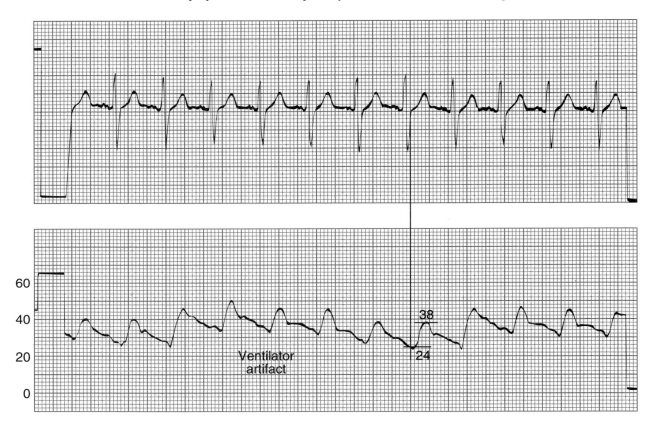

PRACTICE WAVEFORM 8–25. In this waveform obtained from the proximal port, the patient was breathing spontaneously. What is the tracing and the value associated with the waveform?

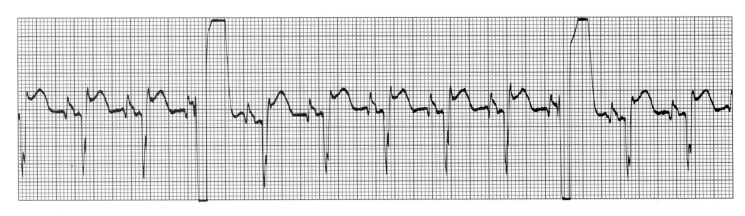

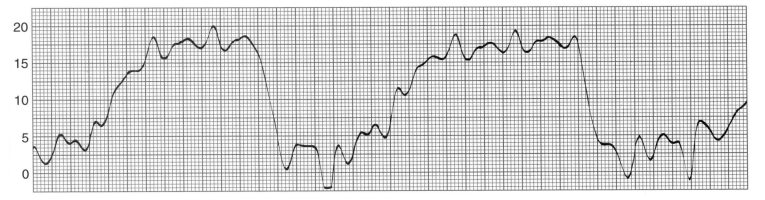

PRACTICE WAVEFORM 8–25. *Analysis:* This is a CVP waveform in a patient with marked inspiratory waveform distortion. End expiration is marked just before the sharp inspiratory dip. CVP value is about 18 mm Hg.

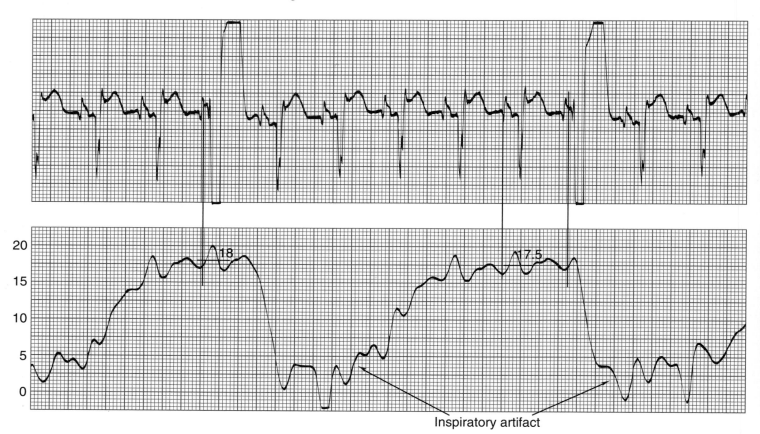

Inspiratory artifact

PRACTICE WAVEFORM 8–26. In this waveform obtained from the distal port, the patient was on assist/control ventilation plus intermittent spontaneous initiation of ventilator breaths. What is the tracing and the value associated with the waveform?

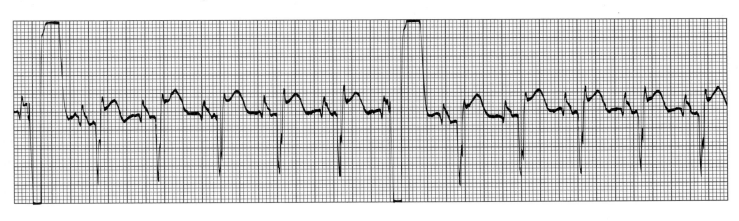

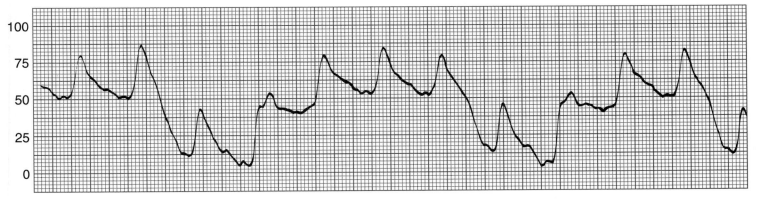

PRACTICE WAVEFORM 8–26. *Analysis:* PA waveform with marked spontaneous inspiratory artifact. End expiration is noted just before the inspiratory dip in the waveform. PA value is about 85/50 mm Hg.

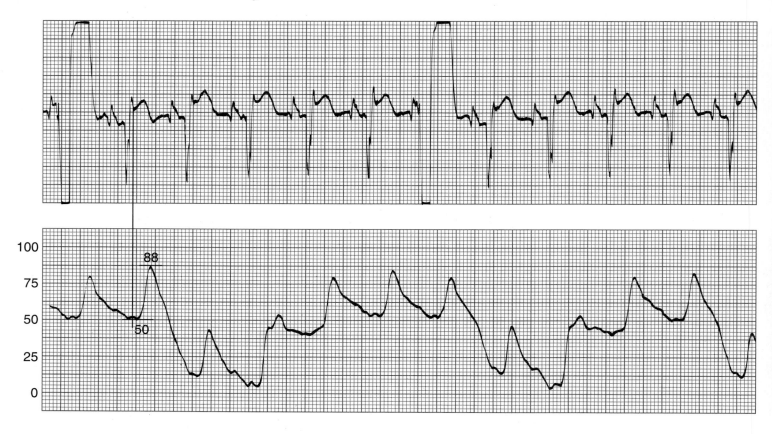

PRACTICE WAVEFORM 8–27. In this waveform obtained from the femoral arterial line, the patient was experiencing cardiopulmonary arrest. This waveform is hard to interpret and requires looking closely at the QRS and waveform. What is the tracing and the value associated with the waveform?

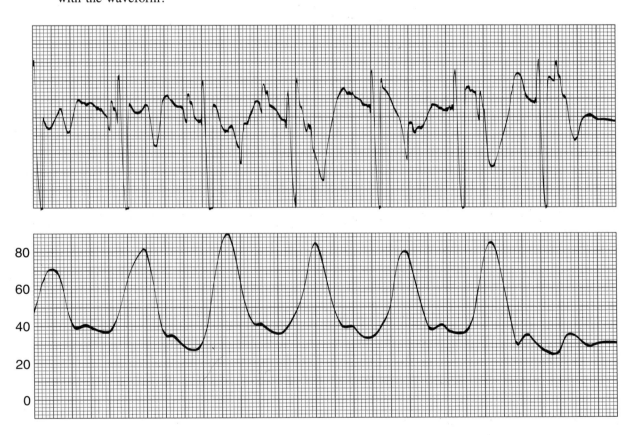

PRACTICE WAVEFORM 8–27. *Analysis:* The waveform obviously must be a femoral arterial waveform but is not generated from the ECG complex. The patient is in electromechanical dissociation as can be seen by the QRS complexes not consistently aligning with the pressure waves. Initially, the arterial value is about 82/32 mm Hg. Note how the waveform decreases during a change in personnel performing compressions.

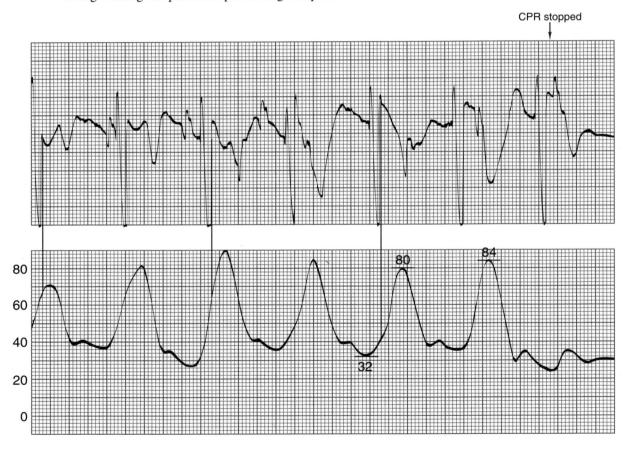

PRACTICE WAVEFORM 8–28. In this waveform obtained from the distal port, the patient was on assist/control ventilation without spontaneous initiation of ventilator breaths. What is the tracing and the value associated with the waveform?

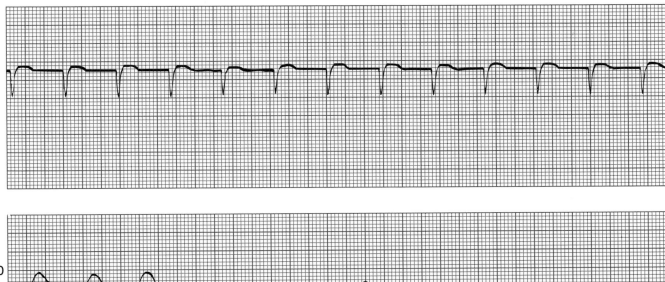

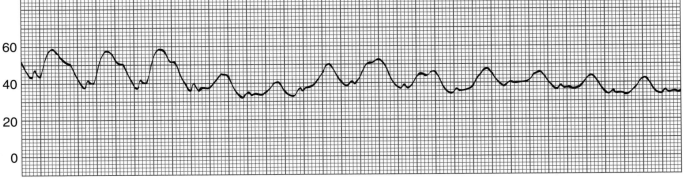

PRACTICE WAVEFORM 8–28. *Analysis:* This is a PA waveform changing to a PCWP waveform. Note the large V waves in the PCWP tracing. PA pressure is about 58/40 mm Hg, with the PCWP about 36 mm Hg.

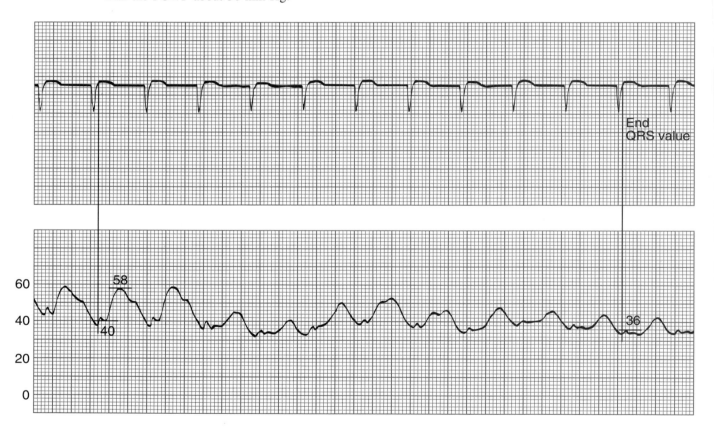

PRACTICE WAVEFORM 8–29. In this waveform obtained from the distal port, the patient was on IMV ventilation without spontaneous breathing. What is the tracing and the value associated with the waveform?

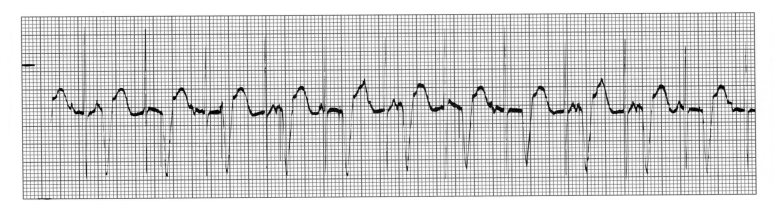

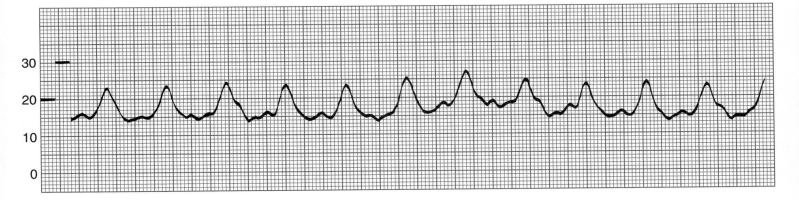

PRACTICE WAVEFORM 8–29. *Analysis:* This is a PCWP waveform in an A-V sequential pacemaker rhythm. This waveform is illustrated by the large V wave late in the T–P interval. PCWP value is about 15 mm Hg.

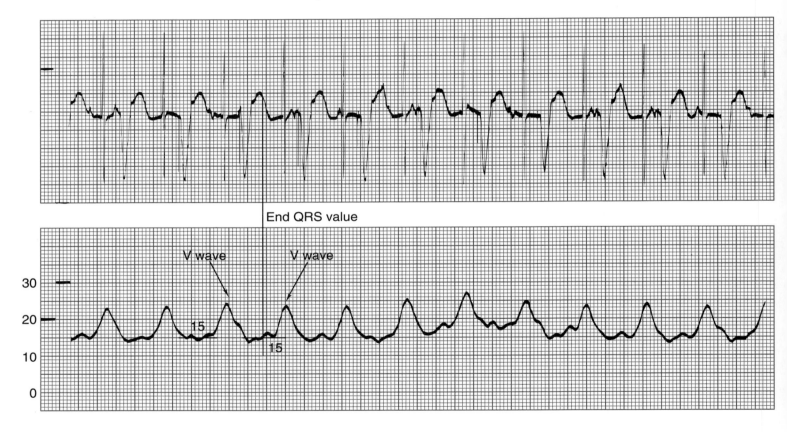

PRACTICE WAVEFORM 8–30. In this waveform obtained from the proximal port, the patient was on assist/control ventilation plus spontaneous initiation of ventilator breaths. What is the tracing and the value associated with the waveform?

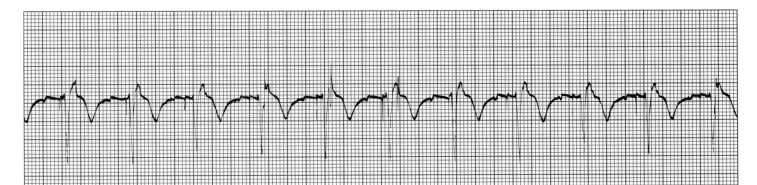

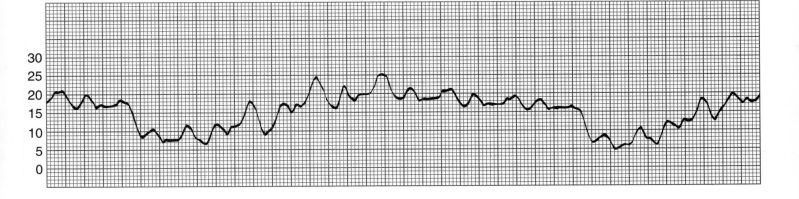

PRACTICE WAVEFORM 8–30. *Analysis:* This is a CVP waveform in an improperly sensing pacemaker ECG pattern. Spontaneous breaths are causing artifact and need to be recognized in order to avoid false low readings. CVP value is about 16–17 mm Hg.

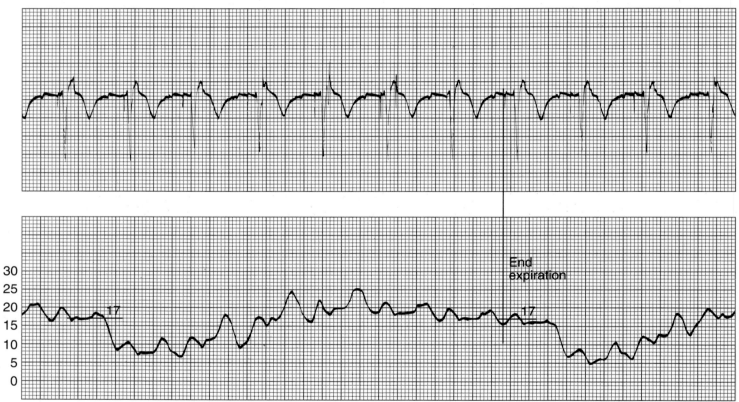

PRACTICE WAVEFORM 8–31. In this waveform obtained from the proximal port, the patient was on IMV ventilation without spontaneous ventilation. What is the tracing and the value associated with the waveform?

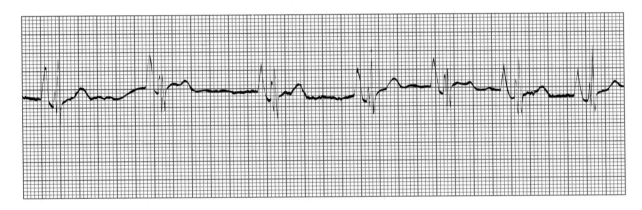

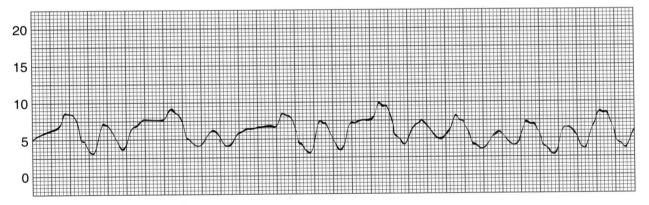

PRACTICE WAVEFORM 8–31. *Analysis:* This is a CVP waveform with clear A and V waves. The change in the waveform is due to change in the heart rate. Note the clear A and V waves, particularly at slower heart rates. CVP value is about 7 mm Hg.

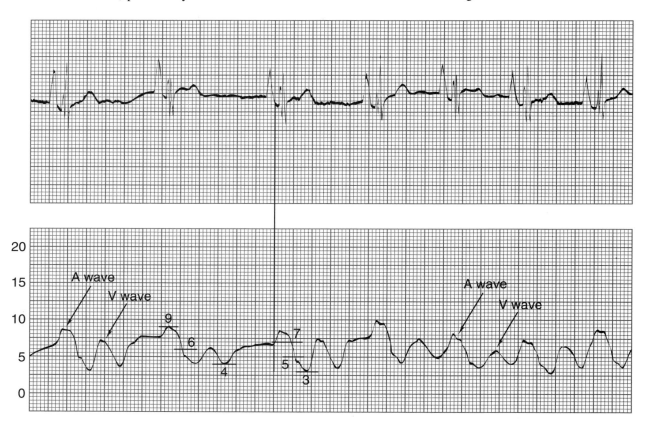

PRACTICE WAVEFORM 8–32. In this waveform obtained from the distal port, the patient was on assist/control ventilation without spontaneous initiation of ventilator breaths. What is the tracing and the value associated with the waveform?

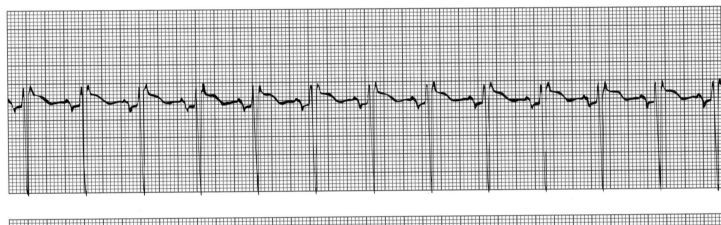

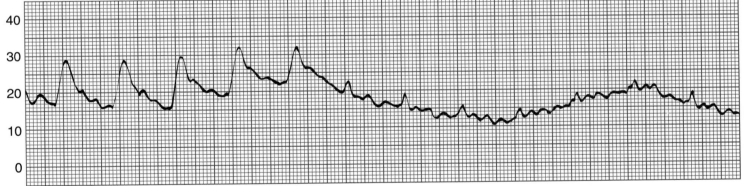

PRACTICE WAVEFORM 8–32. *Analysis:* This is a PA waveform changing to a PCWP tracing. The interesting aspect of this waveform is the large positive pressure artifact produced by the ventilator breath. The peak value is not the correct location to read the PCWP for two reasons: (1) the peak value would produce a PCWP value higher than the PAD pressure; and (2) because no spontaneous breaths are present, the only artifact is from the positive pressure due to the ventilator. The PA pressure is about 29/15 mm Hg, with the PCWP about 12 mm Hg.

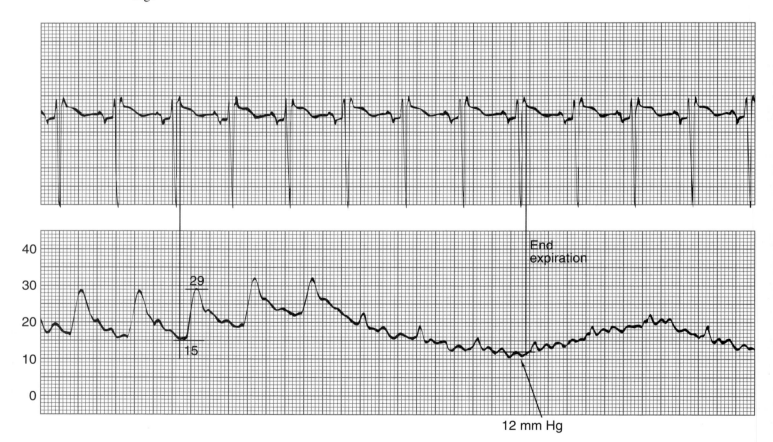

PRACTICE WAVEFORM 8–33. In this waveform obtained from the proximal port, the patient was on IMV ventilation without spontaneous breathing. What is the tracing and the value associated with the waveform?

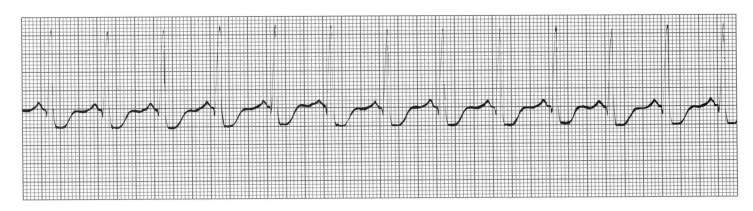

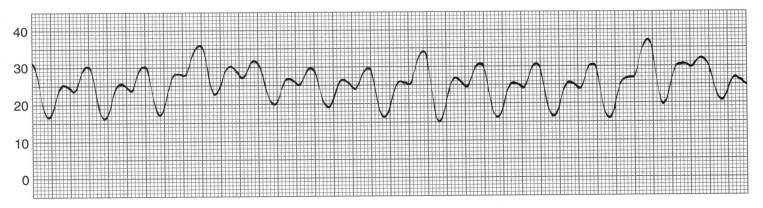

PRACTICE WAVEFORM 8–33. *Analysis:* This is a CVP tracing with a large V wave. The V wave is readily identified owing to the appearance of the large wave during the T–P interval. The mean of the A wave is about 25 mm Hg.

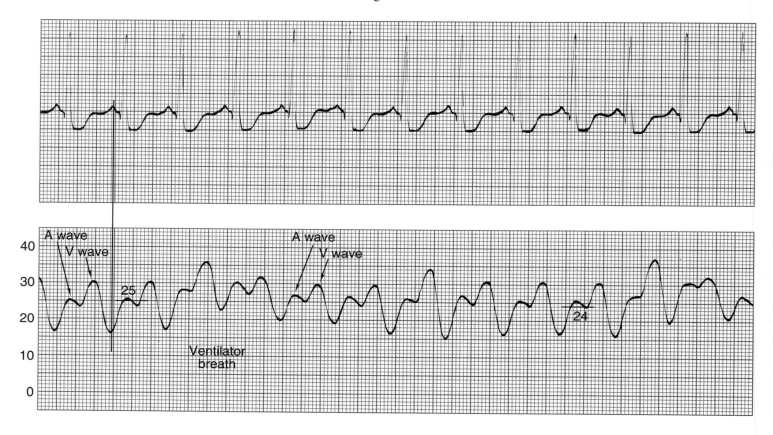

PRACTICE WAVEFORM 8–34. In this waveform obtained from the distal port, the patient was on IMV ventilation without spontaneous breathing. What is the tracing and the value associated with the waveform?

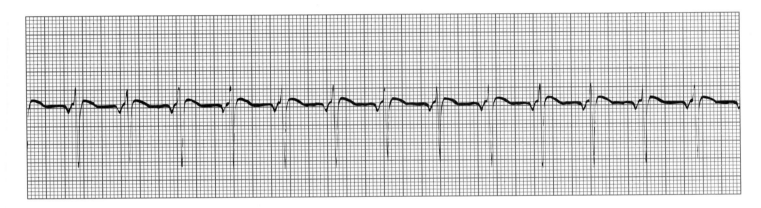

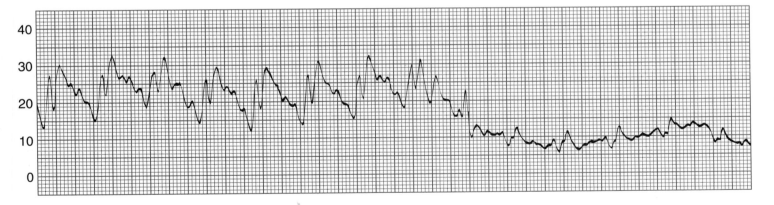

PRACTICE WAVEFORM 8–34. *Analysis:* This is a PA tracing that changes into a PCWP waveform. The PA tracing had multiple distortions due to artifact, with the most difficulty presented in the reading of the diastolic value. PA pressure is about 30/15 mm Hg, with the PCWP about 7 mm Hg.

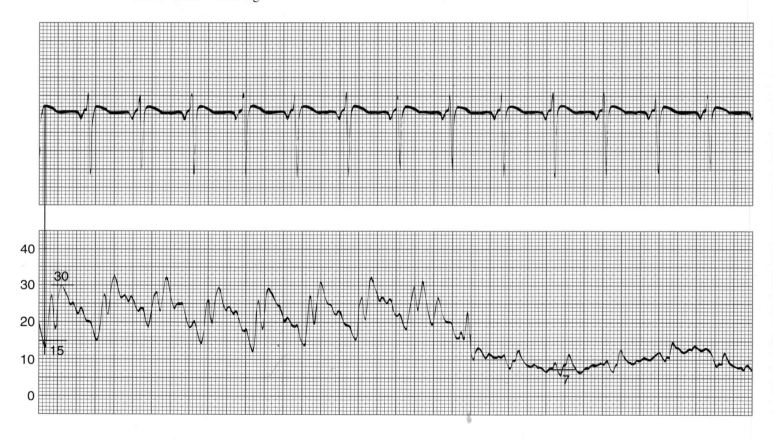

PRACTICE WAVEFORM 8–35. In this waveform obtained from the proximal port, the patient was on assist/control ventilation without spontaneous initiation of ventilator breaths. What is the tracing and the value associated with the waveform?

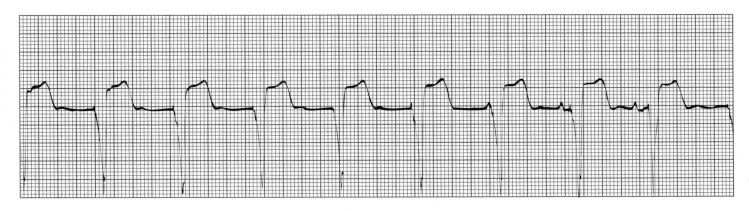

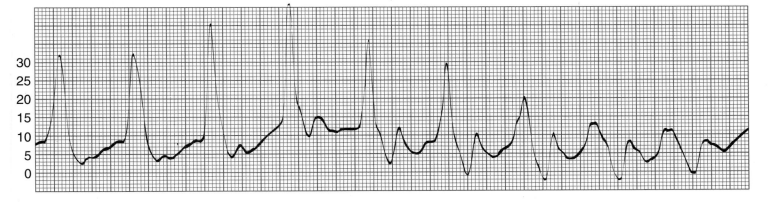

PRACTICE WAVEFORM 8–35. *Analysis:* This is a CVP tracing with giant A waves due to the loss of A-V synchrony. The appropriate A wave value would be read at the 8th or 9th ECG complex, which has a normal P-QRS relationship. The CVP value would be about 6 mm Hg. If this waveform did not have normal A-V synchrony, an end-QRS value could be used. In this case, the value is about 8 mm Hg.

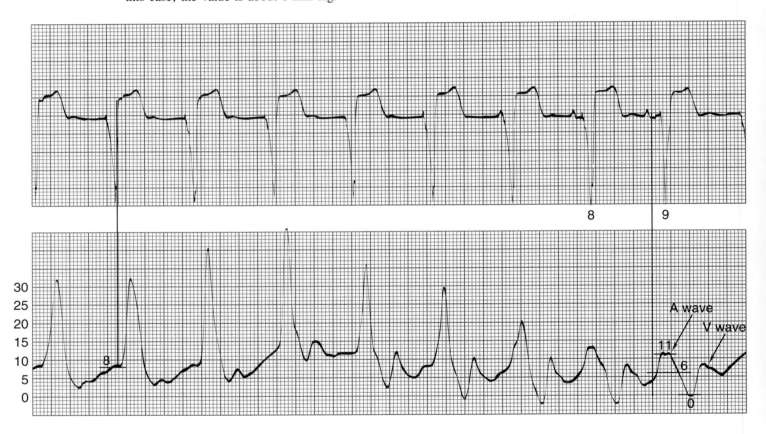

PRACTICE WAVEFORM 8–36. In this waveform obtained from the distal port, the patient was on assist/control ventilation plus spontaneous initiation of ventilator breaths. What is the tracing and the value associated with the waveform?

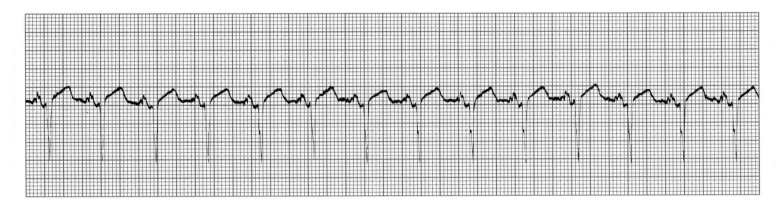

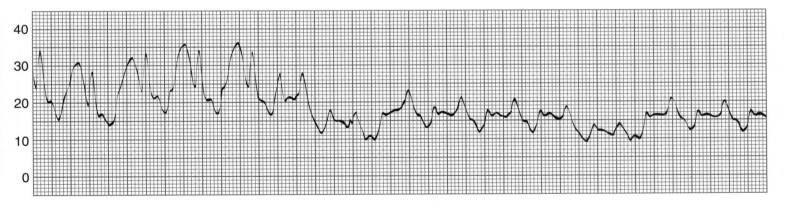

PRACTICE WAVEFORM 8–36. *Analysis:* This is a PA tracing changing to a PCWP wave-form. In the PCWP tracing, the V wave is larger than the A wave and should be avoided when obtaining values. The PA tracing has artifact immediately after the systolic value but is causing no apparent problems in obtaining the PCWP value. PA pressure is about 36/17 mm Hg, with the PCWP value about 16 mm Hg.

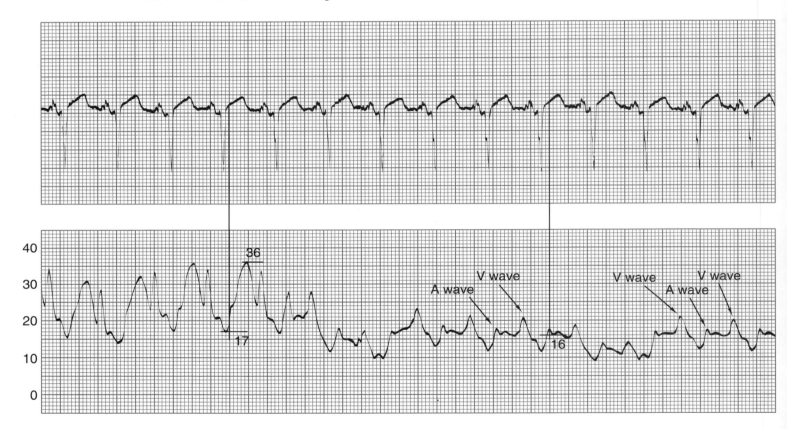

PRACTICE WAVEFORM 8–37. In this waveform obtained from the proximal port, the patient was breathing spontaneously. What is the tracing and the value associated with the waveform?

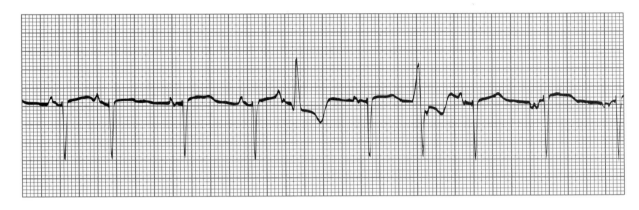

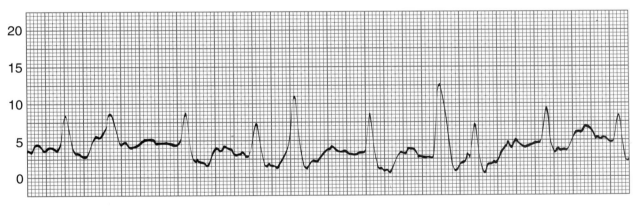

PRACTICE WAVEFORM 8–37. *Analysis:* This is a CVP waveform punctuated with giant A waves from ectopic beats. Obtaining a correct reading requires isolating waveforms with normal ECG intervals. CVP value is about 4 mm Hg.

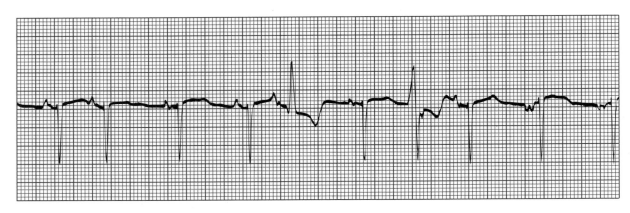

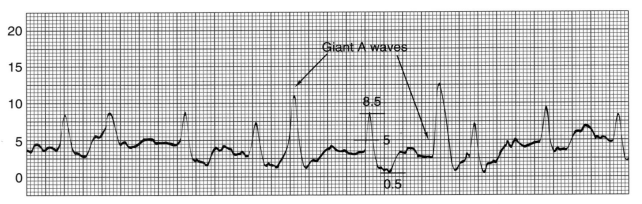

PRACTICE WAVEFORM 8–38. In this waveform obtained from the distal port, the patient was on assist/control ventilation without spontaneous initiation of ventilator breaths. What is the tracing and the value associated with the waveform?

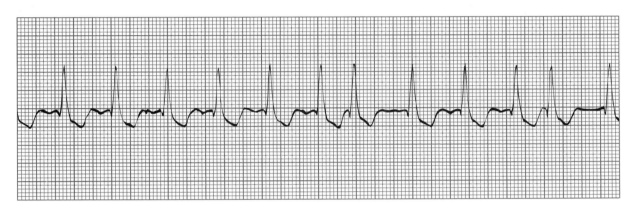

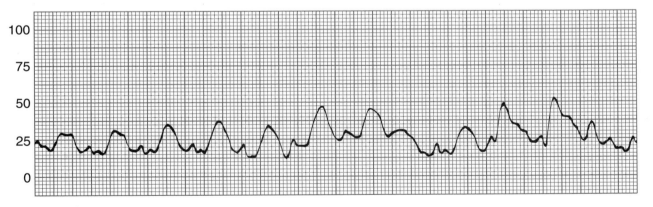

PRACTICE WAVEFORM 8–38. *Analysis:* This is a PCWP tracing changing to a PA tracing. Note the large V waves late in the T–P interval in the PCWP tracing. The small A wave must be located to obtain a correct PCWP tracing. The PCWP value is about 15 mm Hg, with the PA pressure about 50/23 mm Hg.

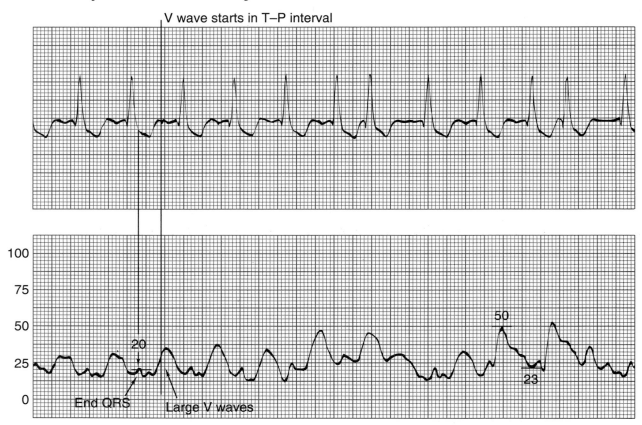

PRACTICE WAVEFORM 8–39. A pulmonary arterial waveform is aligned with an airway pressure curve. The patient is on assist/control ventilation with a PEEP level of 13 cm H_2O (10 mm Hg). Based on the airway pressure curve, identify end expiration, the value associated with the waveform, and if the patient is triggering any of the ventilator breaths.

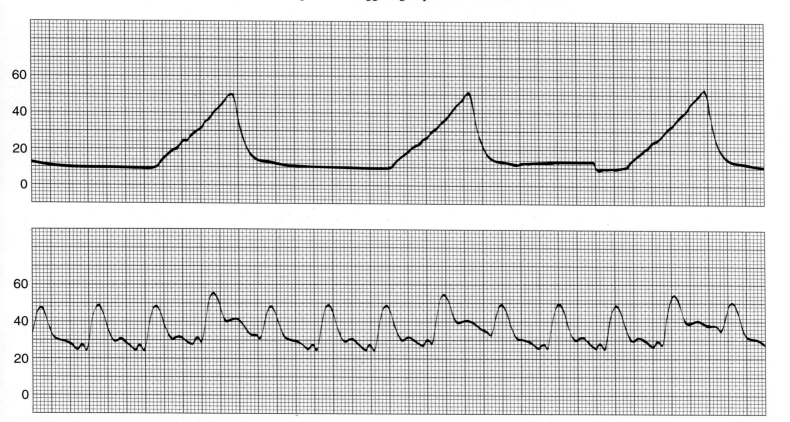

PRACTICE WAVEFORM 8–39. *Analysis:* Ventilator breaths are identified by the upward deflections in the pressure curve. No spontaneous breaths are present as evidenced by the lack of any decrease in the pressure level below 10 mm Hg (the PEEP level). If spontaneous breathing were present, the inspiratory effort would have pulled the pressure below the baseline of 10 mm Hg. End expiration is seen at any point in the airway pressure curve where the reading is 10 mm Hg. The PA pressure is about 50/24 mm Hg.

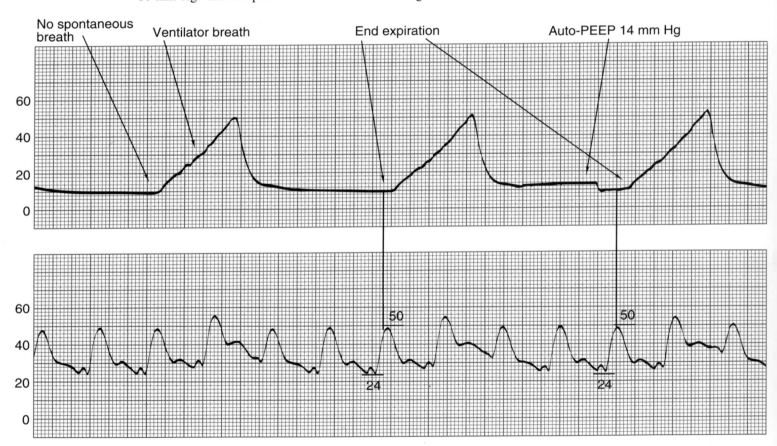

PRACTICE WAVEFORM 8–40. In this tracing from the proximal port of the PA catheter, the patient was receiving IMV without spontaneous breathing. Identify the waveform and the value associated with the tracing.

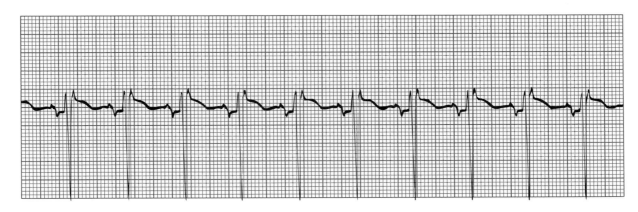

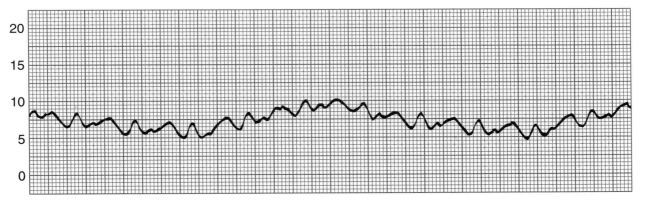

PRACTICE WAVEFORM 8–40. *Analysis:* A CVP waveform with ventilator artifact is evident. End expiration is found in the trough of this waveform. The IMV breath from the ventilator is producing an upward displacement of the waveform. Corresponding ECG complexes that aid in identifying end expiration include the 2nd and 3rd, 8th and 9th, and 11th complexes. The A and V waves are similar in height. The mean of the A wave is about 6 mm Hg.

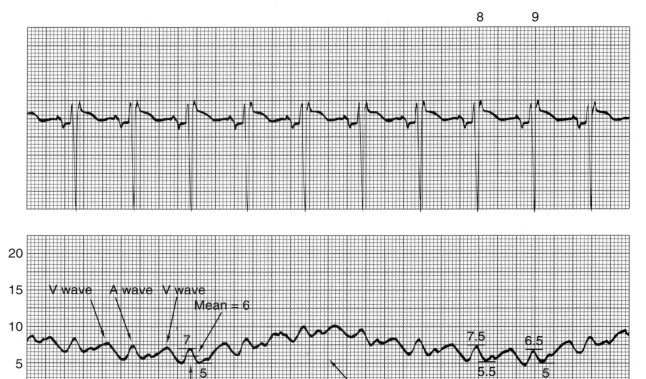

PRACTICE WAVEFORM 8–41. In this tracing from the distal port of the PA catheter, the patient was receiving IMV without spontaneous respirations. An airway pressure tracing is provided to aid in identifying end expiration. Identify the waveform and the value associated with the tracing.

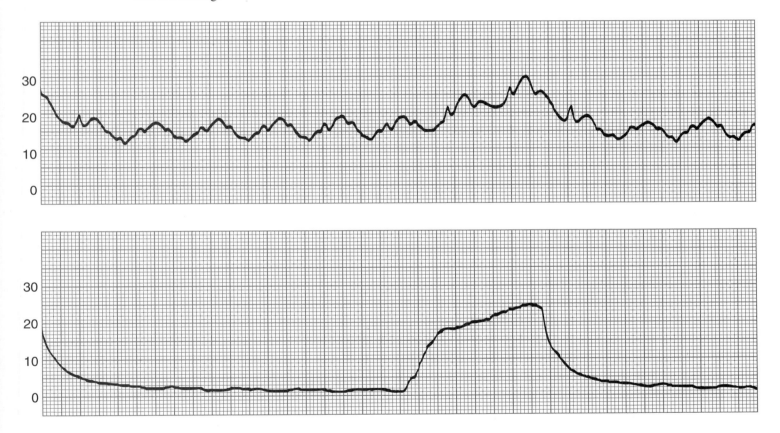

Flow ceases and returns to baseline

PRACTICE WAVEFORM 8–41. *Analysis:* Although no ECG is provided, the pressure tracing appears to be a PA waveform. End expiration is read just prior to the increase in airway pressure. In this tracing, the value associated with the waveform is approximately 20/12 mm Hg. Ventilator artifact is readily identified in this tracing.

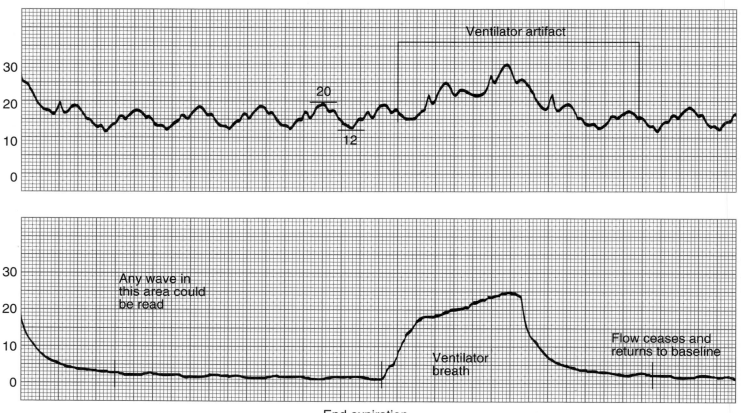

Flow ceases and returns to baseline

PRACTICE WAVEFORM 8–42. In this tracing from the distal port of the PA catheter, the patient was receiving AMV with spontaneous respirations at a rate of about 20 bpm. Identify the waveform and the value associated with the tracing.

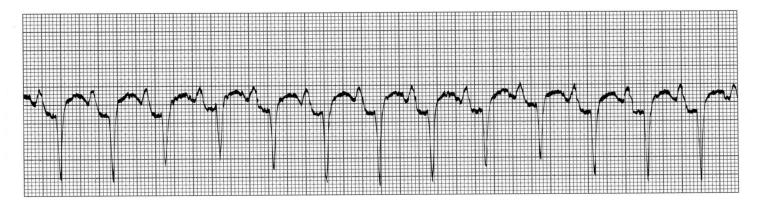

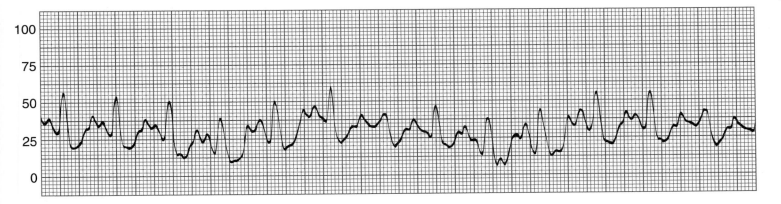

PRACTICE WAVEFORM 8–42. *Analysis:* The waveform is a PA tracing with artifact. The sharp artifact peak is identified primarily through ECG correlation. If this peak were the PAS value, the peak would be immediately after the QRS complex. This peak is too late to be the PAS value because it occurs just before the QRS. The PA pressure in this case is about 37/18 mm Hg.

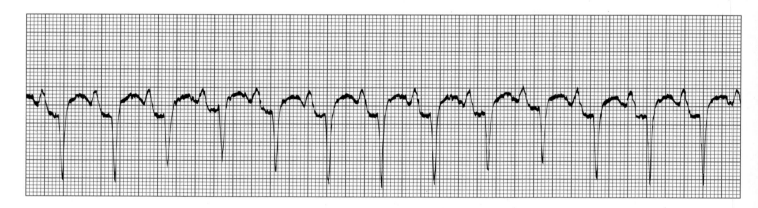

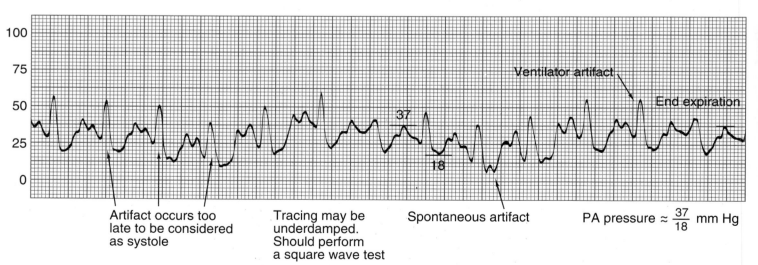

Artifact occurs too late to be considered as systole

Tracing may be underdamped. Should perform a square wave test

Spontaneous artifact

PA pressure $\approx \dfrac{37}{18}$ mm Hg

Ventilator artifact

End expiration

PRACTICE WAVEFORM 8–43. This tracing is from a radial artery line. Based on the square wave test, is the tracing under-, over-, or optimally damped?

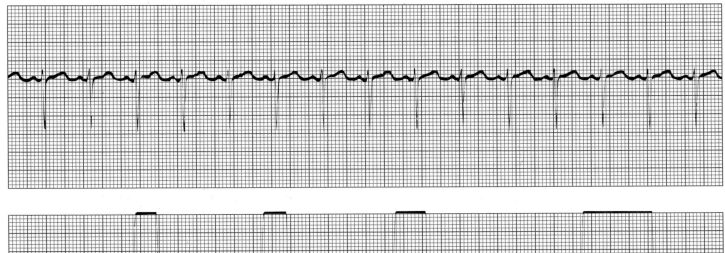

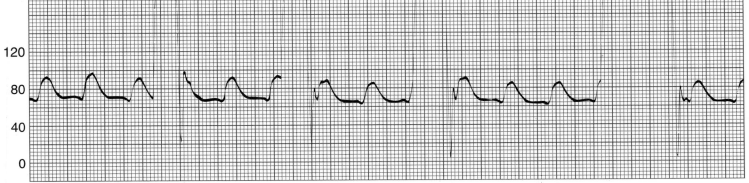

PRACTICE WAVEFORM 8–43. *Analysis:* The tracing is optimally damped based on the frequency response of about 14 Hz and the damping coefficient of 0.54. The BP is about 92/66 mm Hg.

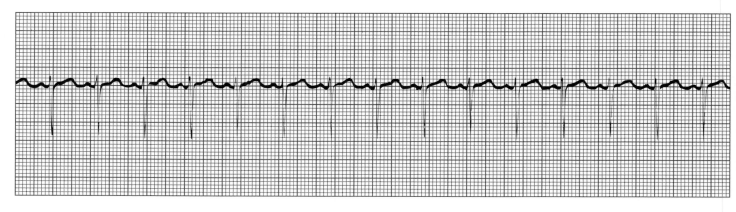

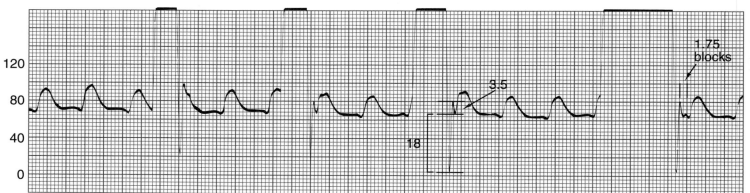

Optimally damped

Frequency response: $\frac{25}{1.75}$ = 14 Hz

Damping coefficient: $\frac{3.5}{18}$ = 0.194 amplitude ratio = 0.54 damping coefficient

PRACTICE WAVEFORM 8–44. This tracing is from the distal port of the PA catheter in a nonintubated patient. The clinician has attempted to place the PA catheter in a PCWP position. Identify the waveforms and the value associated with each waveform.

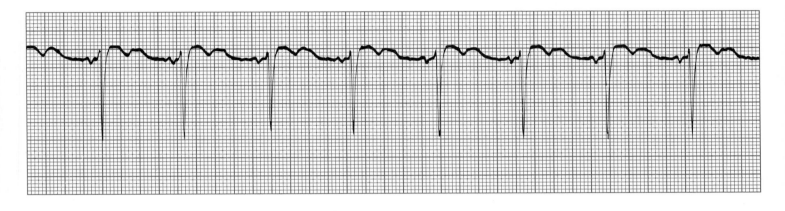

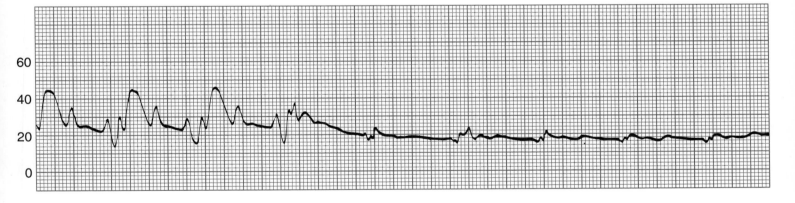

PRACTICE WAVEFORM 8–44. *Analysis:* This waveform is a PA changing to a PCWP wave. The PCWP wave is readily identified with a value of about 18 mm Hg. The PA waveform, however, has diastolic artifact. The PA pressure is about 46/22 mm Hg, based on assuming a continued diastolic pattern. The artifact prior to the PA waveform can confuse interpretation of the waveform, particularly if the monitor is used for the waveform value.

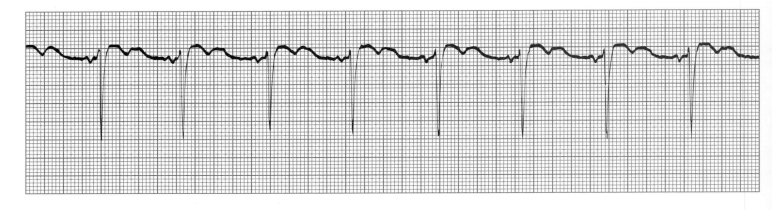

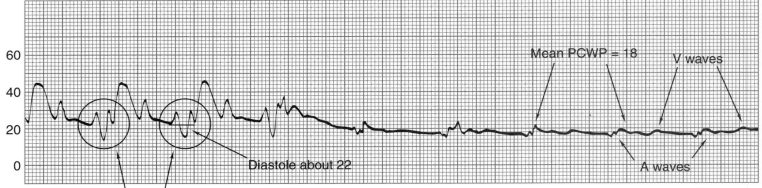

PRACTICE WAVEFORM 8–45. In this tracing from the femoral artery port, the patient was on AMV ventilation at a rate of 20 bpm. Identify the arterial pressure based on the waveform.

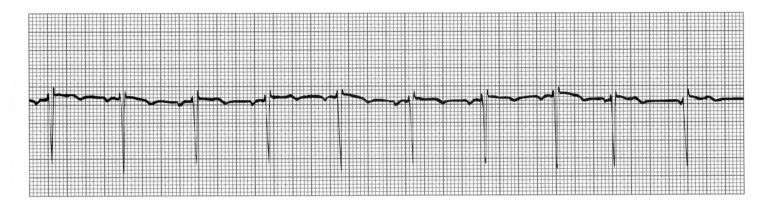

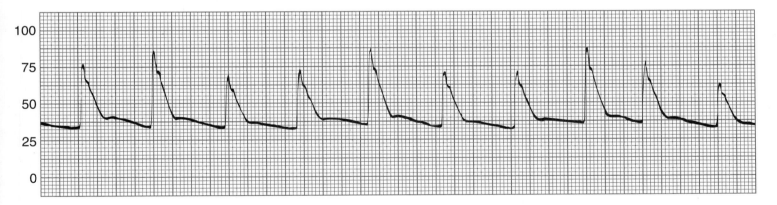

PRACTICE WAVEFORM 8–45. *Analysis:* The pressure fluctuates with each ventilator breath. Averaging the values gives a pressure of about 74/34 mm Hg (averaging pressures over a 6-sec time period). In this case, newer monitors may accurately reflect the correct pressure. Verification still may be necessary with the averaging technique used in this example.

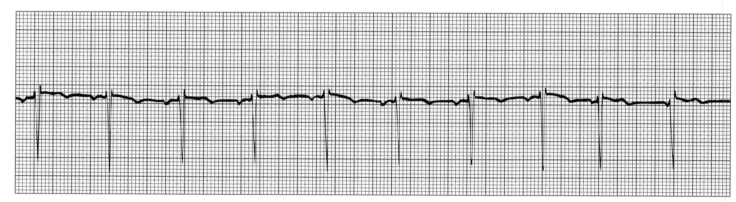

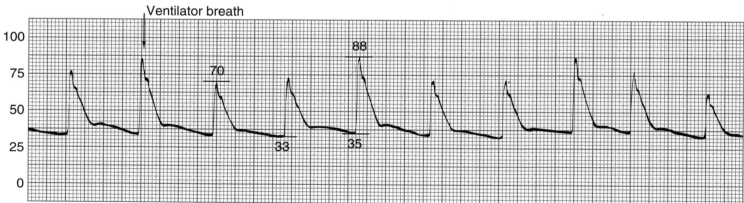

Variations in pressure due to changes in respiration

Respiration rate ≈ 25 bpm

PRACTICE WAVEFORM 8–46. In this tracing from the distal tip of the PA catheter, the patient is on an IMV mode of ventilation at a rate of 12 bpm and is breathing spontaneously at a rate of 30 bpm. The ECG rhythm indicates a supraventricular tachycardia (SVT) rate of 230. What is the waveform and the value associated with the tracing?

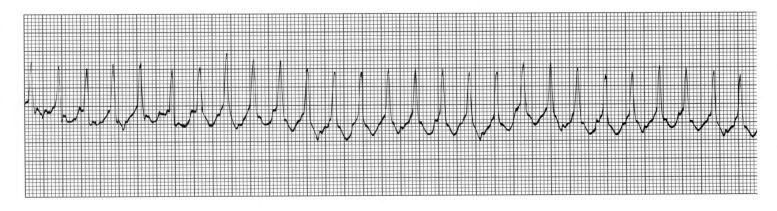

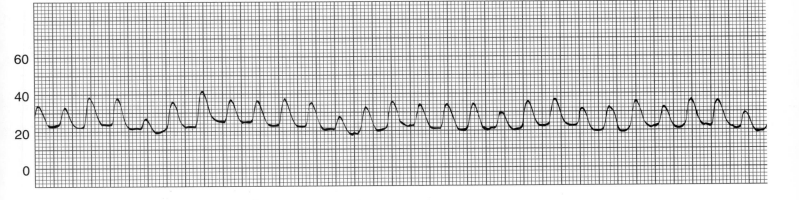

PRACTICE WAVEFORM 8–46. *Analysis:* This is a PA waveform. The waveform illustrates a narrow pulse pressure owing to the lack of diastolic filling time with the rapid heart rate. Read the PA pressure between the 10th and 11th QRS complexes. Also note a spontaneous respiration after the 11th QRS complex and a ventilator breath after the 6th QRS complex. The pressure value is about 33/28 mm Hg.

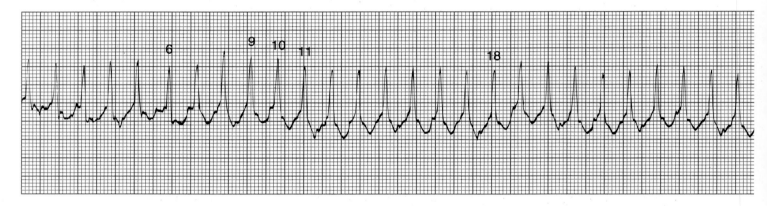

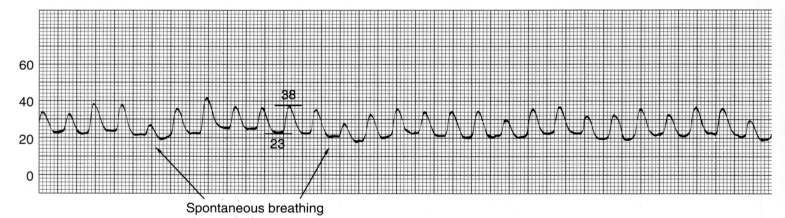

Spontaneous breathing

PRACTICE WAVEFORM 8–47. In this tracing from the distal tip of the PA catheter, the ECG rhythm is sinus changing to an SVT pattern. What is the waveform and the value associated with the wave?

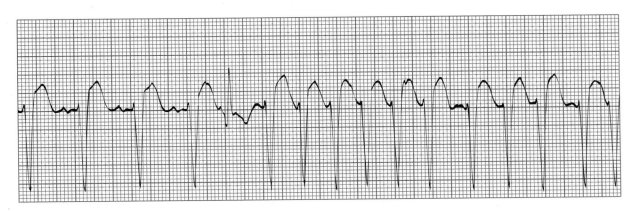

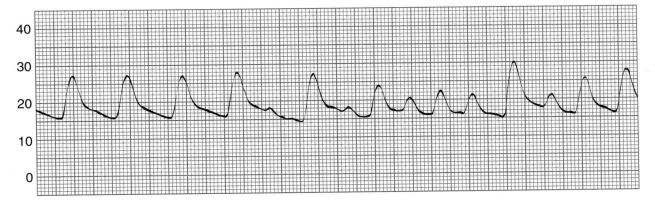

PRACTICE WAVEFORM 8–47. *Analysis:* This is a PA waveform with changing pressures due to the SVT pattern. The pressure changes here are similar to those seen in PRACTICE WAVEFORM 8–46. Note the loss of pulse pressure as the rhythm accelerates. The change in pulse pressure is real, not artifactual. In this situation, reporting the mean pressure rather than systolic/diastolic values may be more helpful in establishing the hemodynamic implications of this dysrhythmia. The approximate PA pressure with the normal sinus rhythm (NSR) is 27/15 and with the SVT 22/16. The mean pressure does not change markedly between the two, i.e., 19 mm Hg during NSR and 18 mm Hg with the SVT.

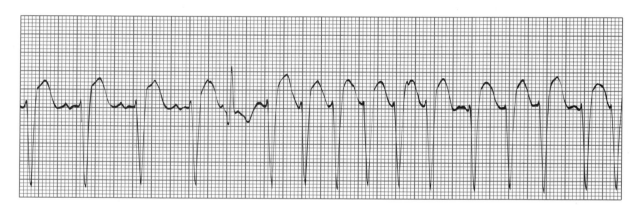

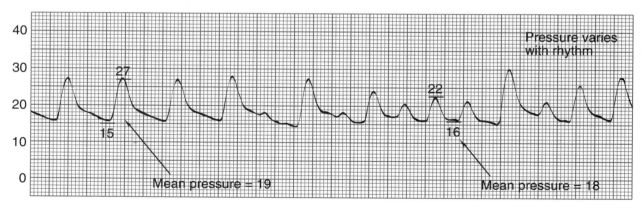

PRACTICE WAVEFORM 8–48. In this tracing from the distal tip of the PA catheter, the patient is breathing spontaneously and is not on the ventilator. What is the waveform and the associated pressure value with the wave?

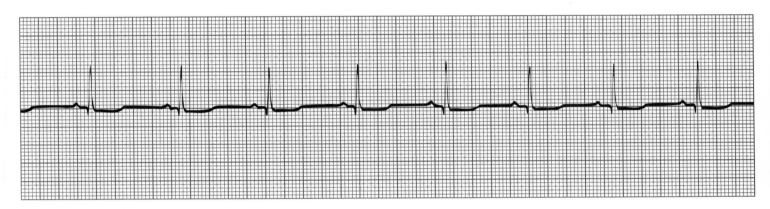

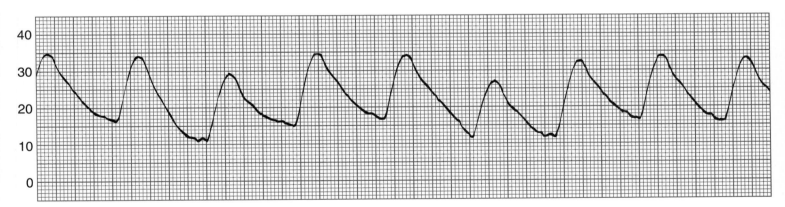

PRACTICE WAVEFORM 8–48. *Analysis:* The PA waveform can be read just before the dip in the waveform baseline. The drop in value is due to the spontaneous inspiration. The PA pressure is about 35/17 mm Hg. Examples of where to read the waveform are present after the 1st, 4th, and 8th ECG complexes.

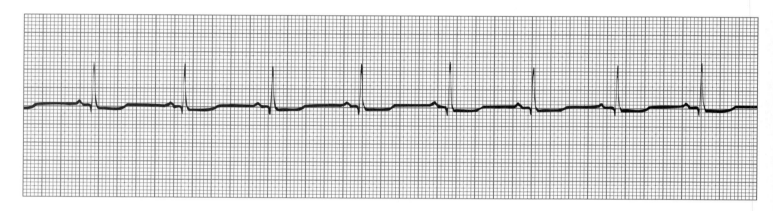

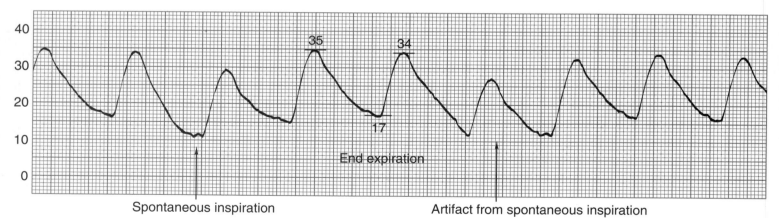

PRACTICE WAVEFORM 8–49. In this tracing from the distal tip of the PA catheter, the patient is on a ventilator in the IMV mode with no spontaneous breathing. What is the waveform and the associated waveform value?

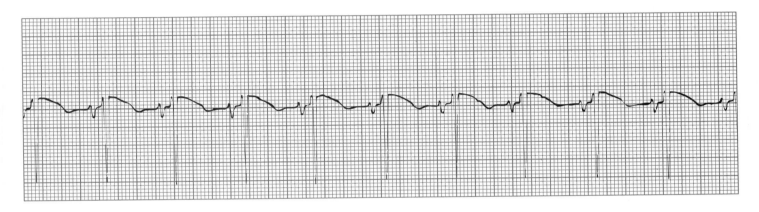

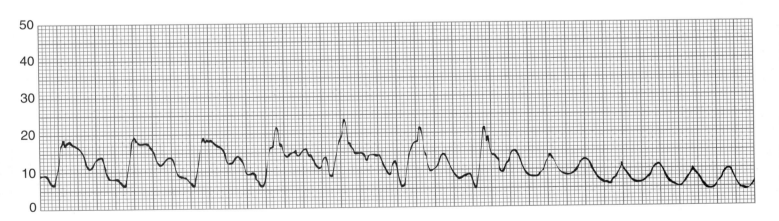

PRACTICE WAVEFORM 8–49. *Analysis:* This is a PA tracing changing to a PA wedge tracing. Reading the PA between the 3rd and 4th QRS complexes gives a pressure value of about 20/6–7 mm Hg. As the PA tracing changes to a PCWP, the ventilator is giving a mechanical breath. End expiration on the PCWP tracing correlates with the 10th QRS complex. This PCWP tracing reveals clear 'a' and 'v' waves. The PCWP is about 7 mm Hg.

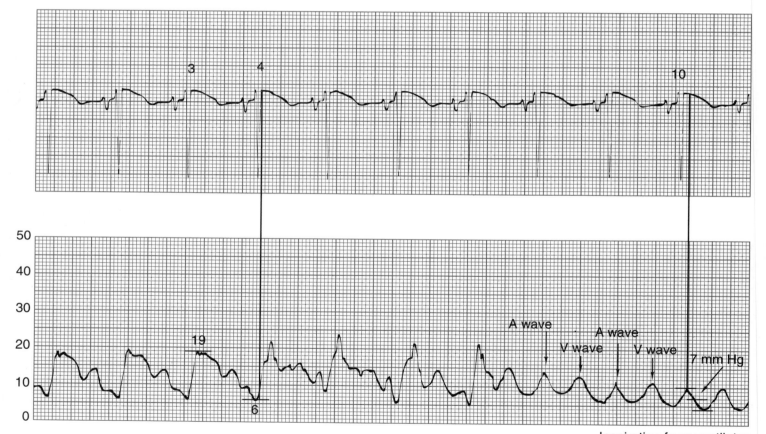

Inspiration from ventilator

PRACTICE WAVEFORM 8–50. In this tracing from the distal tip of the PA catheter, the patient is on AMV at a rate of 12 bpm and is breathing spontaneously at a rate of 20 bpm. What is the waveform and the value associated with the wave?

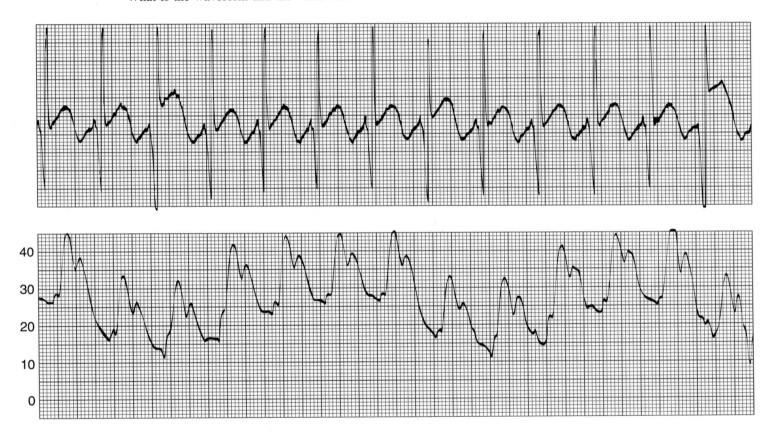

PRACTICE WAVEFORM 8–50. *Analysis:* This is a PA waveform. The end-expiratory value is best read between the 1st and 2nd or the 6th and 7th QRS complexes. The pressure value is about 45/26 mm Hg. Note how the ventilator breath produces minimal change in the waveform. Remember the spontaneous breaths produce the largest distortion in waveform appearance due to a spontaneous breath changing intrapleural pressure to a greater extent than a ventilator breath.

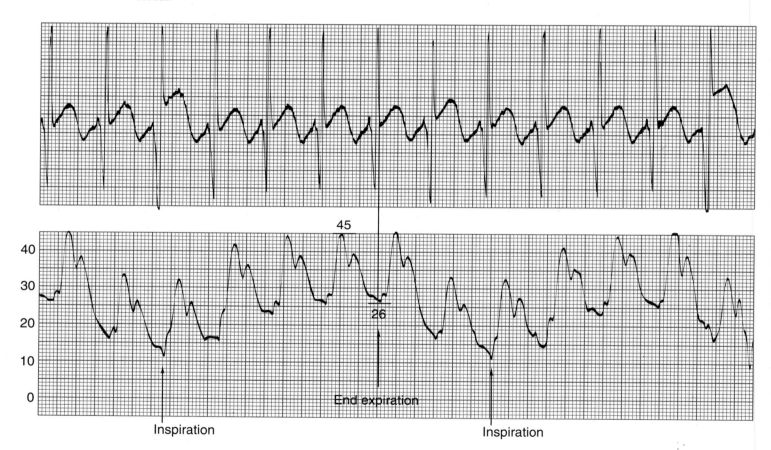

9 : Clinical Scenarios

This chapter includes not only waveforms for your interpretation but also the clinical situation surrounding the waveform procurement. The combination of waveform interpretation and clinical scenario will provide you with the opportunity to test your ability to read waveforms while placing the waveform in the context of actual clinical situations. You will be required to identify information that is relevant to waveform interpretation and discard information that is distracting. After completing this chapter, you should feel more comfortable with your ability to read waveforms in clinical settings. If you are able to interpret the waveforms in this section, you should be able to correctly interpret hemodynamic waveforms in the most common clinical settings. If you still have difficulty, return to the chapters that cover the situations with which you seem to have the most problems.

PRACTICE CLINICAL SCENARIO 9–1. A 58-year-old man is admitted to the unit with the diagnosis of congestive heart failure (CHF). A pulmonary artery catheter is placed to improve management of the CHF. He has a history of valvular disturbances. The patient is intubated and is on IMV with spontaneous breathing. After insertion of the catheter, the nurse caring for the patient calls you because she cannot ''get the catheter to wedge.'' She shows you the following waveform. Do you agree with her interpretation?

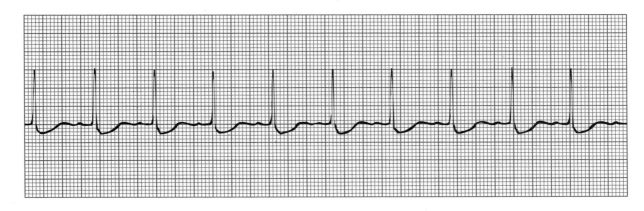

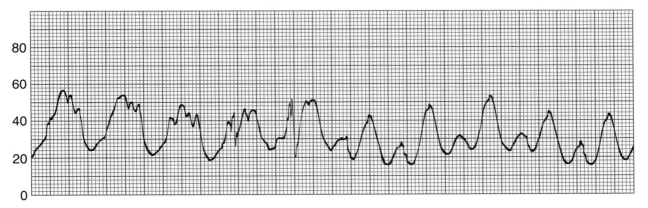

PRACTICE CLINICAL SCENARIO 9–1. *Analysis:* No. Between the 6th and 7th ECG complexes, the PA tracing changes to a PCWP tracing. The PCWP is complicated by a giant V wave and a large A wave. The PA value is about 51/22 mm Hg, with the PCWP value about 26 mm Hg. The higher PCWP than PAD makes this reading suspect with regard to the PCWP accurately reflecting end-diastolic ventricular pressures. The size of the A and V waves may reflect a noncompliant atrium. The actual LVEDP is probably lower than the mean of the A wave in this case.

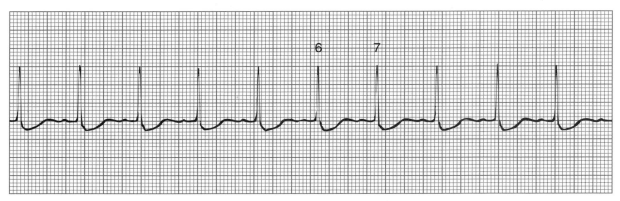

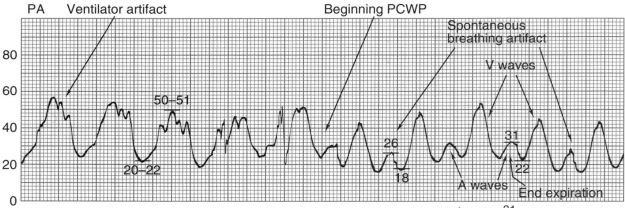

Mean PCWP = $\frac{31}{22}$, or 26–27 mm Hg

PRACTICE CLINICAL SCENARIO 9–2. A 65-year-old man is admitted to the unit with the diagnosis of acute myocardial infarction (anterior wall). He is intubated and is placed on assist/control ventilation with a rate of 12. He is breathing about 20 times/minute, does not complain of shortness of breath, and has a PaO_2 of 168 mm Hg on 50% oxygen. His PvO_2 is 28 mm Hg with a cardiac output of 4.6 liters per minute (LPM), cardiac index of 2.5 L/m^2. You obtain the following waveform from the distal port of the PA catheter. The house officer states that the tracing should be read at the lower values because the patient is on assist/control. He states that the ventilator will push the waveform upward and all high values are ventilator artifact. He believes the PA value is 43/5 mm Hg. Do you agree with that rationale? What type of tracing do you believe is present and what is the value?

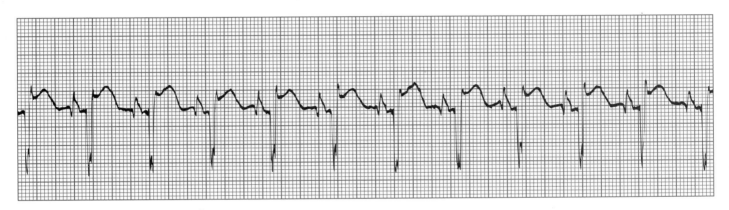

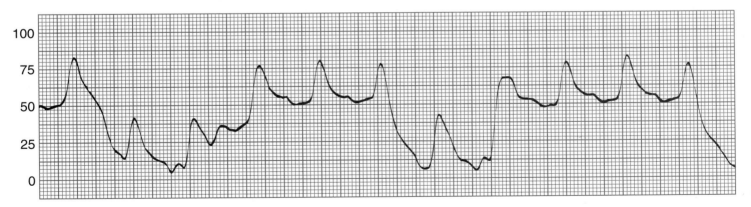

PRACTICE CLINICAL SCENARIO 9–2. *Analysis:* This waveform is a PA tracing with a marked inspiratory artifact. The patient is triggering the ventilator because the respiratory rate is faster than the set assist/control rate. Value read at end expiration is approximately 82/50 mm Hg. Remember, the most disturbance in intrapleural pressure comes from spontaneous breathing and therefore produces the most artifact in a tracing. The ventilator may cause some distortion but not as much as a spontaneous breath. In addition, the inspiratory/expiratory ratio can serve as a guide in this case. Note that the expiratory phase, which is longer than the inspiratory phase, is readily seen at the higher values (3–4 pressure waves during expiration versus 1–2 during inspiration).

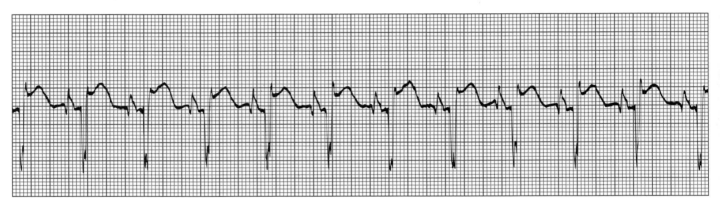

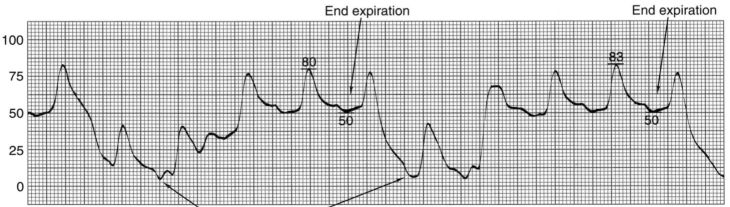

End expiration

End expiration

Spontaneous breathing artifact

PRACTICE CLINICAL SCENARIO 9–3. A 71-year-old man is in the unit with the diagnosis of rule-out myocardial infarction. Nurses on the prior shift have stated that they had trouble obtaining a clear pulmonary artery tracing. When you go to check the tracing, the nurse has informed you that she thinks the catheter is ''wedged.'' Based on the following waveform, what do you think the waveform represents?

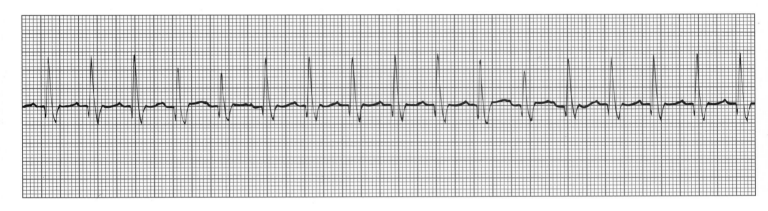

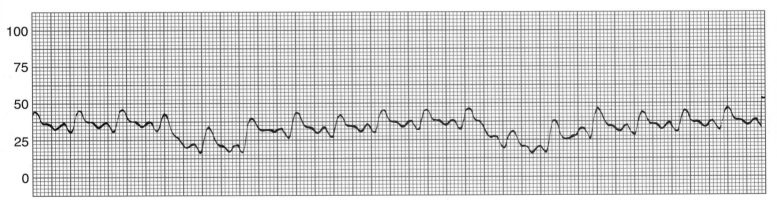

PRACTICE CLINICAL SCENARIO 9–3. *Analysis:* The waveform represents a PA tracing. End-QRS complex aligns well with PAD values. The waveform is small due to the large scale and the fast heart rate.

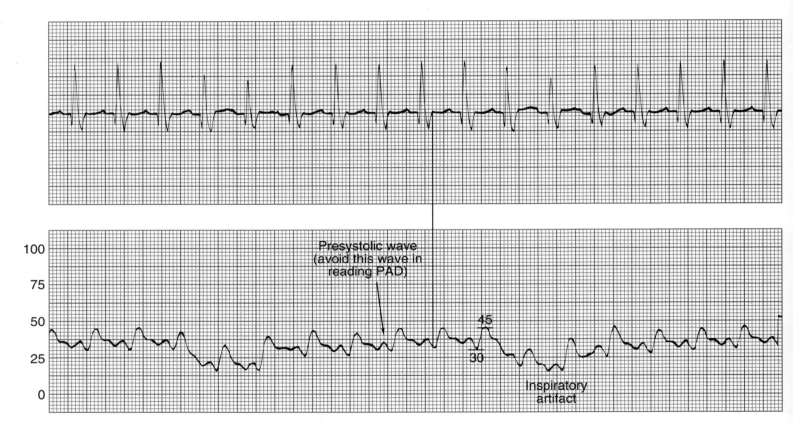

PRACTICE CLINICAL SCENARIO 9–4. When you try to obtain your first set of readings for the shift, you notice the following waveform. During report, you were told the catheter was unable to wedge. What is your interpretation of the following?

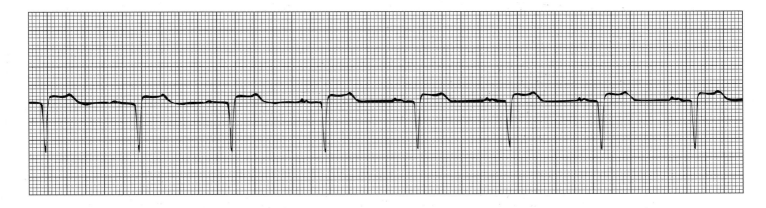

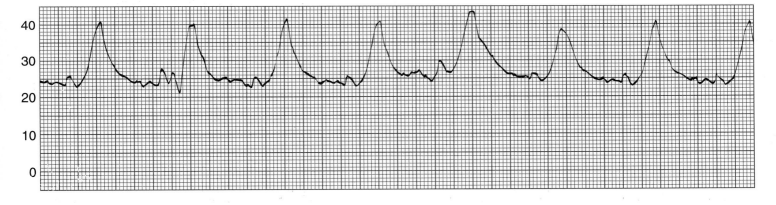

PRACTICE CLINICAL SCENARIO 9–4. *Analysis:* The tracing appears to be a PCWP waveform with a giant V wave. Evidence to support this interpretation includes the large wave starting 0.2 sec after the QRS. PA systolic values normally start closer to the end of the QRS. The small wave in front of the V may be the A wave. The PCWP value is about 24 mm Hg. The catheter needs to be withdrawn out of the wedge position as soon as possible.

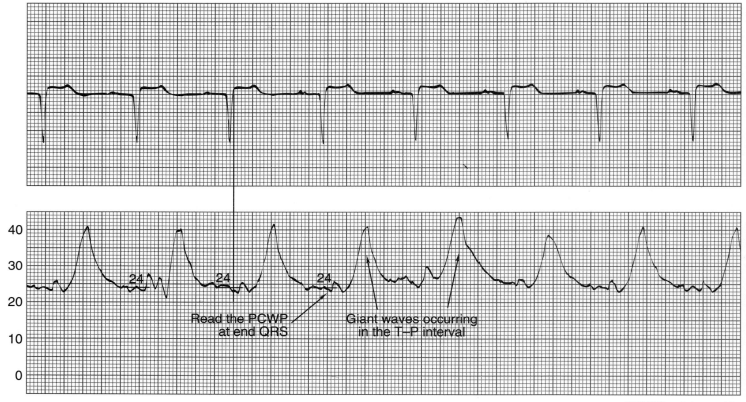

Read the PCWP at end QRS

Giant waves occurring in the T–P interval

PCWP = 24 mm Hg

PRACTICE CLINICAL SCENARIO 9–5. This waveform was obtained from the distal port in a patient breathing spontaneously at a rate of about 22 bpm. A nurse in the orientation program asks you to explain the tracing. In particular, he asks you why the waveform appears to change at regular intervals. What is your interpretation of the waveform and your explanation of the changes in the waveform?

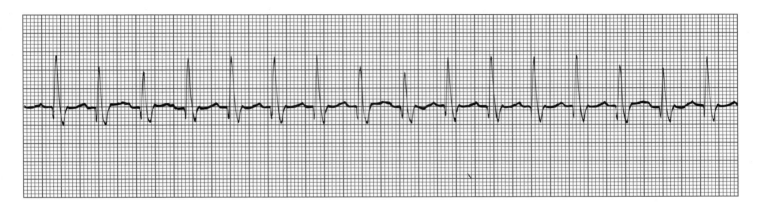

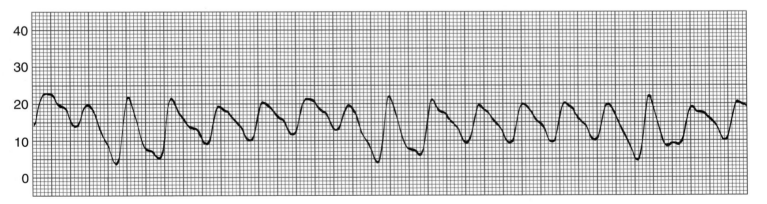

PRACTICE CLINICAL SCENARIO 9–5. *Analysis:* The waveform is a pulmonary artery tracing with regular changes in the baseline when the patient takes a breath. The PA pressure value is about 21/10 mm Hg. The regular changes can easily be verified by watching the patient breathe while recording the waveform.

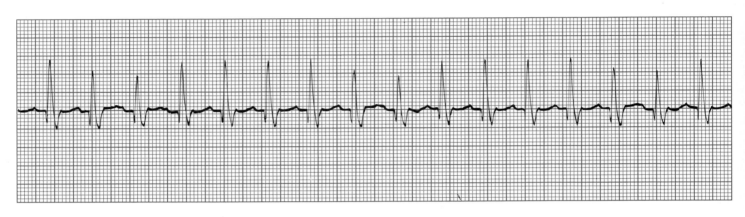

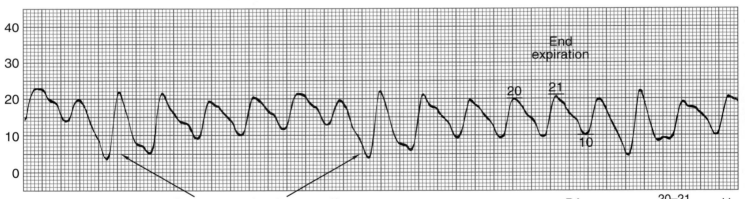

Spontaneous inspiratory artifact

$$\text{PA pressure} = \frac{20\text{--}21}{9\text{--}10} \text{ mm Hg}$$

PRACTICE CLINICAL SCENARIO 9–6. A 48-year-old woman is admitted to the unit with the diagnosis of right ventricular infarction. She complains of shortness of breath with a respiratory rate in the mid 20s. The cardiologist has requested to keep the CVP higher than normal. She states the current value as displayed by the monitor (17 mm Hg) is not high enough. From the following CVP tracing, is the monitor reading the waveform correctly? What would be your interpretation of the CVP value?

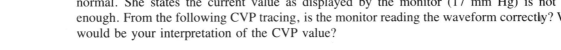

0741 P2 WAVE: 0-40   HR: 89   P1:7677 (41)   P2: 307-5 (17)

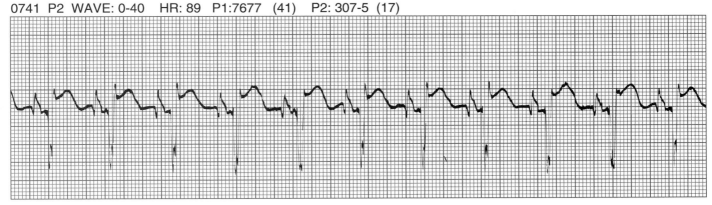

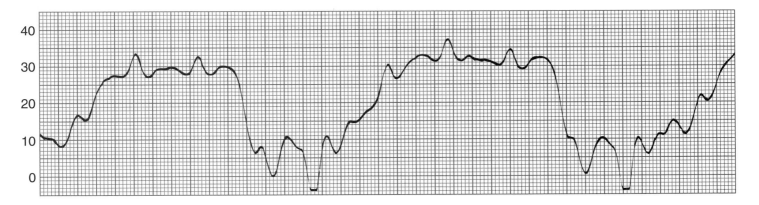

PRACTICE CLINICAL SCENARIO 9–6. *Analysis:* The CVP A wave is clearly seen at the end of expiration just before the inspiratory dip occurs. The CVP value is about 32 mm Hg. In this case, the monitor reading is incorrect and should be disregarded.

0741 P2 WAVE: 0-40   HR: 89 P1:7677 (41)   P2: 307-5 (17)

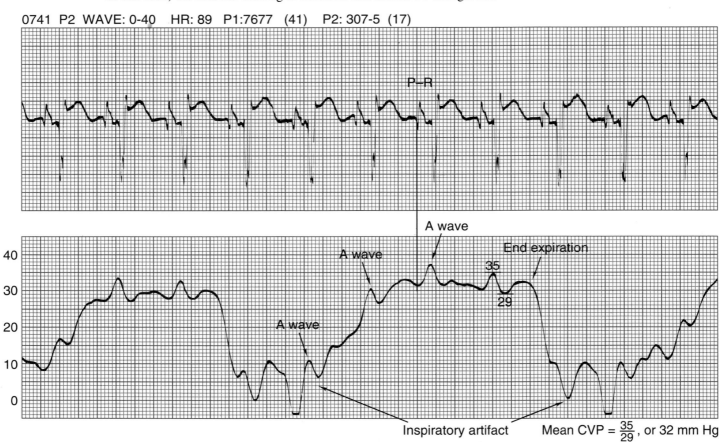

PRACTICE CLINICAL SCENARIO 9–7. A 51-year-old woman with the diagnosis of cardiomyopathy and mitral regurgitation is admitted with acute onset of shortness of breath. She does not require intubation at this point. When you try to obtain a PCWP reading, you note the following waveform. From the waveform, are you able to obtain a PCWP tracing? If so, what is the value of the PCWP and the PA waveform?

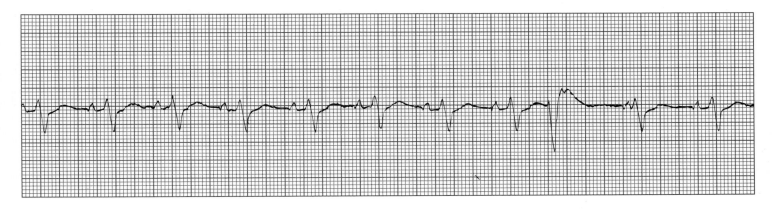

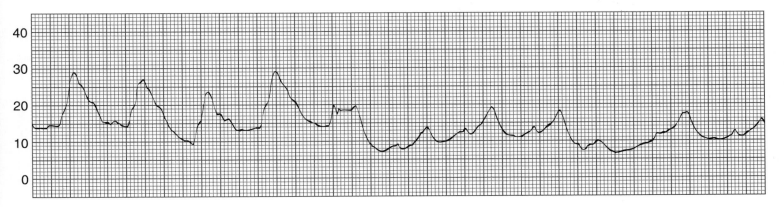

PRACTICE CLINICAL SCENARIO 9–7. *Analysis:* A PCWP waveform with a large V wave is present after the first 6 QRS complexes. The mean of the PCWP A wave is about 12 mm Hg. The PA pressure value is about 29/14 mm Hg. Inspiratory artifact is present as well as the large V wave and requires identification in order to avoid reading the wrong location.

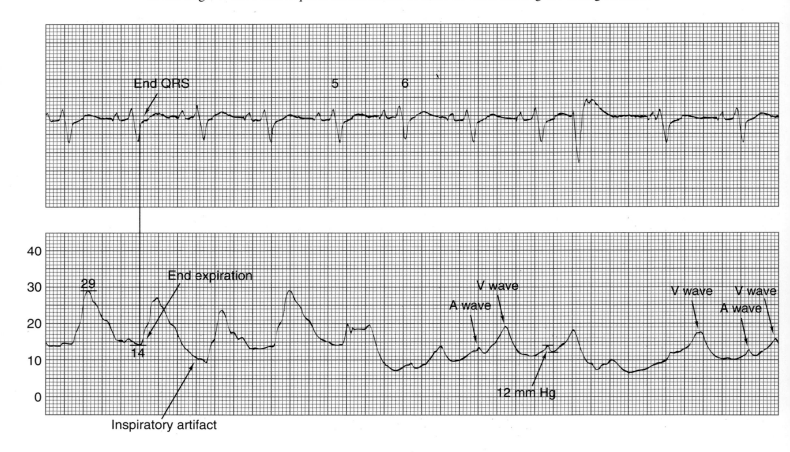

PRACTICE CLINICAL SCENARIO 9–8. A 78-year-old man is admitted to the unit with acute exacerbation of congestive heart failure. He has a past history of sick sinus syndrome and has a pacemaker in place. No clear P waves are present on the ECG. Due to the lack of a clear P wave, questions are present regarding where to read the CVP value. From the strip below, where would you read the waveform?

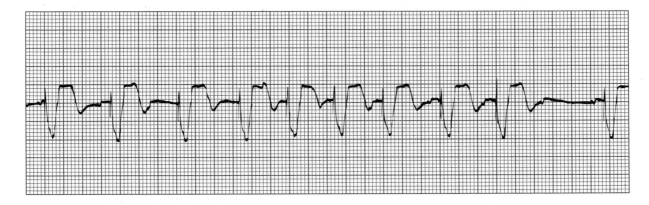

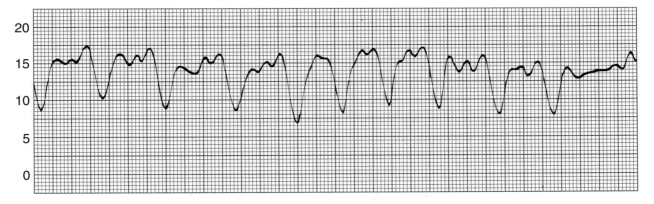

PRACTICE CLINICAL SCENARIO 9–8. *Analysis:* Due to the absence of P waves, read the waveform at the end of the QRS complex. The CVP value at end-QRS complex would be about 15 mm Hg.

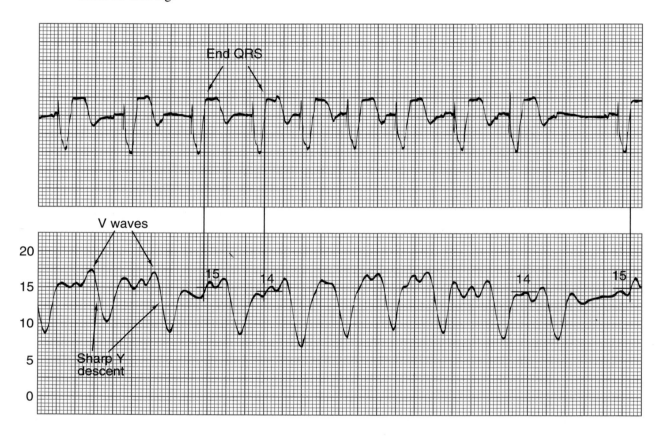

PRACTICE CLINICAL SCENARIO 9–9. Following coronary artery bypass grafting, a 52-year-old man develops chest pain and ECG evidence of a subendocardial myocardial infarction. He currently is in no distress and respiratory rate is about 18 and unlabored. The PA and PCWP tracings are listed below. The physician wants to keep the PCWP below 18 mm Hg. Based on your interpretation, is the following PCWP below 18 mm Hg?

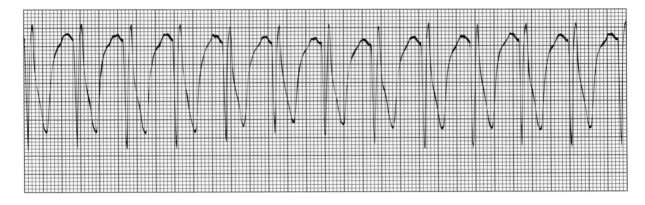

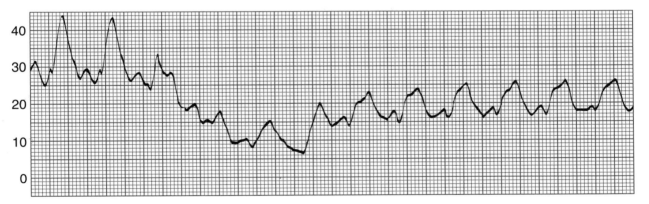

PRACTICE CLINICAL SCENARIO 9–9. *Analysis:* The PA pressure value is about 44/25 mm Hg, with the PCWP about 17 mm Hg. A large V wave could falsely raise the PCWP if it is included in the reading.

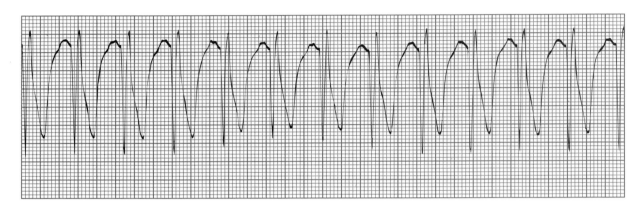

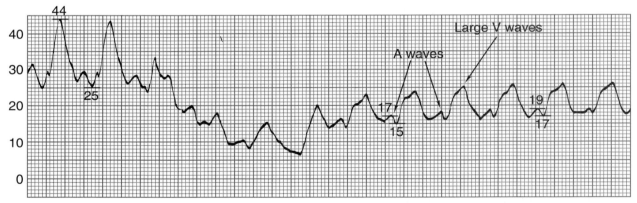

PCWP = 16–18 mm Hg

PRACTICE CLINICAL SCENARIO 9–10. A 27-year-old woman is in the unit following hypovolemic shock from a motor vehicle accident. Following splenectomy, she is in the unit for postoperative stabilization. The pulmonary artery catheter does not wedge and the physician has left instructions to follow the pulmonary artery diastolic value to estimate the PCWP. If the PAD decreases below 6 mm Hg, you are to notify him and start a normal saline fluid bolus. Based on the waveform below, should the physician be notified and saline bolus started?

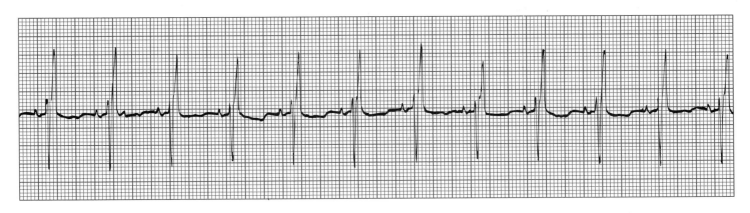

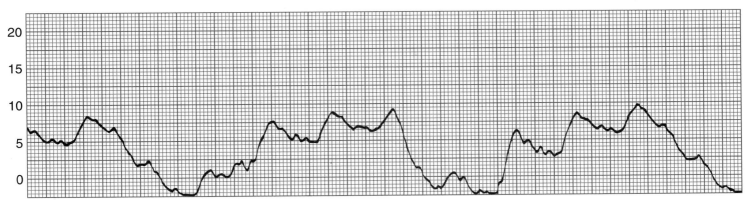

PRACTICE CLINICAL SCENARIO 9–10. *Analysis:* The PA pressure is about 10/7 mm Hg. The PAD is about 7 mm Hg, close but not low enough to call the physician based on the above orders. Other parameters should also be monitored (see Chapters 10 and 11) but the end-expiratory PAD pressure is over 6 mm Hg in this case. These pressures are very low. Check the reading by releveling, rezeroing, and performing a square wave test to check for over-damping.

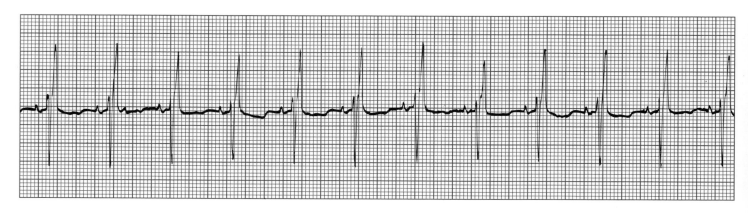

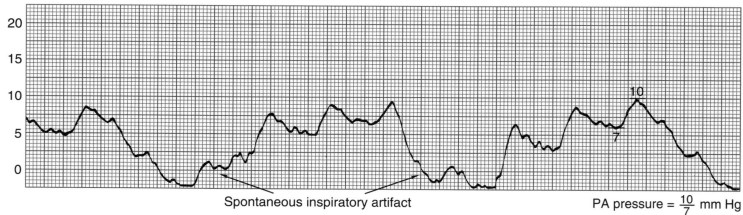

Spontaneous inspiratory artifact

PA pressure = $\frac{10}{7}$ mm Hg

PRACTICE CLINICAL SCENARIO 9–11. In the following PCWP tracing, this 23-year-old man with respiratory failure was very short of breath, tachycardic, and tachypneic. He was on IMV with a set rate of 30 bpm in addition to 20 spontaneous breaths. From the tracing, identify the correct location to read the waveform.

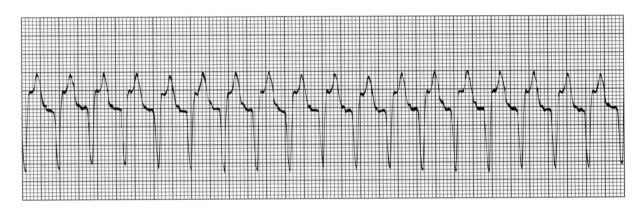

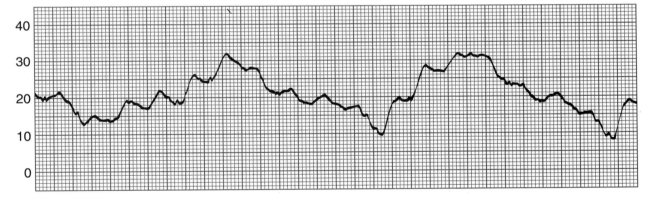

PRACTICE CLINICAL SCENARIO 9–11. *Analysis:* The rapid respiratory rate makes accurate interpretation very difficult. However, end expiration can be noted at three points in this tracing. Two of these points immediately precede a spontaneous breath. These points are located before QRS complexes 9 and 16. The other end-expiratory point follows a spontaneous breath but precedes an IMV breath (QRS complex 4). The approximate value, perhaps artificially elevated due to the rapid rate, is near 18–20 mm Hg.

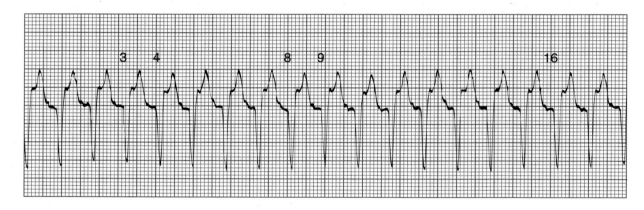

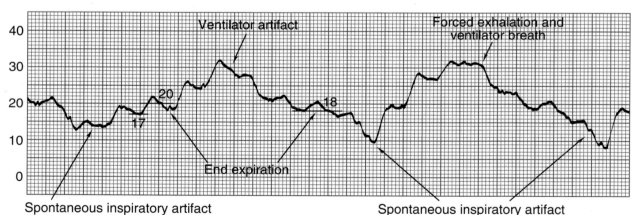

PRACTICE CLINICAL SCENARIO 9–12. When you are making your initial assessment on a 56-year-old man, diagnosis of acute inferior MI, you notice the following waveform from the distal port. The monitor reading is 70/8 mm Hg. The nurse on the prior shift has reported the catheter is unable to "wedge." The physician has left orders to administer a fluid bolus of 200 cc normal saline over 20 minutes if the PCWP drops below 8 mm Hg. Based on the waveform below, what would be your interpretation of the waveform and your recommendations for treatment?

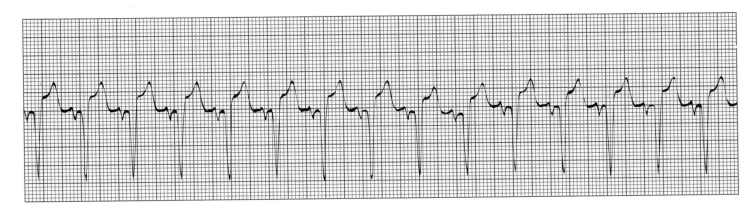

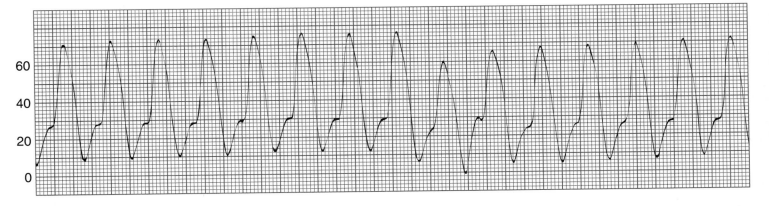

PRACTICE CLINICAL SCENARIO 9–12. *Analysis:* The waveform is a right ventricular waveform, illustrated by the end-diastolic rise at the end of the QRS. The third ECG complex from the left illustrates end-QRS identification of the diastolic value. The actual pressure in the RV is about 70/28 mm Hg. In this case, the patient is not fluid depleted but has fluid overload or right ventricular failure. No fluid bolus should be given.

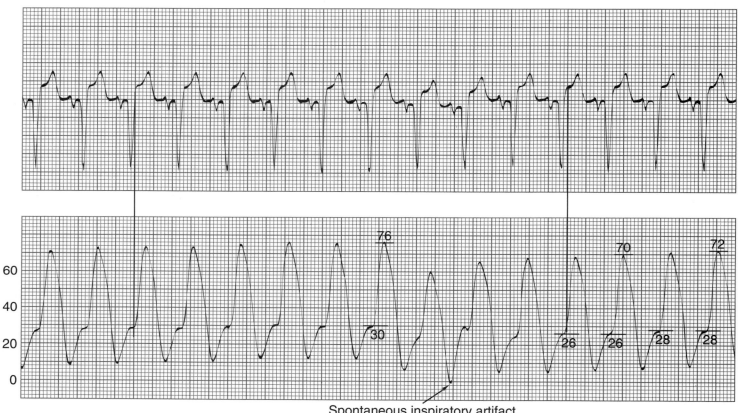

Spontaneous inspiratory artifact

PRACTICE CLINICAL SCENARIO 9–13. The PA catheter in this 69-year-old male, non-intubated patient with congestive heart failure has not been able to wedge for the past 8 hours. The physician asks that the PAD be used to approximate the PCWP. The physician also leaves a request to notify him if the PAD pressure increases over 18 or decreases below 10 mm Hg. The monitor displays a value of 31/7 mm Hg. Based on the following waveform, does the physician need to be notified?

21 MAR 90   0846   P1 WAVE: 0-40   HR:103   P1:31/7 (25)   P2:3/2 (1)

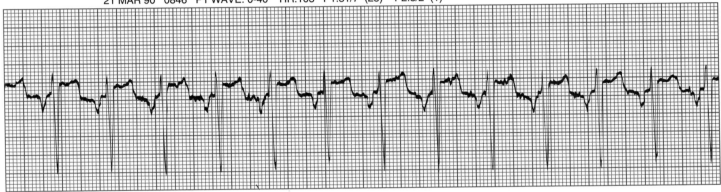

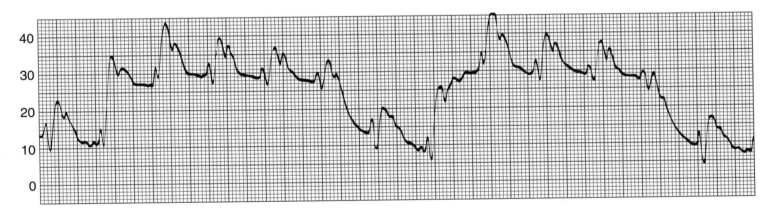

PRACTICE CLINICAL SCENARIO 9–13. *Analysis:* Yes, but not for a low value. The end-diastolic PA pressure value is about 37/28 mm Hg. The physician would need to be notified of the increased PAD pressure value.

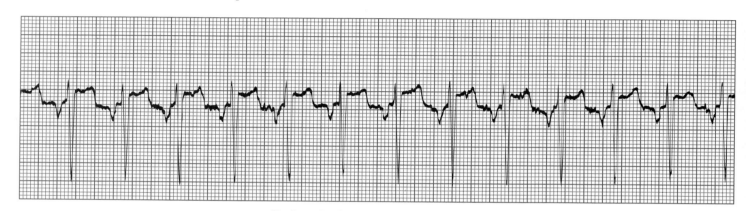

End expiration

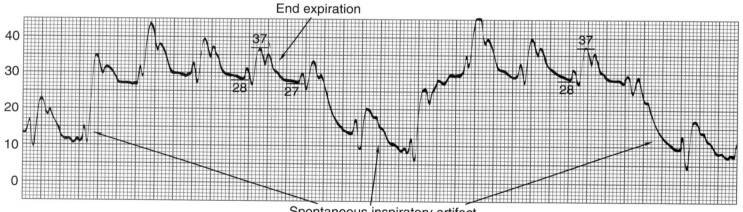

Spontaneous inspiratory artifact

PRACTICE CLINICAL SCENARIO 9–14. A 76-year-old man with the diagnosis of congestive heart failure is admitted to the unit with an exacerbation of the failure. He had had a VVI pacemaker inserted in the past and currently is in atrial fibrillation with intermittent paced beats. He complains of shortness of breath and has inspiratory crackles in both lower lung fields. His CVP reading is listed below. A discussion between the nurses develops over where to read the tracing. One nurse wants to take the monitor value (11 mm Hg). Another agrees, suggesting that because it is not possible to read any clear A waves, taking the monitor value may be the best place to take the reading. Where would you read the tracing?

0208   29 DEC 88   0753 P2 WAVE:0-20   HR:81   P1:67/44 (44)   P2:17/12 (11)

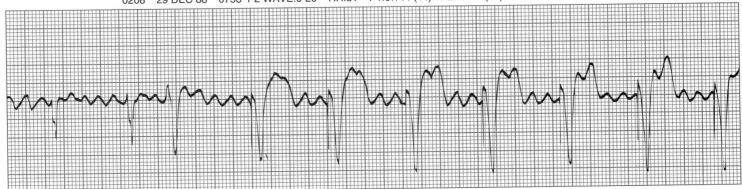

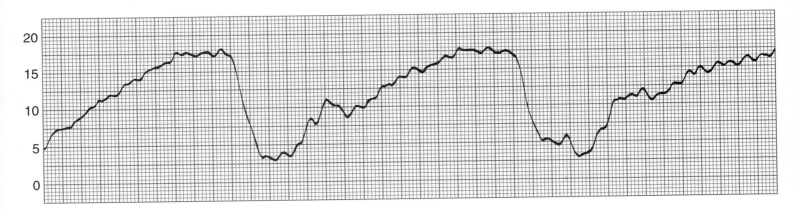

PRACTICE CLINICAL SCENARIO 9–14. *Analysis:* The CVP value is about 17–18 mm Hg. Marked inspiratory artifact is present although clear end-expiratory pauses are visible after the 3rd and 6th QRS complexes. No A waves are present in atrial fibrillation. When this occurs, reading from end QRS will be one method of approximating end-diastolic pressures.

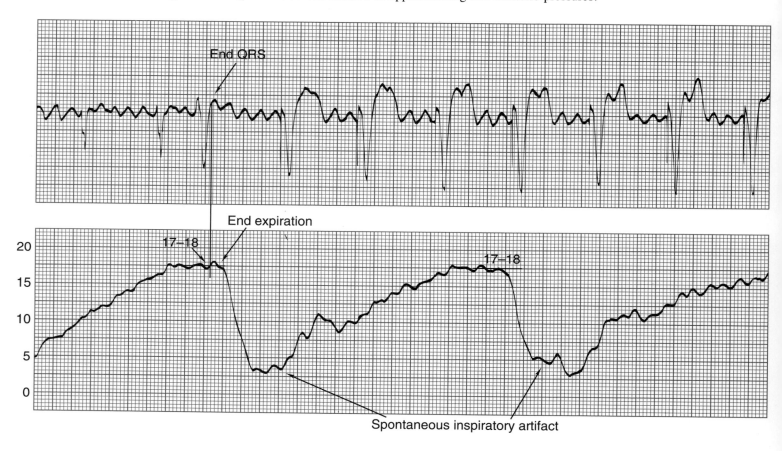

PRACTICE CLINICAL SCENARIO 9–15. The following pulmonary artery tracing is shown to you shortly after the catheter has been inserted. The reported value of the PA pressure is 44/22 mm Hg. Based on the waveform, do you agree with this tracing value?

P1 WAVE: 0-40   HR:128   P1:42/22 (55)   P2:13/10 (13)

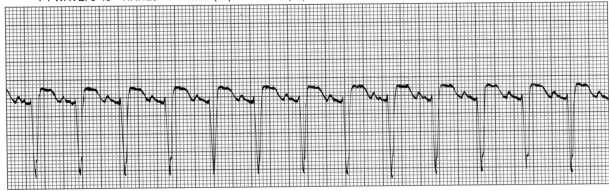

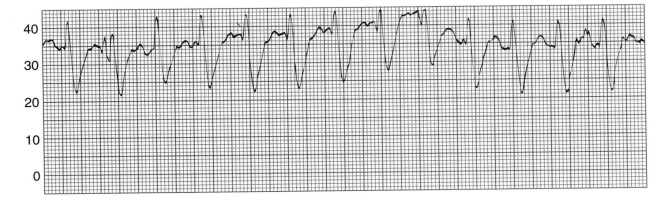

PRACTICE CLINICAL SCENARIO 9–15. *Analysis:* The PA pressure is probably incorrect, based on the peak value occurring too late to represent systole. Note that the peak value is just before the QRS complex, not immediately after the QRS. This most likely represents artifact. Unfortunately, if the artifact is affecting diastole, the diastolic value may also be unclear. The actual systolic PA pressure value is closer to 35 mm Hg. Diastole, when aligned with the end QRS, is about 25 mm Hg.

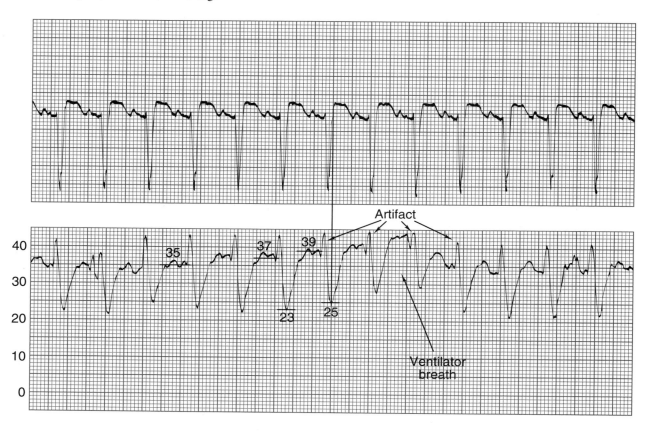

PRACTICE CLINICAL SCENARIO 9–16. At report, you are to care for a 58-year-old man 16 hours post–triple vessel bypass surgery. His blood pressure is reported to you as 109/51 (per the monitor). As you note the waveform value below, does the reported blood pressure agree with the waveform?

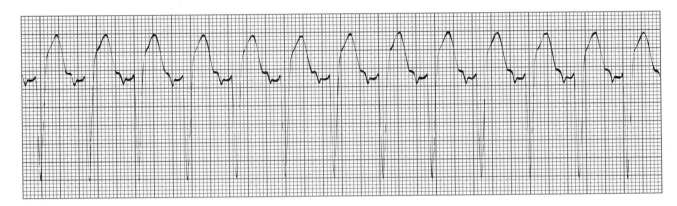

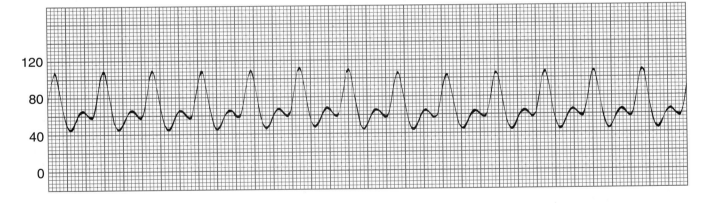

PRACTICE CLINICAL SCENARIO 9–16. *Analysis:* The arterial diastolic pressure is higher than reported. Remember, the arterial diastolic value occurs about 0.2 sec after end QRS in distal arterial lines. In this case, diastole is closer to 60 mm Hg, changing the mean BP from about 70 to 76 mm Hg.

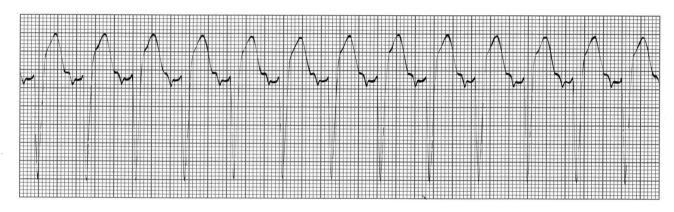

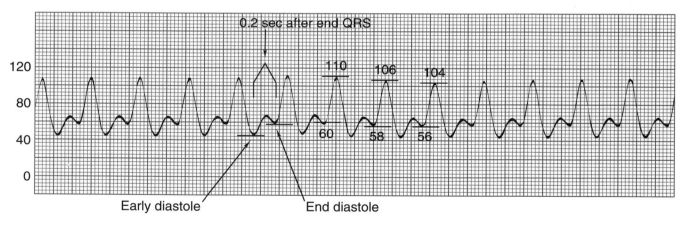

PRACTICE CLINICAL SCENARIO 9–17. The following waveform is given to you by the nurse on the prior shift. She tells you this is the CVP tracing. One of the physicians tells you this cannot be a CVP tracing because it has characteristics of a pulmonary arterial tracing. What do you believe the waveform represents?

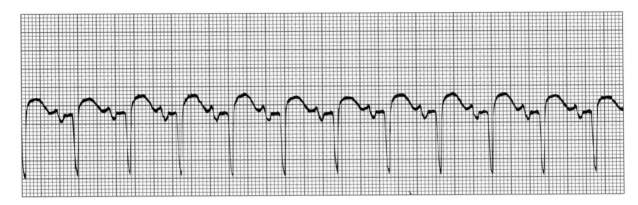

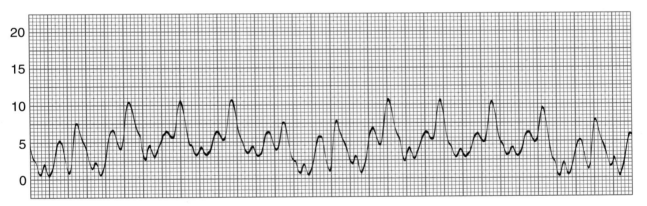

PRACTICE CLINICAL SCENARIO 9–17. *Analysis:* The tracing is a CVP tracing. It looks like a PA waveform due to the large A wave. The tracing could not be a PA waveform because the largest wave (which would be an arterial wave if this were a PA waveform) starts in front of the QRS. Arterial waveforms cannot start until after the QRS complex. The CVP value is about 7 mm Hg.

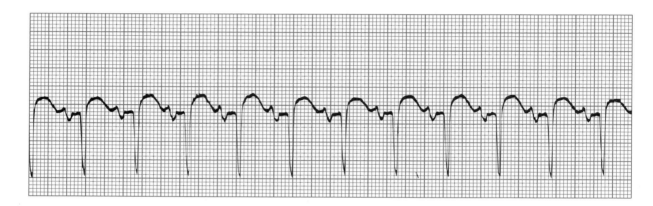

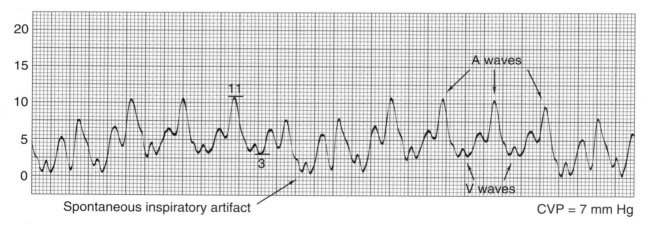

Spontaneous inspiratory artifact

CVP = 7 mm Hg

PRACTICE CLINICAL SCENARIO 9–18. As you are changing shifts, you are giving report to the next nurse. As you are reviewing the hemodynamics, the nurse remarks that the arterial waveform looks overdamped. You have a square wave test to demonstrate, in your opinion, that the waveform is not overdamped. She insists the waveform must be overdamped owing to the appearance of the waveform. Does the square wave test indicate an optimally damped waveform?

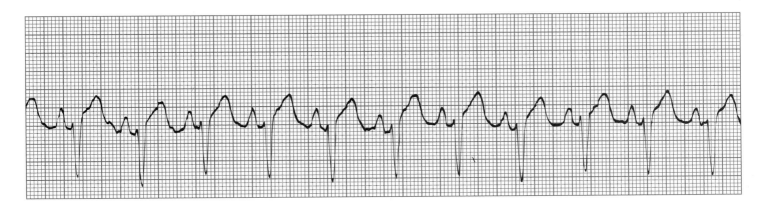

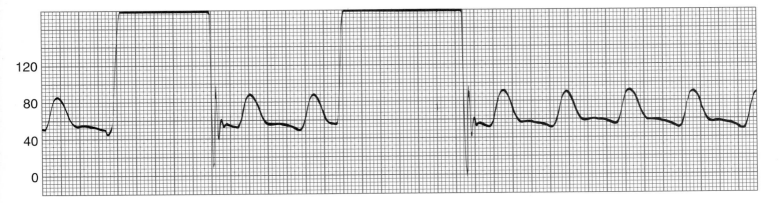

PRACTICE CLINICAL SCENARIO 9–18. *Analysis:* The square wave test indicates an optimally damped waveform. The frequency response is about 20 Hz and the damping coefficient is about 5.5/14 = 0.39 = 0.40. According to Gardner's optimal range responses, this frequency response and damping coefficient place the waveform in the adequate damping range. The waveform appearance is not necessarily a good way to determine if a waveform is optimally damped.

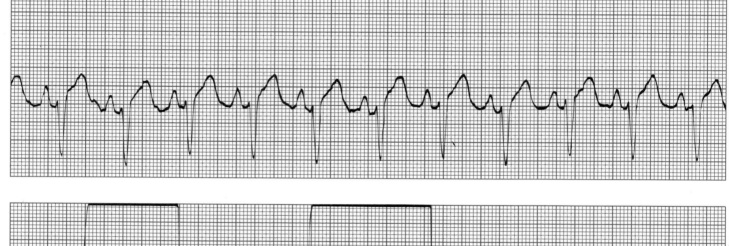

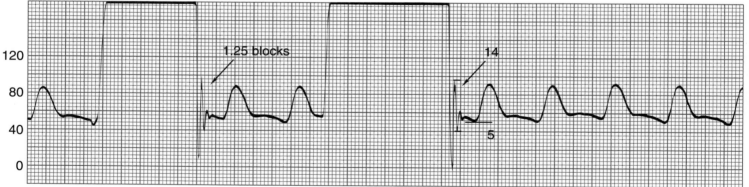

Damping coefficient: $\dfrac{5}{14}$ amplitude ratio = 0.40 damping coefficient

Frequency response: $\dfrac{25}{1.25} \approx 19$ Hz

PRACTICE CLINICAL SCENARIO 9–19. A 42-year-old man is in the unit following multiple gunshot wounds to the chest. Two days postoperative, he is on mechanical ventilation. He is on an IMV of 15 with a total respiratory rate of 40. He is on PEEP of 12 mm Hg (16 cm H_2O). He has an airway pressure transducer in line to help identify end expiration. Based on the airway pressure value, where is end expiration and what is the PA pressure value?

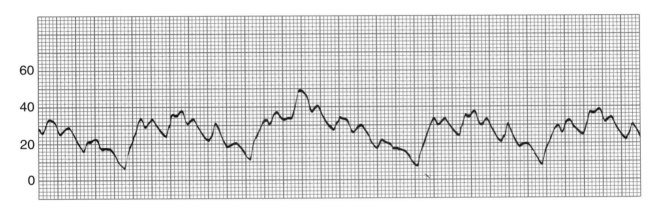

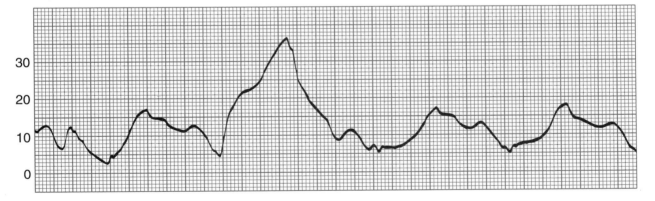

PRACTICE CLINICAL SCENARIO 9–19. *Analysis:* End expiration is found at 12 mm Hg on the airway pressure value. Immediately above these values, end expiration can be identified. The PA pressure value is about 36–38/22 mm Hg.

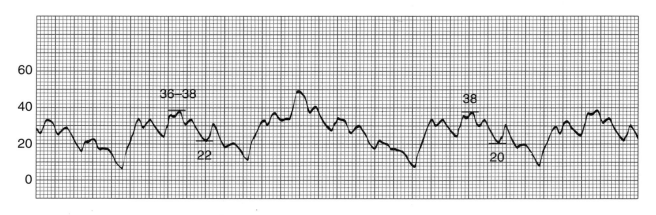

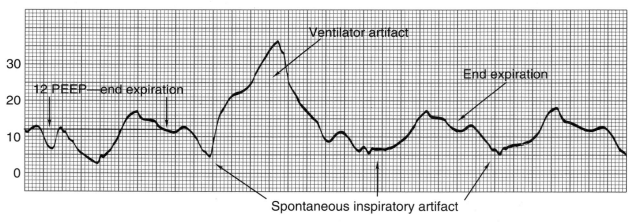

PRACTICE CLINICAL SCENARIO 9–20. A 72-year-old woman is in the unit following an acute MI. She has marked respiratory distress and has poor oxygen gas exchange. She is intubated and receiving mechanical ventilation. Her ventilator is in the assist/control mode of 12, total rate of 30. As you look at her PA tracing, you must eliminate respiratory artifact from the waveform. The physician has left orders to start nitroglycerin if the PCWP rises above 20 mm Hg and is associated with a fall in the cardiac output. Based on the above information and waveform below, does preload reduction with nitroglycerin need to be initiated?

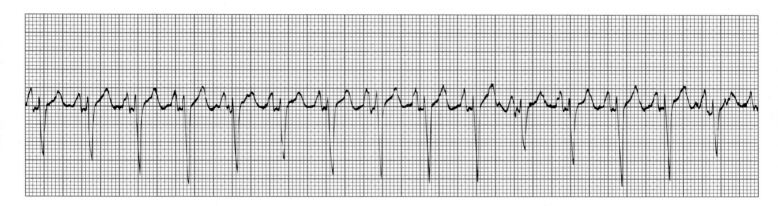

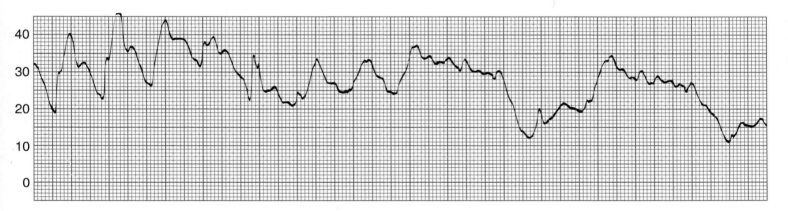

PRACTICE CLINICAL SCENARIO 9–20. *Analysis:* Inspiratory artifact is most noticeable during her spontaneous inspiratory efforts. The PCWP is about 27 mm Hg. Based on these values, in conjunction with examining the cardiac output and stroke volume, preload reduction may be beneficial.

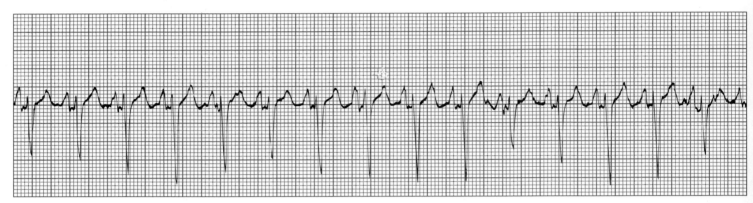

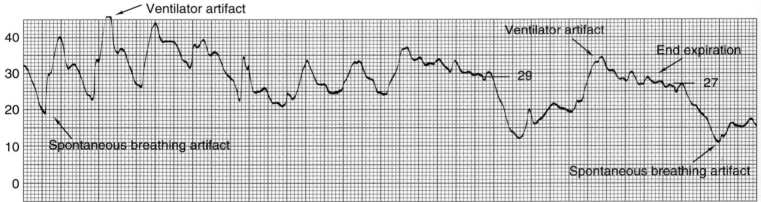

PRACTICE CLINICAL SCENARIO 9–21. A 45-year-old woman is admitted to the unit with acute respiratory failure and hypotension following chemotherapy. She currently is on mechanical ventilation in the assist/control mode. Her respiratory rate is set at 10 but she is triggering the ventilator for a total rate of 20. As you look at her arterial waveform, you notice the blood pressure fluctuate with each ventilator breath. The blood pressure decreases with each ventilator breath and increases with spontaneous breathing. The physician says not to go by the arterial line but to follow the blood pressure cuff, which reports a value of about 90/60 mm Hg. Is this the best method to obtain the blood pressure?

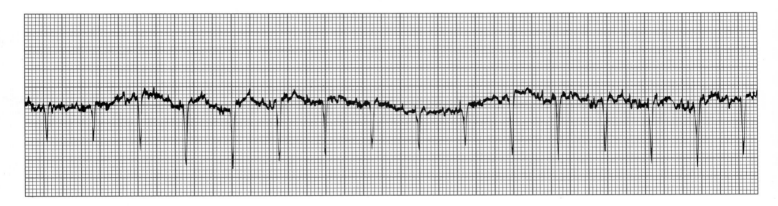

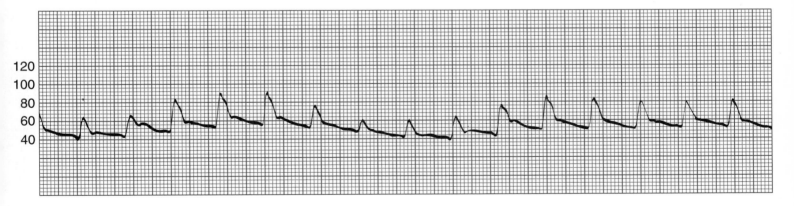

PRACTICE CLINICAL SCENARIO 9–21. *Analysis:* The blood pressure is a combination of all the displayed beats. Use of the blood pressure cuff is not the best method to measure the blood pressure. Either follow the monitor (72/48 mm Hg) or measure a 6-second strip of values and average these (75/49 mm Hg). The blood pressure cuff will only report the value at the time of the measurement, which may be a higher or lower value, depending on which part of the cycle was caught. The decrease in blood pressure during the ventilator breath should be investigated. Auto-PEEP may be present. Increasing the flow rate, decreasing the tidal volume, or sedating the patient may help if auto-PEEP is present.

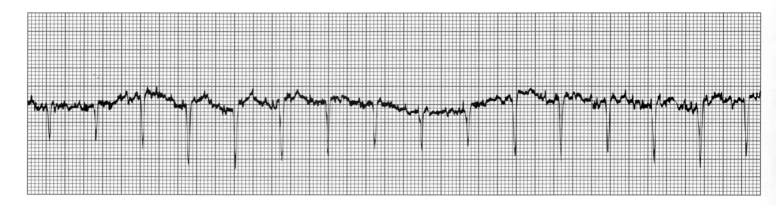

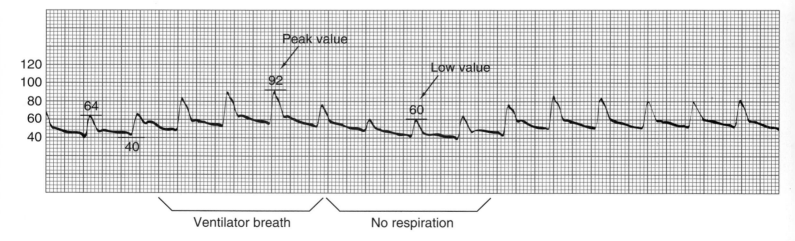

PRACTICE CLINICAL SCENARIO 9–22. During morning rounds, you tell the physician the blood pressure from the arterial line is 108/60 mm Hg. The physician looks at the waveform and states, "That can't be right." The waveform looks to be "damped." When you check the square wave test, you notice the following square waveform. Based on the square wave test, is the waveform overdamped? Should you believe the arterial line?

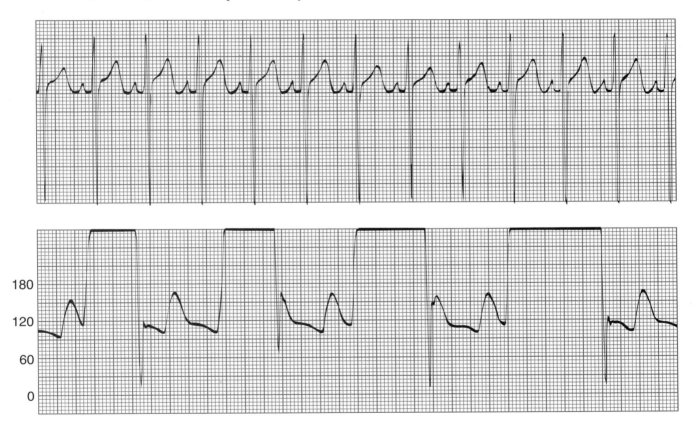

PRACTICE CLINICAL SCENARIO 9–22. *Analysis:* Based on the square wave test, the tracing is optimally damped. The frequency response is about 25 Hz and the damping coefficient is good, about 0.47. The arterial line is accurate and should be believed.

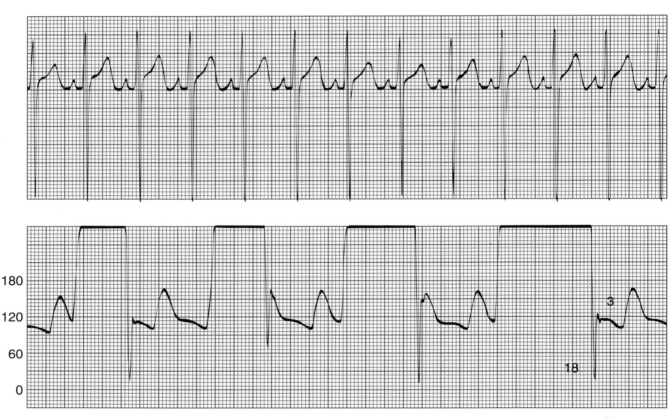

Frequency response: $\frac{25}{1}$ = 25 Hz

Damping coefficient: $\frac{3}{18}$ amplitude ratio = 0.17 = 0.47 damping coefficient

PRACTICE CLINICAL SCENARIO 9–23. A 78-year-old woman is admitted to the unit with congestive heart failure. She is markedly short of breath and appears uncomfortable. A pulmonary artery catheter is placed to aid in treatment determination. Initial hemodynamic readings are as follows:

BP	106/72		PA	38/24
P	108		PCWP	21
CO	3.8		CVP	13
CI	2.0			

Based on the above readings, she was given an infusion of dobutamine (3 μg/kg/min) and a dose of furosemide (Lasix, 20 mg). Her symptoms improved and pulmonary artery pressures decreased. When you come on duty, the catheter cannot be wedged. The physician states that you should track the PAD and if it increases to 18 mm Hg or higher, to notify her. The following pulmonary artery waveform is now present. The time is 0200. The monitor is displaying a value of 40/5 mm Hg. What is your interpretation of the waveform and does the physician need to be called?

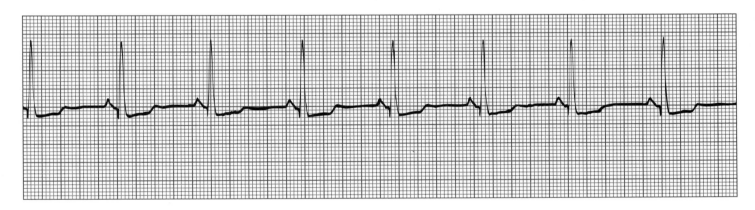

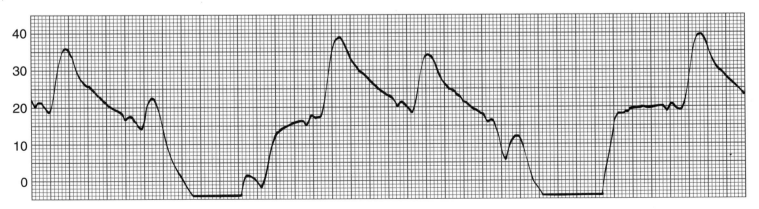

PRACTICE CLINICAL SCENARIO 9–23. *Analysis:* The PA pressure is about 34/20 mm Hg. The physician needs to be called.

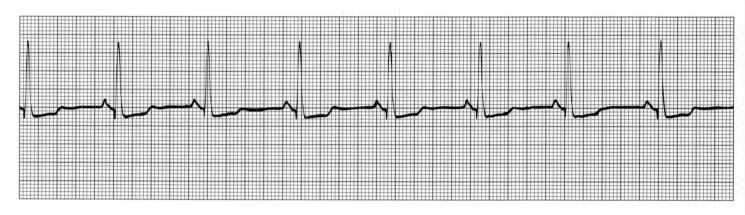

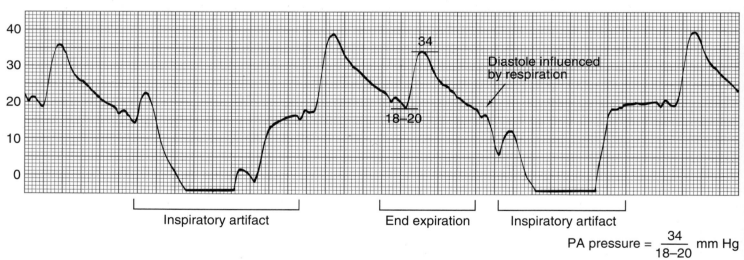

Inspiratory artifact

End expiration

Inspiratory artifact

34

18–20

Diastole influenced by respiration

$$\text{PA pressure} = \frac{34}{18\text{–}20} \text{ mm Hg}$$

PRACTICE CLINICAL SCENARIO 9–24. When you attempt to wedge the PA catheter, you obtain the following waveform. You heard in report that the catheter does not always "wedge." When you try to inflate the balloon, the waveform changes quickly after 1 cc. When you let a small amount of air back out, the waveform changes again. Does the following waveform represent a "wedge" tracing?

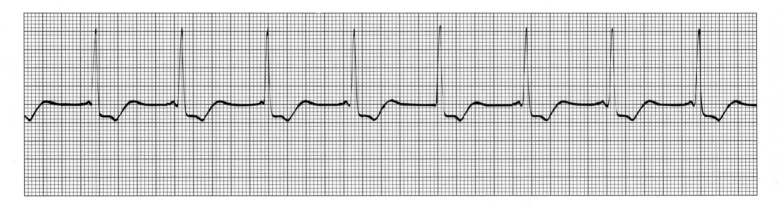

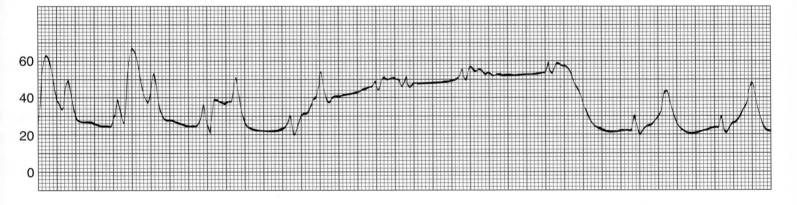

PRACTICE CLINICAL SCENARIO 9–24. *Analysis:* Yes. The initial inflation attempt produced an ''overwedged'' tracing. When the air was slightly reduced, the PCWP tracing with a large V wave became evident. The PCWP value is about 23 mm Hg.

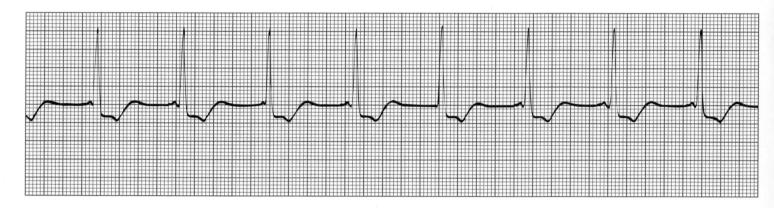

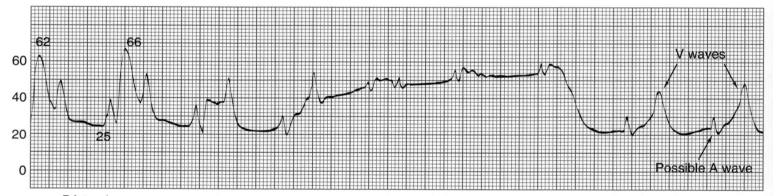

PA tracing

0.5 cc of air allowed to leave balloon—PCWP waveform appears

PCWP ≈ 23 mm Hg

PA pressure = $\dfrac{62\text{–}66}{25}$ mm Hg

PRACTICE CLINICAL SCENARIO 9–25. During the insertion of a pulmonary artery catheter, the cardiology fellow is unable to obtain a wedge waveform. The change in waveform appearance is thought to be due to "damping or stabilizing the PA catheter." He also states he is uncomfortable tracking the PCWP with the PAD inasmuch as the patient may have a pulmonary embolism (causing secondary pulmonary hypertension). When you try to obtain a wedge tracing, you obtain the following waveform. What is your interpretation of the waveform?

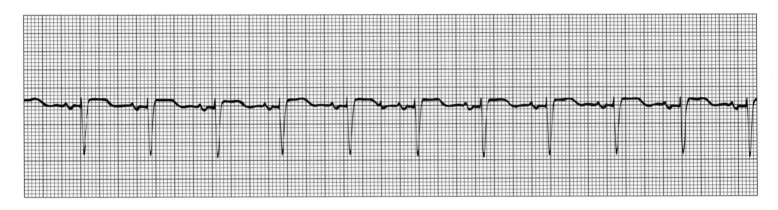

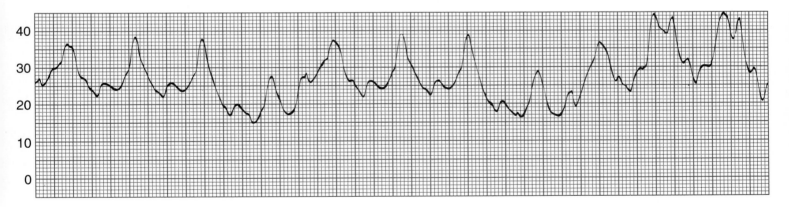

PRACTICE CLINICAL SCENARIO 9–25. *Analysis:* The waveform is a PCWP tracing with a giant V wave. The mean of the A wave is about 25 mm Hg. The PCWP appears to correlate well with the PAD.

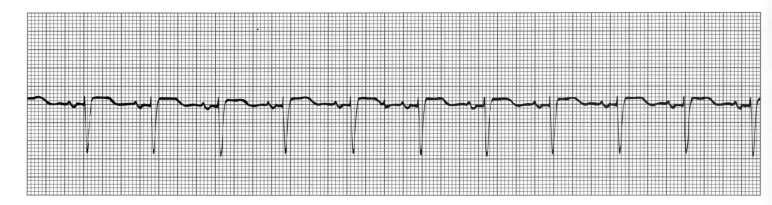

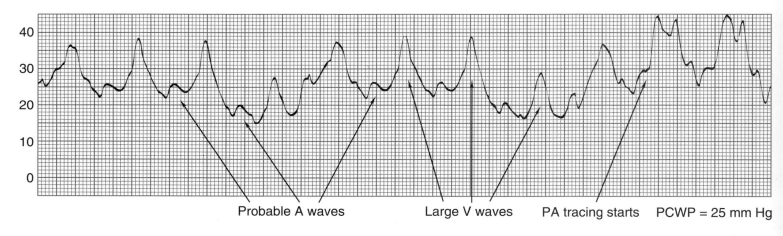

Probable A waves   Large V waves   PA tracing starts   PCWP = 25 mm Hg

PRACTICE CLINICAL SCENARIO 9–26. A 34-year-old man is in the unit following multiple gunshot wounds to the chest and abdomen. Three days postoperatively, he develops a fever, hypotension, and tachycardia. He is on AMV at a rate of 16 bpm but is triggering the ventilator for a total rate of 40 bpm. PEEP is set at 7 mm Hg (10 cm H_2O). An airway pressure waveform is placed next to the pulmonary artery waveform in order to better identify end expiration. Based on the tracing, where would you read the waveform?

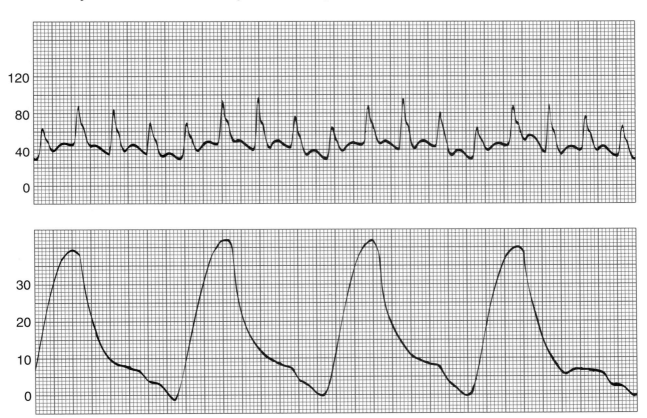

PRACTICE CLINICAL SCENARIO 9–26. *Analysis:* The airway pressure at 7 mm Hg (just before spontaneous inspiratory artifact) indicates a pressure of about 72/36 mm Hg. This tracing indicates the potential value of airway pressure use with pressure values in identifying end expiration. This patient probably would benefit from efforts aimed at slowing respiration before believing these pressures.

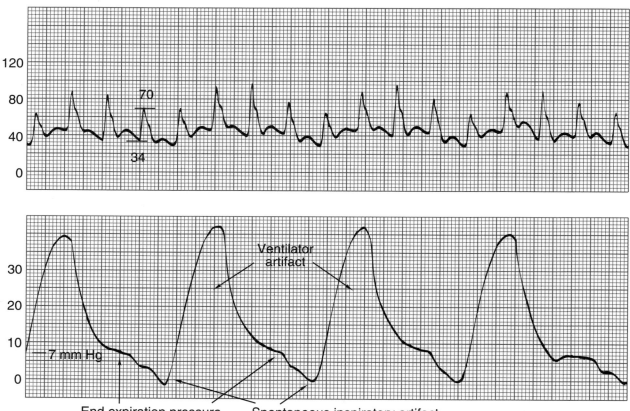

PRACTICE CLINICAL SCENARIO 9–27. A 71-year-old woman is in the unit for rule-out MI. She has no orthopnea although she has inspiratory crackles. She is not intubated and currently is in no distress. Respiratory rate is about 24 bpm. Pulmonary artery pressure values have fluctuated over the past several shifts and several nurses have reported difficulty finding the correct location to read the waveform. Based on the following waveform, what is your interpretation of this PA tracing?

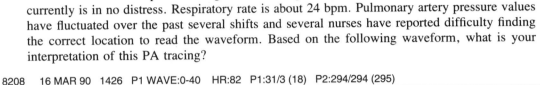

8208   16 MAR 90   1426   P1 WAVE:0-40   HR:82   P1:31/3 (18)   P2:294/294 (295)

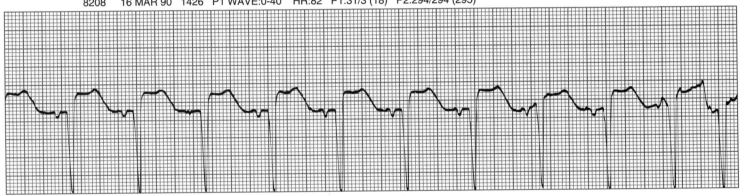

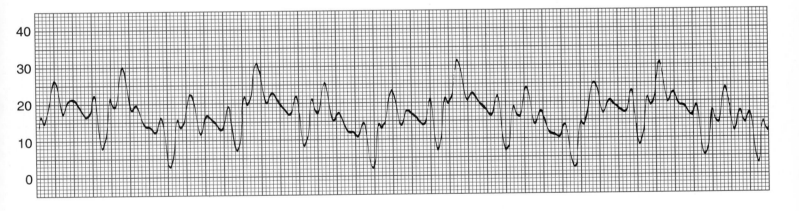

PRACTICE CLINICAL SCENARIO 9–27. *Analysis:* A large diastolic artifact exists, making the tracing difficult to interpret. PA pressure value is about 24/12 based on reading the PA pressure value before inspiratory artifact. This waveform is difficult to read, and correct interpretation would benefit from your checking the square wave test to determine if the waveform is underdamped. If this is the case, a damping device may help improve this waveform's readability.

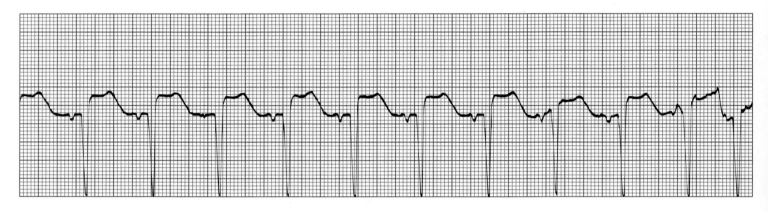

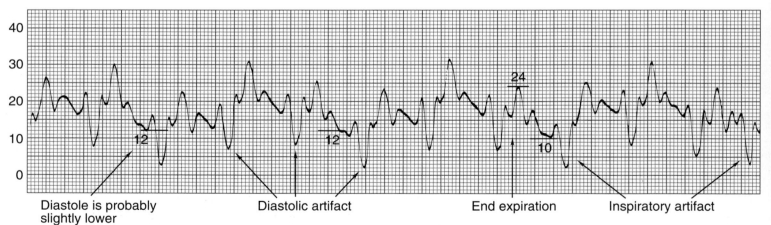

Diastole is probably slightly lower   Diastolic artifact   End expiration   Inspiratory artifact

PRACTICE CLINICAL SCENARIO 9–28. A 29-year-old man is in the unit for acute respiratory failure following chemotherapy for leukemia. He currently is sedated and on AMV with a rate of 20 bpm. The rapid heart rate exists despite attempts to control anxiety and pain. The nurse on the prior shift states that the catheter appears to be wedged and asks your opinion as to whether he should notify the physician. What is your interpretation of this PA tracing?

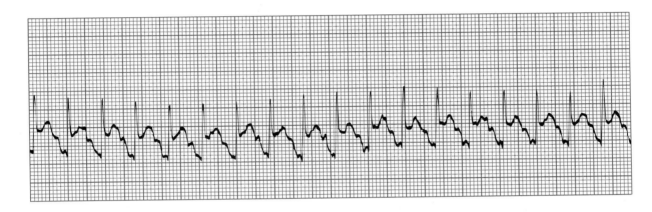

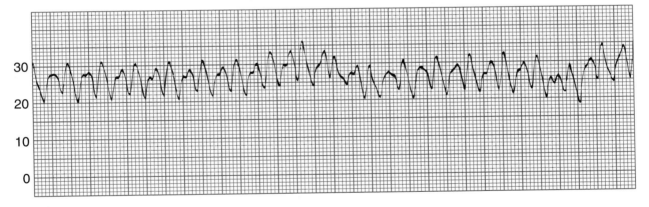

PRACTICE CLINICAL SCENARIO 9–28. *Analysis:* The waveform is a PA tracing that
has a narrow pulse pressure due to the rapid heart rate. In addition, the larger pressure wave
is not the systolic value, based on ECG correlation with peak pressures. The PA pressure is
about 28/21 mm Hg.

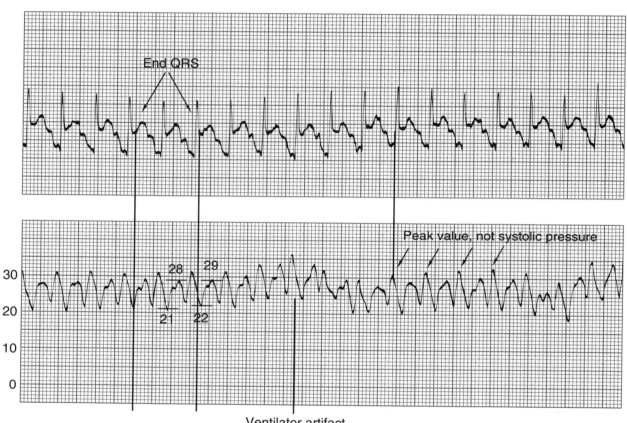

PRACTICE CLINICAL SCENARIO 9–29. A 63-year-old woman is in the unit for treatment of acute respiratory distress syndrome following aspiration of gastric contents. She currently is on inverse-ratio ventilation at a rate of 16 bpm. An airway pressure tracing is placed next to the pulmonary arterial tracing to aid in reading end expiration. Based on the following waveform, where would end expiration be read?

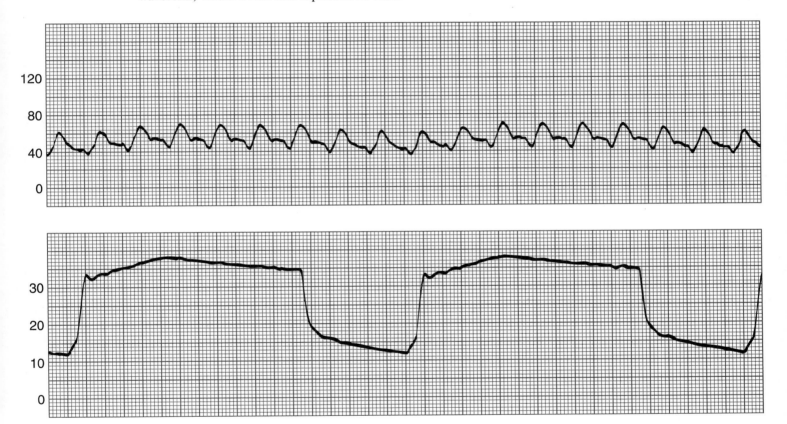

PRACTICE CLINICAL SCENARIO 9–29. *Analysis:* End expiration is identified just prior to the airway pressure increase. The PA pressure at end expiration is about 62/36 mm Hg. Notice how the inverse-ratio ventilation is readily visible in the prolonged inspiratory phase of the airway pressure tracing.

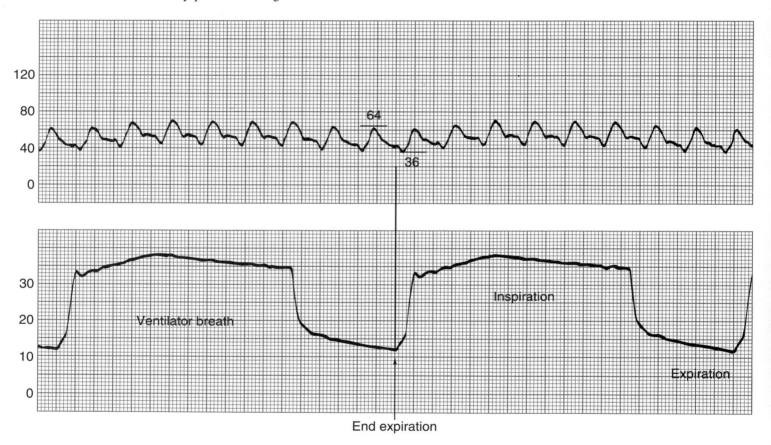

PRACTICE CLINICAL SCENARIO 9–30. A 67-year-old man is in the unit for respiratory distress, hepatic failure, and lymphoma therapy. His pulmonary artery catheter reveals the following tracing. The physician asks if the PCWP value correlates with the PAD. Based on this waveform, what would you say?

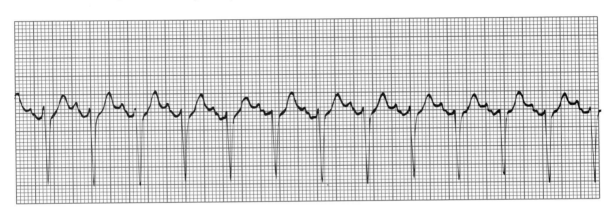

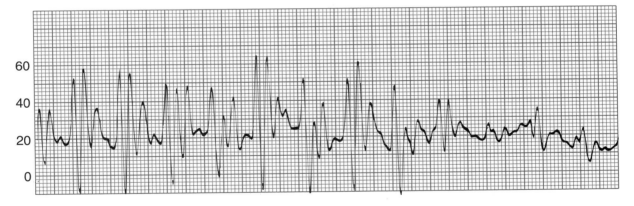

PRACTICE CLINICAL SCENARIO 9–30. *Analysis:* The waveform has marked artifact until the catheter is wedged, which appears to stabilize the tracing. The artifact could be due to underdamping or excessive catheter movement. Insertion of a damping device may be useful, as would possibly repositioning the catheter if underdamping is not present. The systolic PA value is unclear, although the value may be 36/18 mm Hg, with a PCWP of about 18–20 mm Hg. The diastolic value on the PA tracing appears less affected than the reading of the systolic value and correlates well with the PCWP.

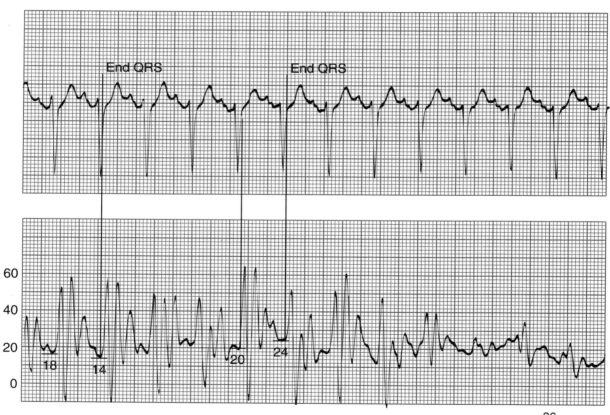

PA pressure $\approx \dfrac{36}{18}$ mm Hg

IV

APPLICATION OF WAVEFORM ANALYSIS

10 Clinical Application of Hemodynamic Data

The mark of a good clinician in terms of hemodynamics is not limited to the ability to correctly analyze hemodynamic waveforms. The clinician must also know how to apply the waveform values in clinical settings. A clinician's ability to understand both the correct interpretation of waveforms and the limitations of waveform values forms the foundation for providing significant benefit to patient assessment and treatment regimens. This chapter focuses on building upon hemodynamic waveform analysis by developing the concepts of hemodynamic interpretation and limitations of pressure analysis. From these goals, the reader should have the foundation to interpret hemodynamic values as well as to apply them to clinical situations.

PRINCIPLES OF HEMODYNAMIC MONITORING

Because the use of waveform values in hemodynamic monitoring requires an understanding of key concepts of blood flow, we will review these concepts before discussing application of waveform values. In addition, a brief review will help to clarify when invasive hemodynamic monitoring is warranted. Not all patients require hemodynamic monitoring, although theoretically a case could be made that many patients would benefit from it. However, studies have not demonstrated how much hemodynamic monitoring changes patient outcome.[73,74] The key limitation to these studies, however, is that they did not assess the appropriate use or interpretation of hemodynamic information.[75] Empirical evidence would suggest that invasive hemodynamic monitoring is necessary due to the limited accuracy in physically assessing patients with abnormal hemodynamics.[76] The primary limitation to physical assessment of hemodynamic disturbances resides in the inability to assess two important hemodynamic parameters, systemic vascular resistance (SVR) and stroke volume (SV), which also represent key components in blood pressure regulation. Table 10–1 provides formulas for calculating these and other hemodynamic parameters.

427

Table 10–1. CALCULATION OF COMMON HEMODYNAMIC PARAMETERS

Parameter	Formula*	Normal Range of Values
Pulmonary Vascular Resistance	$\dfrac{MPAP - PCWP}{CO} \times 80$	40–150 dynes/sec/cm^5
Pulmonary Vascular Resistance Index	$\dfrac{MPAP - PCWP}{CI} \times 80$	200–300 dynes/sec/cm^5/m^2
Systemic Vascular Resistance	$\dfrac{MAP - CVP}{CO} \times 80$	900–1300 dynes/sec/cm^5
Systemic Vascular Resistance Index	$\dfrac{MAP - CVP}{CI} \times 80$	1900–2400 dynes/sec/cm^5/m^2
Cardiac Output	Stroke Volume × Heart Rate	4–8 LPM†
Cardiac Index	Stroke Index × Heart Rate	2.5–4 LPM/m^2
Stroke Volume	$\dfrac{CO}{\text{Heart Rate}} \times 1000$	50–100 cc
Stroke Index	$\dfrac{CI}{\text{Heart Rate}} \times 1000$	25–45 cc/m^2

*MPAP = mean pulmonary artery pressure; PCWP = pulmonary capillary wedge pressure; CO = cardiac output; CI = cardiac index.
†LPM = liters per minute.

Regulation of Blood Pressure

Blood pressure (BP) regulation lies at the heart of hemodynamic monitoring. The concept of blood pressure monitoring is based on the following theoretical equation:

$$BP = \text{cardiac output (CO)} \times \text{systemic vascular resistance (SVR)}$$

Blood pressure is regulated through the interaction of CO and SVR. The cardiac output is comprised of stroke volume (the amount of blood pumped with each contraction) and the heart rate.

The relationship between CO and SVR is usually an inverse one, e.g., if the CO increases, the SVR decreases. The inverse relationship is necessary in order to maintain the blood pressure in an acceptable range. For example, in the patient with a myocardial infarction or hypovolemia, the stroke volume falls and cardiac output may decrease. In order to prevent a fall in blood pressure, the SVR increases to maintain blood pressure. The ability to compensate for a loss of cardiac output makes assessment of the SVR one of the more important hemodynamic goals in monitoring.

The ability of the CO and SVR to compensate for each other limits the use of the blood pressure as the primary mechanism to assess hemodynamics. For example, if the stroke volume falls with hypovolemia, the heart rate will increase to offset the loss of SV. At this point, little change in the blood pressure will occur because the CO is maintained. If the heart rate is unable to compensate for the loss of stroke volume, the CO will fall but the SVR will increase to offset the loss of cardiac output. Again, the change in blood pressure may be small. For the blood pressure to change, both compensating mechanisms (increase in heart rate and SVR) will have to fail. The inability of the blood pressure to reflect early changes in the hemodynamics is one logical reason for the use of hemodynamic monitoring.

Systemic Vascular Resistance

Systemic vascular resistance refers to the resistance facing the left ventricle during contraction. Pulmonary vascular resistance (PVR) refers to right ventricular resistance.[77] Although important clinical differences exist between the use of the SVR and PVR, for the purpose of this section, principles that apply to the SVR also apply to the PVR, with the obvious exception that SVR refers to left ventricular resistance and PVR refers to right ventricular resistance.

SVR has a greater influence in regulating the blood pressure than does CO.[78] Based on this concept, medications that increase SVR, such as norepinephrine, are more likely to elevate the blood pressure than agents that increase the CO, e.g., dobutamine. Although measurement of SVR is difficult, an estimate can be made using an adaptation of Ohm's law:

$$\frac{current - resistance}{flow}$$

which is similar to the SVR formula of:

$$\frac{mean\ arterial\ pressure\ (MAP)\ -\ central\ venous\ pressure\ (CVP)}{CO}.$$

The accuracy of the formula in Table 10–1 in calculating the SVR is limited, partially because not all components of SVR are measured (such as valvular resistance and blood viscosity) and also because the formula is partially comprised of the CO.[79] Changes in the cardiac output will mathematically cause changes in the SVR, although physiologically no change in the SVR may have occurred.

Elevation in the SVR

SVR elevation occurs for one of two reasons. Elevation can occur as a result of vascular disturbances, usually arterial, which cause vasoconstriction. Examples of this type of elevation include situations such as primary hypertension or excessive catecholamine release. SVR elevation in these conditions can produce high resistance levels, e.g., greater than 2000 dynes/sec/cm[5]. Blood pressures under these circumstances are generally elevated.

The second situation causing SVR elevation arises as a compensatory response to reduced CO in an attempt to maintain the blood pressure. Blood pressures in this circumstance are usually normal or reduced. Initial decreases in the CO may not be clinically evident without invasive hemodynamic monitoring because the SVR prevents any marked change in blood pressure. Increases in the SVR as a compensating response are usually less severe, producing SVRs less than 2000 dynes/sec/cm[5].

Two common problems are encountered as the SVR elevates: (1) the workload of the heart increases and myocardial oxygen consumption (MVO_2) rises;[80] and (2) the potential exists for a decrease in the CO through reduction in SV. Avoiding unnecessary increases in the SVR may spare increased myocardial work and improve the stroke volume.

Decreases in the SVR

On the other hand, reduction in the SVR generally decreases myocardial work and raises the potential for an increase in the SV. Assessments of the SVR must be accompanied by an assessment of SV to determine the clinical significance of an altered SVR.

Primary decreases in SVR are due to many potential problems, such as sepsis, portacaval shunting, and neurologically mediated loss of vasomotor tone. Loss of SVR typically causes an increase in the CO to maintain the blood pressure.

Treatment of alterations in the SVR depends on the cause of the SVR change. Medications that alter the SVR are presented in Chapter 11.

Cardiac Output

Cardiac output is frequently the primary focus in assessing and treating hemodynamics. The major goal in assessing the CO is to ensure adequate oxygenation. Assessment of oxygenation parameters, such as mixed venous hemoglobin saturation (SvO_2) and lactic acid levels, should accompany any CO assessment if questions exist regarding the adequacy of the output.

The CO is comprised of two components, heart rate and stroke volume. Understanding the interaction of heart rate and stroke volume is crucial in interpreting hemodynamics.

Heart Rate

The heart rate is easily measured and can serve as a useful assessment tool, particularly if a sinus tachycardia is present. If the CO needs to increase, owing either to increased metabolic rate or to reduction in SVR, the heart rate is the first component to change to meet the increased need. If the SV falls, the heart rate can compensate by increasing and thereby maintain CO. Blood pressure may not be affected by a decrease in stroke volume if the heart rate can increase to compensate for the reduction. A sinus tachycardia can therefore signal one of three potential problems in hemodynamics, i.e., a reduction in stroke volume, an increase in metabolic rate, or a decrease in systemic vascular resistance. Table 10–2 illustrates how an increase in heart rate can mask changes in stroke volume and SVR.

Table 10–2. INCREASES IN HEART RATE MASKING CHANGES IN STROKE VOLUME AND SYSTEMIC VASCULAR RESISTANCE

Hemodynamic Parameter*	Preventing a Fall in CO When SV Decreases			Preventing a Fall in BP When SVR Decreases		
	At 0100 hr	*At 0200 hr*	*Change*	*At 1200 hr*	*At 1400 hr*	*Change*
BP	104/70	106/68	No major change	102/62	100/50	**No major change**
P	100	114	**14% increase**	90	110	**22% increase**
CO	3.7	3.7	**No major change**	4.1	4.9	17% increase
CI	2.3	2.3	No major change	2.4	2.9	17% increase
SV	37	32	**16% decrease**	46	45	No major change
SI	23	20	15% decrease	27	29	No major change
PCWP	16	17	No major change	11	11	No major change
CVP	11	11	No major change	7	7	No major change
SVR				1333	974	**27% decrease**

*BP = blood pressure; P = pulse; CO = cardiac output; CI = cardiac index; SV = stroke volume; SI - stroke index; PCWP = pulmonary capillary wedge pressure; CVP = central venous pressure; SVR = systemic vascular resistance.

Stroke Volume and Stroke Index

Stroke volume and stroke index are the key parameters in assessing most hemodynamic disturbances. The majority of hemodynamic interventions, such as inotropic agents, fluid boluses, and diuretics, are used to improve stroke volume and index. The importance of stroke volume and stroke index can be seen through the components that determine stroke output. For the purpose of this chapter, stroke volume will be primarily discussed although stroke indices should also be computed whenever stroke volumes are measured.

Stroke volume is composed of three factors: preload, afterload, and contractility, which are defined in Table 10–3. Preload of the left and right ventricles is estimated from left and right ventricular end-diastolic pressures. Afterload facing the left and right ventricles is estimated from SVR and PVR. Contractility has no clear clinical parameter by which to measure but can be inferred by changes in stroke volume, as will be discussed over the next several paragraphs.

Preload Assessment

Use of the Pulmonary Capillary Wedge Pressure

Interpretation of the pulmonary capillary wedge pressure (PCWP), along with the central venous pressure (CVP), forms the basis for current assessment of the critically ill patient's cardiac performance. However, the PCWP (for left ventricular assessment) and the CVP (for right ventricular assessment) must never be used in isolation. The purpose of measuring the PCWP is for assessment of preload, one of the components of stroke volume. Because the PCWP tells only about preload, it is important to measure afterload and contractility at the same time as measuring PCWP.

Three reasons exist for the measurement of the PCWP: (1) estimation of left ventricular preload; (2) assessment of extravascular lung water (EVLW) accumulation; and (3) estimation of myocardial oxygen consumption. Estimation of LV preload is the most common use of the PCWP and will receive most of the attention in this section. Estimation of EVLW, the amount of fluid that accumulates in the lung beyond normal, is an imporant adjunct in the clinical application of the PCWP and can generate valuable information. Use of the PCWP to estimate EVLW will be briefly addressed. Myocardial oxygen consumption assessment, a less common application of PCWP, is difficult to measure noninvasively. The PCWP/MVO_2 relationship will be briefly discussed at the end of the section.

The PCWP As an Estimate of Left Ventricular Preload

General Assumptions Relating to PCWP Values. Two key assumptions apply when interpreting the PCWP. Both principles are based on physiologic studies, although the correct application of these assumptions requires an understanding of their physiologic origins. The first assumption is: If the PCWP is low, volume in the left ventricle is low; the second is: If the PCWP is elevated, volume in the LV is increasing.

Table 10–3. DEFINITIONS OF STROKE VOLUME DETERMINANTS

Determinant	Definition
Preload	The maximal stretching of the muscle prior to contraction. Cardiac muscle has maximal stretch at end diastole.
Afterload	The amount of resistance the muscle faces as it contracts. Most of the resistance the heart muscle faces is from the blood vessels, although valves, blood viscosity, and flow patterns can also have an influence.
Contractility	The force or strength of muscle contraction.

Elevated PCWP Values

As the PCWP increases over normal values (8–12 mm Hg), the potential exists for application of Starling's law. Starling's law states: As muscle fibers are stretched, the resulting contraction is more forceful (Figure 10–1).[81] The increasing strength is a compensating mechanism that allows for adaptation to stress on the muscle.

The increased strength of contraction is limited to a certain amount of stretching. As too much stretch occurs, the muscle strength lessens and becomes dysfunctional.

Application of Starling's law to cardiac muscle would indicate as values elevate over normal, i.e., 12 mm Hg, and up to 18 mm Hg, the muscle strength should be improving. In simplistic terms, values in excess of 18 mm Hg could indicate loss of strength. Generally, two reasons account for the increase in PCWP, either excessive vascular fluid or loss of muscle strength due to myocardial failure. Loss of muscle strength is the most common cause of increased PCWP. Table 10–4 illustrates the clinical implications of the PCWP in hemodynamics.

Although increasing PCWP can signal an initial gain followed by a loss of contractility strength, too simplistic an application of the PCWP can result in clinical errors. If Starling's law applied directly to clinical situations, an increase in the PCWP up to 18 mm Hg should be correlated with an improvement in SV (reflecting an increased contractile strength of the heart). Values in excess of 18 mm Hg should show a decrease in SV (reflecting a loss of contractile strength).

In theory, each patient's values should follow a predictable left ventricular function curve. Table 10–5 illustrates theoretical PCWP/SV relationships.

Just as increasing PCWP pressures have theoretical effects, low PCWP pressures also have theoretical predictable relationships with cardiac performance. As the PCWP falls below normal (less than 8 mm Hg), ventricular filling is inadequate. Inadequate ventricular filling produces decreases in SV. Table 10–6 illustrates the normal effect of decreases in PCWP on the stroke volume.

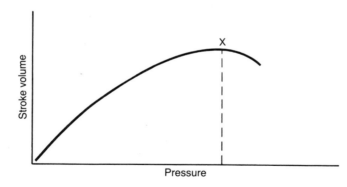

Figure 10–1. Theoretical relationship of Starling's law between muscle response and change in pressure. As pressure increases up to a point in the left ventricle, stroke volume also increases (X). After this point, further increases in pressure cause a reduction in stroke volume.

Table 10–4. CLINICAL IMPLICATIONS OF PCWP VALUES

PCWP Value	Clinical Implication
Below 8 mm Hg	Potential hypovolemia
Between 8 and 12 mm Hg	Normal
Between 12 and 18 mm Hg	Gray area, potentially indicating improved contractility as volume overload develops
Greater than 18 mm Hg	Development of LV* dysfunction and LV failure

*LV = left ventricular.

Table 10–5. THEORETICAL NORMAL PCWP/SV RELATIONSHIPS

Hemodynamic Parameter*	During Early PCWP Increases			During Later PCWP Increases		
	At 1400 hr	*At 1500 hr*	*Change*	*At 0600 hr*	*At 0800 hr*	*Change*
BP	96/64	102/68		112/72	110/70	
P	101	96		85	98	
CO	4.0	4.5		4.5	3.9	
CI	2.4	2.7		2.2	1.9	
PAP	19/12	26/19		28/18	35/26	
SV	40	47 ⎫	Increase as	53	40 ⎫	Decrease
SI	24	28 ⎭	PCWP rises	26	19 ⎭	as PCWP rises
PCWP	10	16		14	23	
CVP	5	9		10	15	

*BP = blood pressure; P = pulse; CO = cardiac output; CI = cardiac index; PAP = pulmonary artery pressure; SV = stroke volume; SI = stroke index; PCWP = pulmonary capillary wedge pressure; CVP = central venous pressure.

Table 10–6. THEORETICAL NORMAL EFFECT OF DECREASES IN PCWP ON SV

Hemodynamic Parameter*	At 1900 hr	At 2100 hr	Change
BP	116/70	120/74	
P	109	112	
CO	4.7	4.1	
CI	2.3	2.0	
SV	43	37 ⎫	Decrease as
SI	21	18 ⎭	PCWP falls
PCWP	12	5	
CVP	6	2	

*BP = blood pressure; P = pulse; CO = cardiac output; CI = cardiac index; SV = stroke volume; SI = stroke index; PCWP = pulmonary capillary wedge pressure; CVP = central venous pressure.

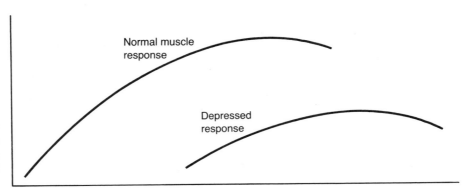

Figure 10–2. Variations in Starling's relationship between pressure and stroke volume. In contractile depressed states, e.g., chronic heart failure, the curve is shifted down and to the right. This results in higher pressures being necessary to achieve improved stroke volumes.

Normal muscle response

Depressed response

Variations in Normal PCWP Interpretation

Studies have demonstrated that Starling's law has variations in the failing heart.[82] In the contractile depressed muscle, higher pressures are required to achieve an improvement in SV (Figure 10–2). In this type of patient, values in excess of 22 mm Hg may be required to achieve the same change in stroke volume a normal person may achieve with a PCWP of 18 mm Hg. Table 10–7 gives an illustration of a patient with a depressed contractile state.

Table 10–7. CHRONICALLY DEPRESSED MYOCARDIUM INCREASING
OPTIMAL PCWP PRESSURE

Hemodynamic Parameter*	At 2300 hr	At 0100 hr	Change
BP	86/52	98/60	
P	114	104	
CO	3.1	4.3	
CI	1.6	2.4	
PAP	30/17	40/25	
SV	27	41 ⎫	Increase despite PCWP ele-
SI	14	23 ⎭	vations beyond normal
PCWP	15	22	
CVP	8	12	

*BP = blood pressure; P = pulse; CO = cardiac output; CI = cardiac index; PAP = pulmonary artery pressure; SV = stroke volume; SI = stroke index; PCWP = pulmonary capillary wedge pressure; CVP = central venous pressure.

Limitations to the PCWP

PCWP is not the only contributor to muscle stretching. Volume has as much of a role as does pressure, and the PCWP does not measure volume. Concern over pressure being used as a sole or primary contributor to ventricular assessment was a concern even before the advent of bedside pulmonary artery catheterization.[83,84] A common clinical error is to assume changes in the PCWP equal volume changes, a point physics indicates is incorrect. For example, when inflating a balloon for the first time, the balloon requires large pressures to overcome the resistance of the balloon. After the balloon has been inflated several times, the resistance is very low and the pressure required to inflate the balloon is markedly reduced. In both instances, however, upon initial inflation and also after multiple inflations, the volume required to inflate the balloon does not markedly change.

In other words, initially, high pressures were required to inflate the balloon with the same volume lower pressures were later able to accomplish. The same principle applies to the heart muscle. In patients with compliant left ventricles, such as cardiomyopathy, large volume changes can occur without large pressure changes.[85] On the other hand, in patients with noncompliant ventricles (acute myocardial infarction), small volume changes may produce large pressure changes. One patient could have marked changes in ventricular volume without PCWP changes although another may have small volume changes with large pressure changes.

Use of Stroke Volume with the PCWP

In order to make clinical sense out of the PCWP, the clinician should correlate changes in the PCWP with SV. Inasmuch as the PCWP is measured because it serves as an estimate of left ventricular preload, SV can be used as a marker of the importance of PCWP values. Although measurement of SV via thermodilution technique is a right ventricular measurement, a strong relationship is generally present between right and left ventricular stroke volumes.[86] The relationship is not perfect; however, assuming that right ventricular stroke volumes reflect left ventricular stroke volumes is generally clinically safe.

Stroke volume is not a perfect indicator of the implications of a PCWP change. Other parameters, such as ejection fraction, end-diastolic volumes, and continuous stroke volume measurement, would be valuable adjuncts in assessing PCWP values. New parameters are rapidly being introduced into clinical practice as technology increases the information available to the clinician. For the present time, stroke volume is the only commonly available parameter to correlate with PCWP values. As more information is available, an improved assessment of the PCWP with other parameters in addition to the stroke volume will occur.

Preload is measured because it is one of three factors that affect the stroke volume.

Therefore, changes in the preload (PCWP) are important primarily if they affect stroke volume. Table 10–8 illustrates the importance of noting the PCWP in conjunction with the stroke volume.

Notice that in the right hand portion of Table 10–8, no optimal PCWP appears to exist. The lack of determining an optimal wedge pressure is more the rule than the exception. Be very cautious in using the PCWP as the primary guide to treating hemodynamics. PCWP values are only useful when used in conjunction with other hemodynamic information. To use the PCWP as the primary indicator for therapies runs the risk of employing unnecessary or inappropriate therapies.

Use of the PCWP to Estimate EVLW

As the PCWP increases, intravascular hydrostatic pressure also increases. Increased intravascular hydrostatic pressure potentially increases the flow of vascular fluid into the pulmonary interstitial space (Figure 10–3). As pulmonary interstitial space receives increased vascular fluid, the lung water content increases. Initially, pulmonary lymphatics will eliminate the increased lung water.[87] As the pulmonary lymphatics become overwhelmed, increased lung water will cause impaired gas exchange. The primary clinical symptoms will be the pulmonary symptoms of shortness of breath, dyspnea on exertion, and orthopnea. Blood gases will illustrate an increasing intrapulmonary shunt. The primary blood gas affected is the arterial oxygen tension (PaO_2). The PaO_2 will diminish due to the increased intrapulmonary shunt, and the patient will require increasing amounts of oxygen therapy. If the intrapulmonary shunt becomes severe, mechanical ventilation and positive end-expiratory pressure therapy may be necessary.

The point where the PCWP causes an increased EVLW is unclear although theoretically the point is in the low 20s mm Hg. It is useful to measure the intrapulmonary shunt in order to estimate the effect of the PCWP on EVLW. Table 10–9 contains the formula for measuring the intrapulmonary shunt.

The intrapulmonary shunt measurement requires a mixed venous blood gas value and may not be practical for all patients. The use of estimates of intrapulmonary shunt with oxygen-

Table 10–8. IMPORTANCE OF NOTING PCWP IN CONJUNCTION WITH SV

Hemodynamic Parameter*	Increase in PCWP Without Change in SV			Fluctuation in PCWP Without Correlation with SV			
	At 0400 hr	*At 0500 hr*	*Change*	*At 0900 hr*	*At 1100 hr*	*At 1300 hr*	*Change*
BP	88/54	90/58		122/72	114/68	130/76	
P	106	108		103	92	90	
CO	3.5	3.7		3.8	4.1	4.2	
CI	2.1	2.2		2.3	2.5	2.6	
SV	33	34	Unchanged as PCWP increases; the change in PCWP is not clinically important	37	45	47	
SI	20	20		22	27	28	
PCWP	15	22		21	25	16	
CVP	12	15		13	17	9	Changes in PCWP do not correlate well with SV
PAP	28/17	34/24	36/23	42/27	32/19		

*BP = blood pressure; P = pulse; CO = cardiac output; CI = cardiac index; SV = stroke volume; SI = stroke index; PCWP = pulmonary capillary wedge pressure; CVP = central venous pressure; PAP = pulmonary artery pressure.

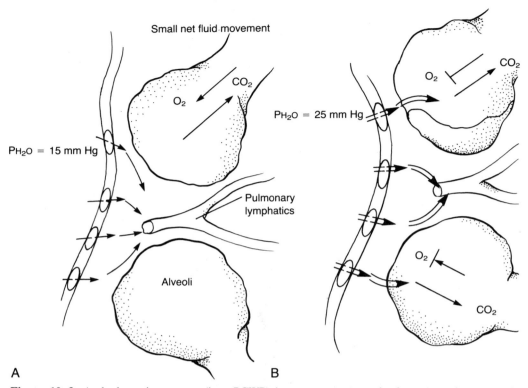

Figure 10–3. As hydrostatic pressure (i.e., PCWP) increases, extravascular lung water increases. *A,* Initial increases in fluid movement out of the capillaries and into the pulmonary interstitial space are initially drained by the pulmonary lymphatics. *B,* As fluid flow increases, the pulmonary lymphatics are overwhelmed and fluid leaks into the alveoli.

Table 10–9. MEASURING INTRAPULMONARY SHUNT (Qs/Qt)

Intrapulmonary shunting can be measured by employing the shunt formula:

$$Qs/Qt = \frac{Cc_{O_2} - Ca_{O_2}}{Cc_{O_2} - Cv_{O_2}}$$

where Qs = shunted pulmonary blood flow; Qt = total pulmonary blood flow; Cc_{O_2} = pulmonary capillary oxygen content; Ca_{O_2} = arterial oxygen content; and Cv_{O_2} = venous oxygen content.

derived tension variables can serve as a clinical substitute for direct intrapulmonary shunt measurement. Five estimates of intrapulmonary shunting exist, including the respiratory index, arterial/alveolar ratio, Pa_{O_2}/Fi_{O_2} ratio, the alveolar-arterial (A-a) gradient, and the estimated shunt. Formulas for each of these estimates are included in Table 10–10.

Each of these formulas is a reasonable estimate of the intrapulmonary shunt, although actual measurement of the shunt is preferable. The least accurate of the estimates is the A-a gradient. The other values are similar in accuracy. The easiest to use is the Pa_{O_2}/Fi_{O_2} ratio. The Pa_{O_2}/Pa_{O_2} is the easiest to explain and will be the example used to correlate the PCWP with the EVLW.

As lung water increases, less alveolar oxygen can diffuse into the pulmonary capillaries.

Table 10–10. ESTIMATES OF
INTRAPULMONARY SHUNTING

Hemodynamic Parameter	Normal
Pao_2/Fio_2 ratio	>300
Arterial/alveolar ratio (Pao_2/Pao_2)	>60%
Respiratory index $\dfrac{(Pao_2 - Pao_2)}{Pao_2}$	<1
Alveolar − arterial gradient ($Pao_2 - Pao_2$)	<20 mm Hg
Estimated shunt $\dfrac{Cco_2 - Cao_2}{3.5 + (Cco_2 - Cao_2)}$	3.5–5.0

Table 10–11. EFFECTS OF INCREASED PCWP ON EVLW*

Hemodynamic Parameter†	At 0500 hr	At 0600 hr	Change
BP	102/58	98/60	
P	88	104	
CO	5.1	4.2	
CI	2.8	2.3	
SV	58	40	
SI	32	22	
PCWP	15	24	Increase produces worsening gas exchange
CVP	11	14	
Pao_2	87	64	
Pao_2 (from alveolar air equation)	237	242	
Fio_2	0.40	0.40	
$Paco_2$	38	34	
a/A	0.37	0.26	Increase produces worsening gas exchange

*EVLW = extravascular lung water.
†BP = blood pressure; P = pulse; CO = cardiac output; CI = cardiac index; SV = stroke volume; SI = stroke index; PCWP = pulmonary capillary wedge pressure; CVP = central venous pressure; Pao_2 = partial arterial pressure of oxygen; Pao_2 = alveolar pressure of oxygen; Fio_2 = fraction of inspired oxygen; $Paco_2$ = partial arterial pressure of carbon dioxide; a/A = Pao_2/Pao_2.

The decreased diffusion of oxygen produces a larger gradient between alveolar and arterial oxygen levels. Normally, about 60–100% of alveolar oxygen reaches the arteries, producing an arterial/alveolar ratio in excess of 60%. As increased lung water occurs, the percent of oxygen reaching the arteries diminishes and produces a decreased Pao_2/Pao_2 ratio.

If a PCWP increase causes an increased EVLW, the Pao_2/Pao_2 ratio should decrease. Table 10–11 illustrates the expected effect of an increase in PCWP on the Pao_2/Pao_2 ratio (a/A).

Table 10–12 illustrates a change in the PCWP that does not correlate with an increase in EVLW. In this situation, despite the increase in the PCWP, no substantial increase in EVLW occurred. The clinical significance of the change in the PCWP is limited under the above conditions.

Table 10–12. INCREASED PCWP WITH NO EFFECTS ON EVLW*

Hemodynamic Parameter†	At 0700 hr	At 0900 hr	Change
BP	124/66	112/64	
P	105	100	
CO	5.3	4.9	
CI	2.9	2.7	
SV	50	49	
SI	28	27	
PCWP	13	25	Increase does not change gas exchange
CVP	10	16	
PaO_2	87	84	
PAO_2	237	234	
FIO_2	0.40	0.40	
$PaCO_2$	38	41	
a/A	0.37	0.36	Increase does not change gas exchange

*EVLW = extravascular lung water.

†BP = blood pressure; P = pulse; CO = cardiac output; CI = cardiac index; SV = stroke volume; SI = stroke index; PCWP = pulmonary capillary wedge pressure; CVP = central venous pressure; PaO_2 = partial arterial pressure of oxygen; PAO_2 = partial alveolar pressure of oxygen; FIO_2 = fraction of inspired oxygen; $PaCO_2$ = partial arterial pressure of carbon dioxide; a/A = PaO_2/PAO_2.

PCWP and MVO_2

Increases in left ventricular wall tension have been shown to correlate with myocardial oxygen consumption. PCWP, as a reflector of left ventricular pressure, can be a factor in MVO_2.[88] As the PCWP increases, MVO_2 is potentially increased. Clinically, measurement of MVO_2 is difficult and correlation with the PCWP is limited. Estimates of MVO_2 such as the rate pressure product (RPP) have limited accuracy in the critical care setting. Due to the limited assessment of MVO_2, keeping the PCWP as low as possible is one clinical goal to avoid increased MVO_2.

INTERACTION OF PARAMETERS DETERMINING STROKE VOLUME

The three parameters that determine stroke volume interact in a dynamic manner. A fourth parameter affecting stroke volume—heart rate—also interacts in a dynamic manner. The effect of heart rate on stroke volume can be seen in Table 10–2. According to Starling's law, if preload increases slightly, contractility improves. In a patient with an elevated SVR, reducing the SVR would act to increase the stroke volume by improving contractility. The clinician must evaluate the three stroke volume parameters together when making any hemodynamic assessment. Observing one value in isolation increases the likelihood of making an error in assessment.

SUMMARY

Interpretation of the waveform values depends on understanding the clinical application of values. Inasmuch as the waveforms generate only information regarding pressures, the clinician must incorporate other factors regulating hemodynamics in order to make a complete hemodynamic assessment. Because of the interaction of all parameters, such parameters as the PCWP must never be used in isolation when making a clinical assessment. This chapter provided an introduction to key concepts necessary to apply in conjunction with waveform analysis for appropriate clinical decision making in hemodynamic monitoring. As improved technology increases the amount of hemodynamic information, such as ejection fractions and continuous cardiac outputs, the limitations of using pressures in isolation will become even more apparent. Until this time, use all available information in addition to pressures in the assessment of hemodynamics.

PRACTICE CLINICAL SCENARIOS

The following practice clinical scenarios will give you opportunity to practice performing the integrated assessment necessary for hemodynamic interpretation.

PRACTICE CLINICAL SCENARIO 10–1. A 72-year-old man is admitted to the unit with the diagnosis of congestive heart failure. Due to initial hypotension, a pulmonary artery catheter is placed. Initial readings at 0300 are listed below. Based on these readings, dobutamine is started at 4 μg/kg/min. The 0400 readings demonstrate the values listed below. Based on this information, did an improvement in the clinical status occur?

Hemodynamic Parameter*	at 0300 hr	at 0400 hr
BP	92/56	94/58
P	112	110
CO	3.8	4.4
CI	2.1	2.4
SV	34	40
SI	18.8	22
PAP	34/21	36/22
PCWP	18	20
CVP	13	14

*BP = blood pressure; P = pulse; CO = cardiac output; CI = cardiac index; SV = stroke volume; SI = stroke index; PAP = pulmonary artery pressure; PCWP = pulmonary capillary wedge pressure; CVP = central venous pressure.

PRACTICE CLINICAL SCENARIO 10–2. A 61-year-old woman with an acute anterior myocardial infarction becomes hemodynamically unstable (hypotensive) on your shift and requires pulmonary artery catheter insertion. She has the following set of hemodynamic values:

Hemodynamic Parameter*	at 1800 hr	at 1900 hr	at 2000 hr
BP	90/60	88/54	94/62
P	110	108	106
CO	4.2	4.4	4.1
CI	2.5	2.6	2.44
SV	38	41	39
SI	23	24	23
PAP	30/16	40/24	36/20
PCWP	14	21	17
CVP	11	16	12

*BP = blood pressure; P = pulse; CO = cardiac output; CI = cardiac index; SV = stroke volume; SI = stroke index; PAP = pulmonary artery pressure; PCWP = pulmonary capillary wedge pressure; CVP = central venous pressure.

Based on the above sets of readings, was the PCWP elevation at 1900 hours clinically significant?

PRACTICE CLINICAL SCENARIO 10–1. *Analysis:* The dobutamine action was effective based on the above situation. The improved stroke volume was reflecting the inotropic action of dobutamine. Although the PCWP did not improve, the improved contractility caused an improvement in stroke volume. This example demonstrates the need to look at both contractility and PCWP (preload) in order to determine changes in hemodynamic performance.

PRACTICE CLINICAL SCENARIO 10–2. *Analysis:* From the lack of change in stroke volume, the change in the PCWP was not clinically significant. This observation is further supported by the 2000 readings, which indicate a stability in the stroke volume. This example illustrates how preload changes, i.e., the PCWP increase, do not by themselves indicate clinical significance. The increased PCWP without change in the stroke volume could reflect a non-compliant ventricle that has large pressure changes with small volume changes.

11 : Treatment for Hemodynamic Disturbances

TREATMENT GUIDELINES

No universal consensus exists regarding the treatment of hemodynamic disturbances. Treatment guidelines are based on the principles influencing one of the parameters in blood pressure regulation, either cardiac output or systemic vascular resistance. Treatment of the components of blood pressure regulation can be further subdivided. Cardiac output can be treated through each component that determines output—stroke volume and heart rate. Stroke volume itself can be further segmented by identifying the two most common features influencing it—volume and loss of contractility. The principles of treatment in hemodynamic alterations can be better understood through isolating these aspects of blood pressure regulation.

The following section will provide theoretical and clinical examples of how treatment principles are generally employed in improving hemodynamics. Many variations of the treatment scenarios presented in this chapter are possible, but this chapter should give a foundation for understanding the principles involved in treating abnormal hemodynamics.

DECREASE IN STROKE VOLUME SECONDARY TO LOSS OF CONTRACTILITY

Low stroke volumes accompanied by high pulmonary capillary wedge pressures (PCWPs) usually require improvement in contractility. Contractility improvement can take place through one of three mechanisms, i.e., reduction in preload, reduction in afterload, or improvement in contractility.

Reduction in Preload

Preload reduction is achieved by reducing vascular volume (diuretics) or causing venodilation. Treatment with agents that alter preload is summarized in Table 11–1. In theory, the reduction in preload moves the ventricular muscle stretching to a more optimal point on Starling's curve.[89] Whichever treatment modality is employed in an attempt to reduce the preload, success is measured by the improvement in cardiac performance. Cardiac performance can be assessed by parameters such as the stroke volume or ejection fraction.

Reduction in Afterload

Reduction in afterload can theoretically improve stroke volume by easing the work the ventricle faces in contraction.[90] Many agents, through both oral and intravenous routes, are available to reduce afterload. Again, in order to determine that afterload reduction is effective, the clinician must measure improvement in parameters of cardiac performance. Treatment with agents that reduce afterload is summarized in Table 11–2.

Improving Contractility (Inotropic Support)

Increasing contractility in the acute care setting is one of the most common treatments in the hemodynamic disturbances. Controversy exists regarding the role of an inotropic agent in treating a chronic failing heart, although the role in acute failure is well accepted.[91,92] Although acute and chronic left ventricular failure is primarily due to reduced muscle strength, simple inotropic support does not seem to achieve optimal results when used in isolation. Acute ventricular failure appears to respond well to inotropic support, but current theory points more toward afterload reduction to improve cardiac output in chronic cardiac failure.

Acute cardiac failure employs inotropes as one of the mainstays in treatment. Indications for the use of inotropes center on low stroke volume and increased left ventricular filling pressures (as reflected in the PCWP). Treatment with agents that increase contractility is summarized in Table 11–3.

Dobutamine is probably the most common inotrope.[93] In addition to being an excellent agent to improve contractility, dobutamine also produces a slight reduction in systemic vascular resistance (SVR) through its action in beta receptor stimulation. Dobutamine is usually the drug of choice to increase the stroke volume when the PCWP is elevated.

Dopamine, in mid-dose regions (3–10 μg/kg/min), acts as a strong inotrope. However, due to both alpha and beta receptor stimulation, dopamine increases both SVR and contractility.[94] During the increase in SVR and contractility, myocardial oxygen consumption (MVO_2) can

Table 11–1. TREATMENT WITH PRELOAD REDUCING AGENTS

Drugs of Choice	Dose	Route
Vasodilators		
Diltiazem (Cardizem)	180–360 mg/day q 6–8 hr	Oral
Nifedipine (Procardia)	40–240 mg/day q 6–8 hr	Oral
Nitroglycerin (Nitrostat)	10–400 μg/min	IV
Diuretics		
Furosemide (Lasix)	10–600 mg/day divided doses	IV/Oral
Ethacrynic acid (Edecrin)	50–150 mg/day 2–3 times daily	IV/Oral
Bumetanide (Bumex)	0.5–10 mg/day	IV/Oral
Chlorothiazide (Diuril)	1000–2000 mg/day	Oral
Zaroxolyn (Matolazone)	5–20 mg/day	Oral

Table 11–2. TREATMENT WITH AFTERLOAD REDUCING AGENTS*

Drugs of Choice	Dose	Route
Vascular Smooth Muscle Relaxants		
Sodium nitroprusside (Nipride)	0.5–10 µg/kg/min	IV
Hydralazine (Apresoline)	40–200 mg/day	Oral
	10–40 mg	IV
Diazoxide (Hyperstat)	50–100 mg bolus	IV
Nitroglycerin	10–400 µg/min	IV
Alpha Inhibitors		
Clonidine (Catapres)	0.2–0.6 mg/day (divided doses)	Oral
Phentolamine (Regitine)	0.1–2 mg/min	IV
Methyldopa (Aldomet)	500–2000 mg/day (divided doses)	Oral
	250–1000 mg/dose (every 6 hours)	IV
Trimethaphan (Arfonad)	starts at 3–4 mg/min up to 6 mg/min	IV
Prazosin (Minipress)	1–20 mg/day (divided doses)	Oral
Angiotensin Converting Enzyme (ACE) Inhibitors		
Captopril (Capoten)	25–150 mg/day bid or tid	Oral
Enalapril (Vasotec)	5–40 mg/day bid	IV and Oral
Beta Blocking Agents		
Metoprolol (Lopressor)	15 mg loading (in 3 doses, 2 min apart)	IV
	100–400 mg daily	Oral
	50–100 mg q day–qid	
Propranolol (Inderal)	1–3 mg	IV
	120–240 mg/daily (divided doses)	Oral
Labetalol (Trandate)	0.25 mg/kg initial	IV
	50–200 mg total	
	400–2400 mg (divided doses)	Oral
Calcium Channel Blocking Agents		
Diltiazem (Cardizem)	180–360 mg/day q 6–8 hr	Oral
Nifedipine (Procardia)	40–240 mg/day q 6–8 hr	Oral

*All dosages should be individualized per patient; dosages listed are common clinical guides but may vary among patients.

Table 11–3. TREATMENT WITH INOTROPIC (CONTRACTILITY) AGENTS

Drugs of Choice	Dose	Route
Dobutamine	1–20 µg/kg/min	IV drip
Dopamine	1–5 µg/kg/min (renal + +)*	IV drip
	5–15 µg/kg/min (contractility +)†	
	>15 µg/kg/min (vasopressor)	
Amrinone	0.75 mg/kg (loading dose)	IV push
	5–10 µg/kg/min	IV drip

*+ + = moderate.
†+ = mild.

markedly increase. Dopamine is not the first drug of choice for low stroke volumes with elevated PCWP values. Dopamine is superior, however, to dobutamine in raising the blood pressure, owing to the increased SVR effect of dopamine. In the hypotensive patient with low stroke volumes and high filling pressures, dopamine may achieve better results at improving the blood pressure than dobutamine. Dobutamine and dopamine can be given together to achieve a combination of inotropic and afterload increases.

Because amrinone acts as a phosphodiesterase inhibitor rather than primarily by sympathetic stimulation, it provides a useful alternative to dobutamine or dopamine.[95] Evidence exists that in chronic cardiac failure, sympathetic sites are depleted.[96] Agents such as dobutamine and dopamine will not be effective in such a situation; however, agents such as amrinone would potentially still be effective. As other phosphodiesterase inhibitors become available, this category of drug may see increased use in the acute and chronic treatment of cardiac failure. If the patient does not increase the stroke volume with the use of dobutamine, amrinone would be a logical alternative.

INCREASING PRELOAD

Treatment of Hypovolemia

Increasing preload is the treatment of choice when encountering any unknown cause of hypotension.[97] The primary question surrounding preload augmentation is the type of agent that would work best. Controversy over crystalloid vs colloidal solutions has raged for decades.[98–100] The primary question regarding agent type centers on which fluid compartment is being treated. If the vascular compartment alone is to be expanded, colloidal agents are likely more effective.[101] Colloidal agents, due to their large molecular weight, remain in the vascular compartment much more effectively than crystalloidal agents. The osmotic effect of the colloidal agents causes a rapid expansion of the vascular compartment. Expansion can take place with only about 20% of the fluids necessary to achieve the same expansion with crystalloids. Colloidal agents are commonly used in the acute hypovolemic state (trauma, postoperatively).

If the interstitial and cellular compartment also needs expansion, crystalloids may be more effective.[102] Because crystalloidal agents can more effectively leave the vascular space (only about 200 cc of 1000 cc remain in the blood vessels), the interstitial space is more actively reexpanded. Crystalloidal agents are more likely to be used in chronic hypovolemia, unknown cause for hypotension, and mild acute hypovolemia.

Concern over the use of colloidal agents is due to more potential complications, primarily an increase in extravascular lung water.[103] A second concern is in the cost of colloidal agents, usually much more expensive than crystalloids. Regardless of the type of volume expander employed, monitoring hemodynamics is the best method to assess the effectiveness of the therapy. Treatment with agents that increase preload is summarized in Table 11–4.

ELEVATING THE SVR

Increasing the SVR is possible through the use of several vasoconstricting agents. Treatment with agents that increase the SVR is summarized in Table 11–5. The primary circumstances for elevating the SVR are related to situations that cause loss of vasomotor tone, such as sepsis and neurogenic injuries. When the SVR decreases, the cardiac output will usually increase to offset the loss of resistance.[104] In addition, as the SVR decreases, the preload also frequently

Table 11–4. TREATMENT WITH AGENTS THAT INCREASE PRELOAD

Crystalloids	Colloids
Normal saline	Albumin
Lactated Ringer's	Hetastarch (Hespan)
Dextrose in water (D5W)	Whole blood
Advantages	*Advantages*
1. Less costly.	1. Less fluid necessary to expand vascular space.
2. Less likely to increase lung water.	2. More rapid response blood pressure response.

Table 11–5. TREATMENT WITH
AGENTS THAT INCREASE
AFTERLOAD

Drug	Dose
Norepinephrine (Levophed)	1–20 μg/min
Dopamine (Intropin)	>5 μg/kg/min
Phenylephrine (Neo-Synephrine)	1–20 μg/min

falls.[105] The loss of vasomotor tone frequently requires a combination of vasopressors and fluid administration (preload augmentation).[106] Inotropes are of less value, but may still be required, in improving hemodynamics when the SVR is reduced.

Perhaps the most important concept to consider when the SVR falls is that the use of hemodynamic agents such as vasopressors is only a temporary support until the problem causing the SVR to fall is identified. Unless the cause of the low SVR is identified, the use of vasopressors and fluid administration may not be sufficient to maintain adequate blood pressures. Use of agents to increase afterload should be assessed for their effectiveness through noting improvement in both afterload and other hemodynamics, e.g., blood pressure, preload (PCWP), stroke volume, and heart rate.

SUMMARY

The treatment of hemodynamics was briefly addressed in this chapter, with the emphasis being given to practical application and assessment of the impact of the therapies. Many excellent references are available that address treatment of hemodynamics in more depth than provided here. This chapter, however, provides applicable guidelines in the treatment of hemodynamics through general principles used in assessment and interventions associated with hemodynamics.

PRACTICE CLINICAL SCENARIOS

The following clinical scenarios provide an opportunity to assess your understanding of the effectiveness of therapies in the treatment of hemodynamic disturbances. Practice Clinical Scenarios 11–1 and 11–2 provide illustrations of the effectiveness and lack of effectiveness of changes in preload. Practice Clinical Scenarios 11–3 and 11–4 provide examples of afterload reduction interventions and the assessment of their effectiveness. Practice Clinical Scenarios 11–5 and 11–6 illustrate the use of inotropes in acute cardiac failure. Practice Clinical Scenarios 11–7 and 11–8 provide situations for analysis when volume expanders have been used. Practice Clinical Scenario 11–9 provides an example of successful use of afterload increasing agents.

PRACTICE CLINICAL SCENARIO 11–1. A 72-year-old man is in the unit with the diagnosis of congestive heart failure. At 1200, he begins to complain of mild shortness of breath. By 1400, the dyspnea has not improved and his urine output is 35 cc for the past hour. He has crackles along his posterior lung border. He has the following hemodynamic data available at 1400. Based on these data, the physician elects to administer a diuretic (Lasix 20 mg). At 1600, he has the hemodynamics listed below. His symptoms of shortness of breath remain, lung sounds are unchanged, but the urine output is up to 50 cc in the last hour. Based on the 1600 readings, has the diuretic been effective in improving the cardiac performance?

Hemodynamic Parameter*	at 1400 hr	at 1600 hr
BP	108/72	110/70
P	106	108
CO	3.8	3.9
CI	2.3	2.3
SV	36	36
SI	22	21
PAP	37/19	33/16
PCWP	18	14
CVP	11	8

*BP = blood pressure; P = pulse; CO = cardiac output; CI = cardiac index; SV = stroke volume; SI = stroke index; PAP = pulmonary artery pressure; PCWP = pulmonary capillary wedge pressure; CVP = central venous pressure.

PRACTICE CLINICAL SCENARIO 11–2. A 52-year-old man is admitted to the unit with an acute anterior myocardial infarction. He is unresponsive at this time and pulmonary auscultation reveals dependent crackles and expiratory wheezing. He has the hemodynamics listed below at 2230, for which the physician orders nitroglycerin as a preload reducing agent. At 2330, he remains unresponsive, and dependent crackles are still present although expiratory wheezing has diminished. Based on the 2330 readings, was the nitroglycerin effective?

Hemodynamic Parameter*	at 2230 hr	at 2330 hr
BP	128/78	130/82
P	108	96
CO	4.2	4.5
CI	2.4	2.6
SV	39	47
SI	22	27
PAP	35/23	31/19
PCWP	20	17
CVP	10	6

*BP = blood pressure; P = pulse; CO = cardiac output; CI = cardiac index; SV = stroke volume; SI = stroke index; PAP = pulmonary artery pressure; PCWP = pulmonary capillary wedge pressure; CVP = central venous pressure.

PRACTICE CLINICAL SCENARIO 11–1. *Analysis:* Inasmuch as the CO, CI, SV, and SI did not change, the reduction in the PCWP did not achieve optimal effects. The pressures are not markedly elevated at 1600 and may signal the need to try another treatment modality, such as an inotrope. Preload reduction in this case did not achieve the desired outcome.

PRACTICE CLINICAL SCENARIO 11–2. *Analysis:* Based on the above improvements in CO, CI, SV, and SI, the reduction in preload appears to have been effective. Remember it is not the amount of PCWP change that is important, but the effect on the cardiac performance.

PRACTICE CLINICAL SCENARIO 11–3. An 81-year-old woman is in the unit following an episode of left ventricular failure secondary to systemic hypertension. She currently complains of dyspnea on exertion. On cardiac auscultation, you hear a loud S_2, an S_3, and systolic murmur. Her urine is concentrated with a urinary osmolality of 910. Her initial hemodynamics are recorded at 1130. Based on these hemodynamics and symptoms, the physician orders captopril at 6.25 mg. At the 1230 reading, has any significant improvement in hemodynamics occurred?

Hemodynamic Parameter*	at 1130 hr	at 1230 hr
BP	190/108	172/96
P	82	78
CO	3.7	4.0
CI	2.4	2.6
SV	45	51
SI	29	33
PAP	34/21	32/18
PCWP	19	15
CVP	10	6

*BP = blood pressure; P = pulse; CO = cardiac output; CI = cardiac index; SV = stroke volume; SI = stroke index; PAP = pulmonary artery pressure; PCWP = pulmonary capillary wedge pressure; CVP = central venous pressure.

PRACTICE CLINICAL SCENARIO 11–4. A 67-year-old man is in the unit following three-vessel coronary artery bypass grafting. The physician notes the elevated PCWP at 1700 and requests starting nitroprusside at 25 μg/min (.5 μg/kg/min). She states the Nipride should decrease the PCWP by reducing the work on the heart. Based on the following readings, is the addition of the nitroprusside necessary?

Hemodynamic Parameter*	at 1300 hr	at 1500 hr	at 1700 hr
BP	144/88	138/98	142/80
P	101	98	96
CO	4.4	4.7	5.1
CI	2.3	2.5	2.7
SV	44	48	53
SI	23	26	28
PAP	40/24	30/17	38/22
PCWP	21	14	20
CVP	12	5	11

*BP = blood pressure; P = pulse; CO = cardiac output; CI = cardiac index; SV = stroke volume; SI = stroke index; PAP = pulmonary artery pressure; PCWP = pulmonary capillary wedge pressure; CVP = central venous pressure.

PRACTICE CLINICAL SCENARIO 11–3. *Analysis:* Based on the above parameters, the reduction in SVR has produced an increase in stroke volume/index. The addition of the captopril appears to have been effective at this point. Further reduction may be needed and can be monitored via stroke volume changes.

PRACTICE CLINICAL SCENARIO 11–4. *Analysis:* Based on the above set of readings, the PCWP does not seem to correlate with changes in cardiac function (stroke volume). Addition of the nitroprusside does not seem warranted based on the above set of data. The nitroprusside might have been indicated at 1300 although the hemodynamics appeared to improve without any interventions.

PRACTICE CLINICAL SCENARIO 11–5. A 69-year-old woman is admitted to the unit with the diagnosis of congestive heart failure. She currently is short of breath, has crackles in both lungs, and has dependent edema. Based on physical assessment and pulmonary artery catheter information at 2100, dobutamine is started at 3 μg/kg/min. At 2230, she still has crackles but is less short of breath. Based on the results, was the dobutamine therapy successful?

Hemodynamic Parameter*	at 2100 hr	at 2230 hr
BP	96/66	104/72
P	110	108
CO	3.1	4.5
CI	2.1	3.0
SV	28	42
SI	19	28
PAP	42/23	43/23
PCWP	21	21
CVP	11	12

*BP = blood pressure; P = pulse; CO = cardiac output; CI = cardiac index; SV = stroke volume; SI = stroke index; PAP = pulmonary artery pressure; PCWP = pulmonary capillary wedge pressure; CVP = central venous pressure.

PRACTICE CLINICAL SCENARIO 11–6. A 56-year-old man with the diagnosis of cardiomyopathy is admitted to the unit with an exacerbation of CHF followed by a cardiac arrest. On admission, he is tachypneic (38 bpm) and has bilateral crackles in the posterior lung fields. He is unresponsive to verbal stimuli and has a Glasgow coma score of 7. Urine output is low and appears concentrated. A pulmonary artery catheter is inserted and dobutamine (2 μg/kg/min) and dopamine (5 μg/kg/min) are started based on the initial values. By 1600, he is less tachypneic (32 bpm) although crackles are still present. Urine output is 30 cc/hr and still appears concentrated. Based on the information below, was the dobutamine therapy effective?

Hemodynamic Parameter*	at 1500 hr	at 1600 hr
BP	82/52	94/62
P	108	118
CO	3.9	4.3
CI	2.1	2.3
SV	36	36
SI	19	19
PAP	36/22	38/23
PCWP	22	20
CVP	13	14

*BP = blood pressure; P = pulse; CO = cardiac output; CI = cardiac index; SV = stroke volume; SI = stroke index; PAP = pulmonary artery pressure; PCWP = pulmonary capillary wedge pressure; CVP = central venous pressure.

PRACTICE CLINICAL SCENARIO 11–5. *Analysis:* The dobutamine accomplished one key objective in increasing the stroke volume. The PCWP did not decrease as desired but the increase in stroke volume without increasing the heart rate would make this therapy successful.

PRACTICE CLINICAL SCENARIO 11–6. *Analysis:* Although some improvement in the blood pressure has occurred, no substantial change in the stroke volume is present. The action of the dopamine may account for the increased blood pressure. Both the dopamine and dobutamine may have contributed to the increased heart rate. At this point, the dobutamine may need to be increased or changed to amrinone. The therapy has not achieved adequate results at this point.

PRACTICE CLINICAL SCENARIO 11–7. A 67-year-old man returns to the unit following coronary bypass surgery. Initial vital signs and hemodynamics are given at 1430. He remains stable over the next 8 hours. He has increased his core temperature to normal and is extubated by 2200. When you come in to make an initial assessment at 2330, he has the hemodynamics listed below. The patient does not complain of any discomfort or respiratory distress. Based on the decreased pressures at 2330, the physician orders a bolus of 500 cc of hetastarch (Hespan). After administering the hetastarch, you repeat the hemodynamic values at 0015. Based on the hemodynamics, was the hetastarch administration effective?

Hemodynamic Parameter*	at 1430 hr	at 2200 hr	at 2330 hr	at 0015 hr
BP	108/76	98/70	88/62	96/70
P	103	96	100	90
CO	4.1	4.5	3.7	4.3
CI	2.4	2.6	2.2	2.5
SV	40	47	37	48
SI	23	27	22	28
PAP	32/21	34/20	24/10	23/9
PCWP	20	18	6	6
CVP	11	12	9	7

*BP = blood pressure; P = pulse; CO = cardiac output; CI = cardiac index; SV = stroke volume; SI = stroke index; PAP = pulmonary artery pressure; PCWP = pulmonary capillary wedge pressure; CVP = central venous pressure.

PRACTICE CLINICAL SCENARIO 11–8. A 48-year-old woman is admitted to the unit following initial chemotherapy for breast cancer. She has mild shortness of breath and is on a 40% face mask. She currently has the hemodynamics listed below. Based on the 0930 readings, the physician orders 300 cc of normal saline to be given over 15 minutes. Based on the response as obtained by the 1000 readings, was the treatment effective?

Hemodynamic Parameter*	at 0930 hr	at 1000 hr
BP	82/48	88/50
P	126	130
CO	3.1	3.2
CI	1.9	2.0
SV	25	25
SI	15	15
PAP	22/11	26/16
PCWP	7	10
CVP	2	5

*BP = blood pressure; P = pulse; CO = cardiac output; CI = cardiac index; SV = stroke volume; SI = stroke index; PAP = pulmonary artery pressure; PCWP = pulmonary capillary wedge pressure; CVP = central venous pressure.

PRACTICE CLINICAL SCENARIO 11–7. *Analysis:* Based on the increase in stroke volume and cardiac output the fluid bolus with hetastarch appears to be effective. The pressures did not increase as expected but the key parameters to monitor are the overall hemodynamics. The blood pressure increased slightly, the heart rate decreased, and, as mentioned, the cardiac output parameters improved. Perhaps more fluid may be helpful but the patient appears to be more stable at this point.

PRACTICE CLINICAL SCENARIO 11–8. *Analysis:* Although the PCWP and CVP slightly improved, the lack of improvement in the stroke volume and cardiac output indicates the fluid bolus was not adequate. A further fluid challenge may be indicated to obtain a more adequate hemodynamic picture.

PRACTICE CLINICAL SCENARIO 11–9. A 41-year-old woman admitted to the unit following hypotension after a bone marrow transplant has the following hemodynamics at admission. The physician orders norepinephrine at 3 μg/min and normal saline at 150 cc/hr until an improvement in her hemodynamics occurs. Did her hemodynamics improve from 1800 to 1900?

Hemodynamic Parameter*	at 1800 hr	at 1900 hr
BP	90/50	92/56
P	122	108
CO	9.7	8.0
CI	6.1	5.0
SV	80	74
SI	50	46
PAP	38/25	33/20
PCWP	9	12
CVP	7	9

*BP = blood pressure; P = pulse; CO = cardiac output; CI = cardiac index; SV = stroke volume; SI = stroke index; PAP = pulmonary artery pressure; PCWP = pulmonary capillary wedge pressure; CVP = central venous pressure.

PRACTICE CLINICAL SCENARIO 11–9. *Analysis:* Based on the above hemodynamics, the SVR increased from 465 dynes/sec/cm^5 to 590. The above therapy appears to have been partially successful in maintaining the blood pressure with less myocardial work.

12 : Intra-Aortic Balloon Pumping

The intra-aortic balloon was first described by Moulopulas and associates in 1962[107] and was first used clinically in 1968 by Kantrowitz.[108] The intra-aortic balloon pump (IABP) has subsequently gained widespread acceptance as a treatment option for various patient populations needing temporary mechanical assistance.

The assessment of IABP augmentation and its resultant effect on the patient's hemodynamic status is frequently the responsibility of the nurse. Therefore, the nurse must have an in-depth understanding of counterpulsation physiology and its effect on the arterial pressure waveform.

The primary focus of this chapter is to provide the clinician with the physiologic basis of counterpulsation and to provide information for the analysis of the augmented arterial waveform and balloon waveform. The integration of waveform analysis and the corresponding physiologic events has been emphasized, not only to provide the clinician with a technical skill but also to equip the clinician with the ability to effectively communicate and explain the scientific basis for implementing the skill.

It is beyond the scope of this chapter to address specifically each balloon console available today. All manufacturers provide operating instructions and reference literature on the use of their specific pump. Before assuming the responsibility of caring for a patient requiring an IABP, clinicians should thoroughly study the information relevant to that particular balloon pump.

GENERAL DESCRIPTION

The IABP is a volume displacement device. The results of this volume displacement are twofold: (1) circulation is augmented or increased; and (2) ventricular workload is reduced.

Upon balloon inflation, the aortic blood volume is displaced locally (toward the coronary and carotid arteries) and systemically (toward the renal and peripheral arteries) (Fig. 12–1A). As the name denotes, the IABP lies within the ascending thoracic aorta with the tip approximately 2 cm distal to the left subclavian artery. This provides a strategic location to displace the aortic blood volume locally without occluding any of the great vessels branching off the ascending

459

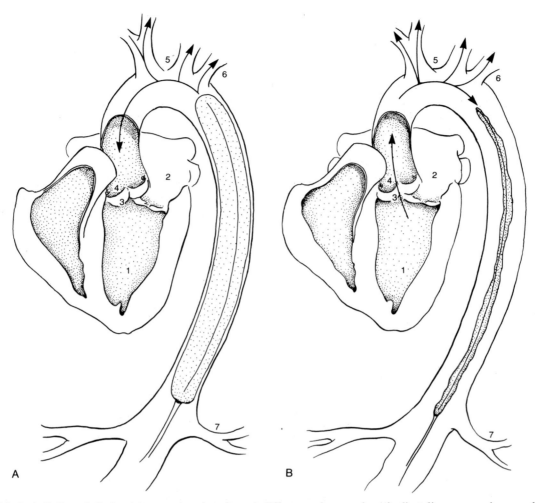

Figure 12–1. *A*, Balloon inflation (upon aortic valve closure). Effects are increased aortic diastolic pressure; increased coronary perfusion; and increased systemic perfusion. *B*, Balloon deflation (prior to aortic valve opening). Effects are decreased aortic pressure; decreased afterload; decreased isovolumetric contraction time; decreased myocardial oxygen consumption; and increased stroke volume. (Anatomy: 1 = left ventricle; 2 = left atrium; 3 = aortic valve; 4 = origin of coronary arteries; 5 = great vessels; 6 = left subclavian artery; 7 = renal arteries.)

aorta; it also provides augmentation of peripheral circulation without obstructing the renal arteries (Fig. 12–1*A*). An increase in the displaced blood volume translates into an increased perfusion pressure to the central and peripheral circulation.[109]

IABP augmentation provides an increase in the pulse rate without increasing the heart rate. An extra perfusion pressure beat is provided by the IABP while the heart is resting. The term counterpulsation refers to this extra perfusion beat upon balloon inflation during diastole. After the volume of blood has been displaced and balloon deflation has occurred, the aortic blood volume is less than the aortic volume prior to balloon assistance (Fig. 12–1*B*). A decreased aortic volume translates into decreased resistance that the heart must overcome to perform ventricular ejection, thereby reducing the ventricular workload.[110,111]

IABP PHYSIOLOGY

The Cardiac Cycle and IABP Interplay

In order to lay a basic foundation for the explanations of IABP physiology and the analysis of the augmented arterial waveform, the left ventricular cardiac cycle must be described (Fig. 12–2).

Intracardiac pressure gradients evoke valvular and mechanical responses that produce the different phases of the cardiac cycle.

Diastole begins with aortic valve closure and ends with mitral valve closure. The diastolic phase of the cardiac cycle involves three events. The first event includes isovolumetric relaxation, which occurs when all the valves are closed and there is no movement of blood through the heart chambers. The second event involves mitral valve opening and the rapid, but passive, filling of the ventricles. The last event of diastole is atrial contraction, which adds 15–30% to the total ventricular volume (atrial kick).

The objective of counterpulsation is to have the intra-aortic balloon (IAB) inflated during the entire diastolic phase, ensuring optimal volume displacement. Therefore, IAB inflation will begin upon aortic valve closure. Aortic valve closure is denoted on the arterial waveform as the dicrotic notch (see Fig. 12–2). Balloon inflation during diastole provides an extra perfusion pressure beat by displacing the aortic blood volume just delivered to the aorta via ventricular ejection. Balloon inflation during systole must be avoided, as it will cause early closure of the aortic valve and incomplete emptying of the left ventricle. The end of diastole is identified as the lowest diastolic point on the arterial waveform just prior to the next systolic beat. This is

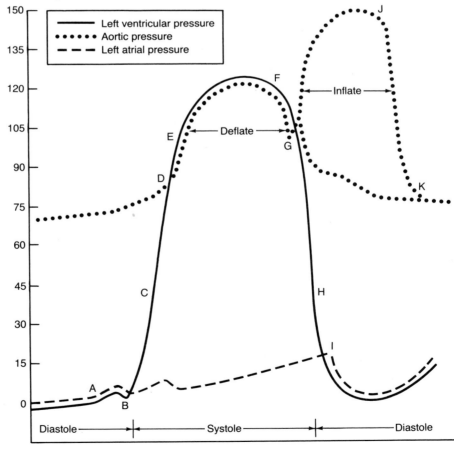

Figure 12–2. Left ventricular cardiac cycle with the augmented aortic (arterial) waveform superimposed. (A = atrial contraction; B = mitral valve closure; C = isovolumetric contraction; D = aortic valve opening and aortic end-diastolic pressure; E = rapid ejection; F = reduced ejection; G = dicrotic notch and balloon inflation point; H = isovolumetric relaxation; I = mitral valve opening; J = peak diastolic pressure or augmented diastole with balloon inflation; K = balloon-assisted end-diastolic pressure.)

the point where balloon deflation should occur. Balloon deflation has "cleared the way" for the next systolic beat by providing a lower resistance in the aorta against which the left ventricle must pump.[110,111]

The systolic aspect of the cardiac cycle begins with mitral valve closure and ends with aortic valve closure. Upon mitral valve closure, isovolumetric contraction (IVC) begins. Actin-myosin filaments of the myocardial muscle fibers overlap and shorten to create intraventricular tension. With this increased muscular tension, the intraventricular pressure increases to produce enough force to open the aortic valve and eject the stroke volume from the ventricle. Isovolumetric contraction requires 85–90% of the myocardial oxygen consumption (MVO_2) to generate this force. The shorter the IVC period, the smaller the demand for oxygen. The relevance of proper IABP timing, with respect to IVC, is very important. If the balloon remains inflated during IVC, the IVC period is lengthened and MVO_2 is increased dramatically and will be detrimental to the patient.

As soon as an intraventricular pressure that exceeds the aortic pressure is generated, the aortic valve opens and rapid ejection begins. Seventy percent of a patient's stroke volume (the volume of blood the left ventricle ejects per beat) is ejected at this time. A period of reduced ejection immediately follows and adds the other 15–30% to the patient's stroke volume. Closure of the aortic valve follows when the aortic pressure exceeds the intraventricular pressure.

Stroke Volume Determinants, Heart Failure, and IABP Interplay

In order to understand the treatment of heart failure with the IABP, the various determinants of stroke volume must be discussed (Table 12–1). Specific medical treatment for heart failure without IABP is provided in Chapter 11.

Table 12–1. INTERPLAY OF HEART FAILURE AND IABP INTERVENTION

Heart Failure	With IABP
Increased Afterload	*Decreased Afterload*
Vasoconstriction	Increased systolic unloading
Sodium retention	Decreased MVO_2
Increased MVO_2	
Increased Preload	*Decreased Preload*
Venoconstriction	Increased forward flow
Sodium retention	Decreased wall tension
Increased myocardial wall tension	Decreased filling pressures
Increased backward pressure	
Increased intracardiac filling pressures	
Decreased Contractility	*Increased Contractility*
Decreased stroke volume	Increased stroke volume
Decreased renal perfusion	Increased renal perfusion
Increased Na retention	
Increased vasoconstriction	
Increased Heart Rate	*Decreased Heart Rate*
Increased sympathetic stimulation	Increased forward flow
Increased preload and atrial stretch	Decreased atrial stretch
	Increased stroke volume
	Decreased need for sympathetic stimulation

Determinants of Stroke Volume

Afterload

Afterload is the resistance the left ventricle (LV) must pump against to open the aortic valve and eject blood out of the heart. During heart failure, the body initiates compensatory mechanisms in an attempt to protect itself against poor perfusion. With a decrease in cardiac output, mechanisms are instituted to maintain blood pressure or perfusion pressure to the vital organs. The renin-angiotensin-aldosterone compensatory mechanism evokes sodium retention and direct vasoconstriction effects that increase systemic vascular resistance (SVR) and maintain blood pressure. These compensatory mechanisms initially maintain perfusion but eventually become detrimental to the myocardium. Vasoconstriction increases afterload (the resistance the LV must overcome to perform ejection). An elevated afterload necessitates a higher energy level and oxygen consumption by the LV to overcome the impedance. During heart failure, oxygen is in short supply and an imbalance between oxygen supply and consumption ensues.

The value of the IABP is to decrease afterload and SVR. After the aortic blood volume has been displaced by balloon inflation, balloon deflation creates a "potential space" in the aorta, thus directly reducing afterload. The secondary effect that occurs as a result of afterload reduction is systolic unloading.[112] The decreased aortic diastolic pressure means the LV does not need to produce the same intraventricular tension and pressure to open the aortic valve as it did without IABP assistance. This beat has been systolically unloaded via afterload reduction. If less work is exerted by the LV, the myocardial oxygen consumption is lessened and the oxygen supply/demand ratio is equilibrated.

Preload

Preload is the volume of blood in the LV at end diastole or just before systole. This volume of blood induces fiber stretching and initiates a strong contraction (see Chapter 10). In the failing heart, preload builds up to overwhelming proportions due to sodium retention and increased venous return via vasoconstriction. The end-diastolic blood volume and pressure has stretched the muscle fibers beyond their physiologic limit to produce a strong contraction. In this situation, preload needs to be reduced. The IABP intervenes to decrease preload by facilitating the forward flow of blood through the heart. Blood will flow to the areas of least resistance. If an area of least resistance is created in front of the heart (i.e., in the aorta), blood will flow easily to that area upon aortic valve opening. IABP creates an area of least resistance by displacing blood out of the aorta. Blood is moved forward through the heart more efficiently, preventing an increase in preload.

Contractility

Contractility refers to the changes in the force of myocardial contraction and is a function of the interaction between the contractile elements (actin and myosin filaments) or fiber stretching. The actual force of contraction is dependent on the amount of preload and afterload present. As discussed earlier, preload and afterload are disproportionally increased with heart failure owing to compensatory mechanisms. Because the IABP decreases preload and afterload, it increases contractility and stroke volume.

Heart Rate

The first compensatory mechanism that responds to heart failure is an accelerated heart rate. Catecholamine surges and increased right atrial stretch induce tachycardia in an attempt to increase the force and rate of myocardial contractions to maintain an adequate cardiac output.

Initially, tachycardia is effective in maintaining an adequate cardiac output, but over time, the effects of tachycardia become deleterious. A rapid heart rate will shorten the diastolic phase of the cardiac cycle. Coronary perfusion and ventricular filling occur during diastole. If this phase is shortened, myocardial ischemia and a reduced stroke volume ensue. Oxygen supply is decreased and myocardial oxygen consumption is increased.

If the stroke volume of a failing heart can be increased, the need for a faster heart rate is decreased. Through the manipulation of preload and afterload, the IABP can increase the patient's stroke volume and thereby decrease the heart rate.

Other Physiologic Factors

Neurohumoral and Metabolic Factors

Neurohumoral and metabolic factors are also involved in the interplay between the IABP and stroke volume determinants.

The compensatory mechanisms of the body are affected by the increase in perfusion with IABP inflation. Owing to the increased diastolic aortic pressure, baroreceptors in the aortic arch increase their parasympathetic output and cause vasodilation. This physiologic event leads to increased afterload reduction.

As perfusion and forward flow improve, the volumes in the heart chambers decrease. There is less stretch of the atria, which leads to decreased sympathetic stimulation, and subsequent decreases in heart rate and myocardial oxygen consumption. If efforts are made to decrease the heart rate, diastolic perfusion time is also increased. By allowing more diastolic time for balloon inflation, coronary perfusion will increase.

An increased pulse rate with balloon inflation refers to the increase in pulsatile flow, not an increase in heart rate. With this increased pulse rate, capillary perfusion is increased and tissue oxygen extraction and consumption are increased. The metabolic effects of this include increased washout of metabolic waste products and lactic acid and decreased metabolic acidosis due to increased oxygen supply.[112] Acidosis depresses contractility and decreases stroke volume.

Coronary Perfusion

The right and left coronary arteries originate within the sinus of Valsalva in the aorta, immediately distal to the aortic valve. Upon aortic valve closure and IABP inflation, blood is directed toward this area to provide coronary perfusion. During systole, muscle tension creates a rise in coronary vascular resistance and reduces coronary circulation. During diastole, the cardiac muscle relaxes completely and no longer obstructs blood flow. The following equation summarizes the concept of coronary circulation during diastole.

Coronary perfusion pressure = aortic diastolic pressure − myocardial wall tension*

The part of this equation that is directly affected by the IABP is the aortic diastolic pressure. With balloon inflation during diastole, the aortic pressure is increased when the wall tension is low, thus increasing coronary perfusion.

The therapeutic benefit of the IABP is somewhat controversial in regard to its effect on improved myocardial blood flow. In some studies,[113,114] no change in perfusion to ischemic areas was noted with IABP intervention although other studies[115,116] have shown an increased perfusion to the ischemic regions.

The amount of myocardial blood flow is determined by the degree of vasodilatation in the

*Myocardial wall tension is indirectly measured by the pulmonary wedge pressure.

coronary artery beds. Ischemia stimulates the coronary arteries to dilate and thereby increases oxygen delivery to the myocardium. Some investigators have indicated that if the coronary arteries are already optimally dilated, an increase in myocardial perfusion pressure as with balloon inflation will not improve coronary blood flow.[117]

In the presence of atherosclerotic heart disease, autoregulation is impaired and the improved coronary perfusion provided by IABP inflation may improve blood flow through obstructed coronary arteries and via collateral vessels.

The varying degrees of impaired autoregulation may be the determining factor as to why the IABP has a variable effect on coronary blood flow.

ASSESSMENT OF IABP AUGMENTATION

Timing Vs Triggering

To understand how the IABP console functions, we must first define timing and triggering.

Triggering is the electrical signal that the IABP console recognizes as the reference point for balloon activation and deactivation. Although the electrical signal usually originates from the electrocardiogram (ECG), it can also come from the arterial waveform or from an inflate/deflate rate preset by the IABP console itself. Triggering is a part of all IABP consoles as a safety mechanism to protect the patient against extreme errors in IABP timing by the operator.

Timing is the operator-controlled synchronization of balloon inflation and deflation with the appropriate phase of the cardiac cycle, performed by visualizing the arterial pressure waveform. Timing is the "fine tuning" of the IABP augmentation by the operator, whereas triggering gives the IABP console a general idea of where the balloon should inflate and deflate. The normal physiologic electrical/mechanical delay between the patient's ECG and the patient's arterial waveform necessitates the use of the arterial waveform for accurate timing of inflation and deflation. An electrical reference should not be used to "fine tune" a mechanical event (IABP augmentation).

Both timing and triggering are essential to proper IABP augmentation, but both are separate entities and are manipulated in different ways.

Triggering

The primary objective to be met in regard to IABP triggering is to generate a signal that will permit accurate initiation of an organized inflate/deflate cycle. Each of the trigger types has advantages in certain situations and the operator needs to make the best choice based on the patient's circumstances and the knowledge of the particular IABP's trigger recognition criteria.

R Wave Triggering

The patient's ECG is utilized most frequently for triggering. More specifically, the R wave of the QRS complex is the signal recognized by the IABP console as the point for IABP deflation (Fig. 12–3). The R wave denotes the beginning of systole—the point where IABP deflation should occur. The IABP console assumes that systole generally occupies that same amount of time with each beat; thus, IABP inflation is triggered after the premeasured systolic time has elapsed or, in other words, at the beginning of diastole.[118] The IABP console identifies the R wave according to various height or width criteria, or both. Therefore, it is essential that a clean ECG tracing that maximizes the R wave and minimizes the other waves is produced to create a trigger signal capable of initiating an organized inflate/deflate cycle.

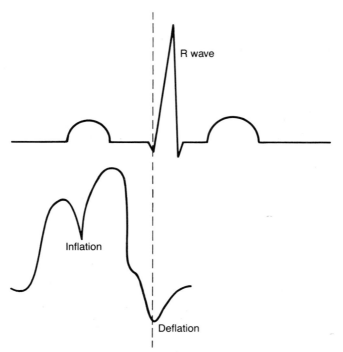

Figure 12–3. Standard R wave deflation.

Pacemaker Spike Trigger

How can a IABP console discriminate between an R wave and a pacemaker spike? This is a situation that involves the use of a pacemaker spike trigger signal. Some IABP consoles use the pacemaker spike for triggering; others utilize a pacemaker spike rejection trigger (Fig. 12–4). In both cases, the rhythm usually must be 100% paced in order for this trigger signal to function consistently.

The pacemaker spike rejection trigger recognizes and rejects the first tall deflection as the pacer spike and assumes that the next tall deflection will then be the R wave.

When the pacemaker spike is utilized as the trigger signal, deflation is induced by the pacer spike, not the R wave. The maximum afterload reduction may not be obtained with this trigger signal due to premature balloon deflation. The different types of pacemakers that the IABP console can detect are atrial, ventricular, and atrioventricular sequential pacers. If the rhythm is not 100% paced, an appropriate ECG lead that minimizes pacer spikes and maximizes R waves should be implemented. The R wave trigger signal can then be utilized.

Arterial Pressure Trigger

The ECG is by far the trigger signal of choice due to its reliability, but there are certain clinical circumstances that make ECG-triggered IAB pumping difficult. Problems with ECG triggering include (1) loss of ECG signal during electrocautery in surgery, (2) poor ECG quality, (3) diaphoretic patient unable to keep ECG electrode on the skin, and (4) excessive pacemaker spike voltage causing distortion of the QRS complex. If these circumstances arise, an arterial pressure trigger is recommended. The primary reference point of the arterial pressure waveform used for deflation triggering is the systolic rise or upstroke.

The arterial pressure trigger should be used with caution. Patients with atrial and ventricular arrhythmias possess an arterial blood pressure that constantly fluctuates, making the reliability of arterial pressure not always optimal (Fig. 12–5).

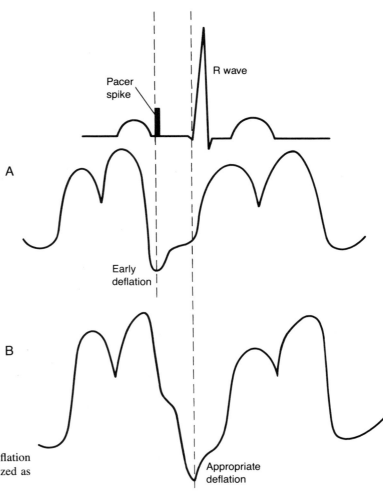

Figure 12–4. *A*, Pacemaker spike recognized as deflation point. *B*, Pacemaker spike rejected. R wave recognized as deflation point.

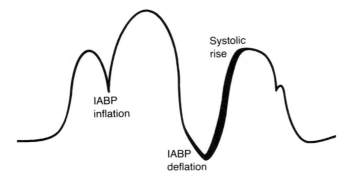

Figure 12–5. Arterial pressure trigger. Systolic rise initiates deflation.

Internal Trigger

An internal trigger is also available. This trigger signal is an electronically generated trigger within the IABP console. The rate for this trigger signal may be set by the console or may be selected by the operator (Fig. 12–6). Use of this type of trigger signal is recommended during cardiopulmonary bypass to simulate pulsatile flow.

The use of the internal trigger during cardiopulmonary resuscitation (CPR) is more controversial. The controversy stems from the following question: *Is it more effective to utilize the*

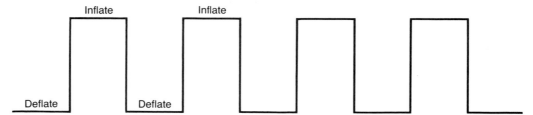

Figure 12–6. Internal trigger. No ECG or arterial pressure is visualized, only internal trigger markers are used.

arterial pressure trigger in hopes of synchronizing balloon inflation/deflation with CPR or to use the internal trigger without regard to CPR synchronization? Theoretically, IABP augmentation can be synchronized with an arterial blood pressure generated by CPR and can assist with the systemic perfusion of vital organs. IABP synchronization with CPR may be difficult to attain and, at present, there is an absence of research demonstrating this practice as being effective.

On the other side of the controversy are those who advocate the use of the internal trigger during CPR. The primary goal with regard to the IAB during a cardiac arrest is to keep the balloon surface moving to prevent thrombus formation. The IABP should never be turned off for more than 20–30 minutes under **any** conditions. Therefore, an internal trigger should be utilized to ensure balloon membrane movement during CPR while the resuscitating personnel concentrate solely on performing adequate CPR. The question to be answered in regard to internal triggering during CPR is: *Can the potential of an inflated balloon against the pressure changes created by CPR be nonproductive in assisting perfusion?* As stated earlier, research is needed to help answer this question.

Irregular Rhythms

Irregular R–R intervals present a problem in efforts to attain consistent, optimal IABP augmentation. The computer software within the IABP consoles monitors the consistency of R–R intervals. If the R–R intervals are regular, effective IABP augmentation can be achieved. When an R wave is detected as being early within the monitored R–R intervals (i.e., atrial fibrillation, atrial flutter, PVCs, etc.), the IABP console immediately deflates the balloon. Many IABP consoles have the availability of automatic R wave deflation with irregular rhythms, which disables operator's deflation control and allows only the IABP console to provide deflation according to the occurrence of a premature R wave. Early R wave balloon deflation does not always guarantee optimal augmentation. In order to facilitate better IABP augmentation, attempts should be aimed toward restoring a regular rhythm.

General Statement Concerning Triggering

No specific trigger mode may work all the time for a specific rhythm or condition on all patients. The clinician must be able to understand the presented rhythm and the triggering capabilities of the institution's particular IABP console to effectively obtain optimal augmentation.

Timing

Properly Timed Augmented Waveform

Landmarks for a properly timed augmented waveform are outlined in Figure 12–7. Because various abbreviations are used by different manufacturers of IABPs, we have provided a key in the legend to explain the abbreviations used.

General rules of timing are listed below:

1. IABP assist ratio (wean control) should be set on a 1:2 mode. Proper assessment of an augmented waveform can only be accomplished by comparing it with an unaugmented waveform.
2. Use the arterial line for assessment and manipulation of timing.
3. Set inflation first, then optimize deflation.

Appropriate Inflation

Inflation should occur during diastole. As stated earlier, diastole begins upon closure of the aortic valve. Aortic valve closure is represented on the arterial waveform by the dicrotic notch (DN). The IABP inflation point should be at the dicrotic notch. Listed below are other general rules to follow for proper inflation.

1. A V-shaped appearance should be present at the inflation point (see D on Fig. 12–7).
2. The dicrotic notch should not be visible at the inflation point (see D on Fig. 12–7).
3. Compare the inflation point of the augmented beat with the dicrotic notch of the preceding beat's dicrotic notch. The inflation point should be within two small boxes of the preceding beat's dicrotic notch on the graphic paper (see C and D on Fig. 12–7).
4. The peak diastolic pressure (PDP) should be higher than the patient's systolic pressure (PSP) (see B and F on Fig. 12–7).

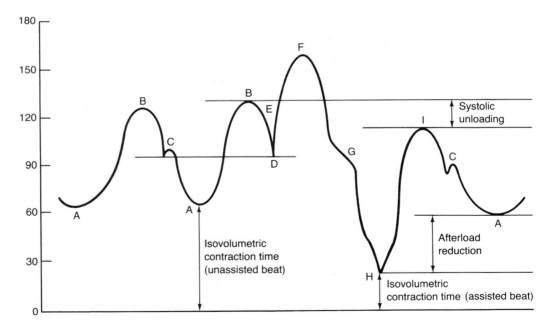

Figure 12–7. Properly timed augmented arterial waveform. (A = patient's aortic end-diastolic pressure [PAEDP]; B = patient's systolic pressure [PSP]; C = dicrotic notch [DN]; D = inflation point [IP]; E = IABP inflation; F = peak diastolic pressure [PDP]; G = IABP deflation with plateau; H = balloon aortic end-diastolic pressure [BAEDP]; I = assisted systolic pressure [ASP].)

Inflation Timing Errors

Early. Early inflation occurs before the aortic valve closes (before the dicrotic notch). This limits the systolic volume ejected from the heart and reduces the amount of aortic volume available for perfusion (Fig. 12–8). This timing error can be unsafe, especially with compromised myocardium at risk. Early inflation can cause premature closure of the aortic valve and incomplete ventricular emptying, thereby reducing an already diminished stroke volume.

Late. If inflation is late, time has allowed the systolic volume (stroke volume) to run off into the periphery, which decreases the potential aortic blood volume to be displaced. Although this situation is not detrimental to the patient, the therapeutic effect of balloon inflation during the entire diastolic phase is reduced (Fig. 12–9).

Appropriate Deflation

Rules for appropriate balloon deflation are as follows:

1. A V-shaped appearance should be present at the balloon aortic end-diastolic pressure (BAEDP) point (see H on Fig. 12–7).
2. The BAEDP should be lower than the patient's aortic end-diastolic pressure (PAEDP) (see H and A on Fig. 12–7).
3. If the above is correct, the assisted systolic pressure (ASP) should be lower than the PSP (see I and B on Fig. 12–7).

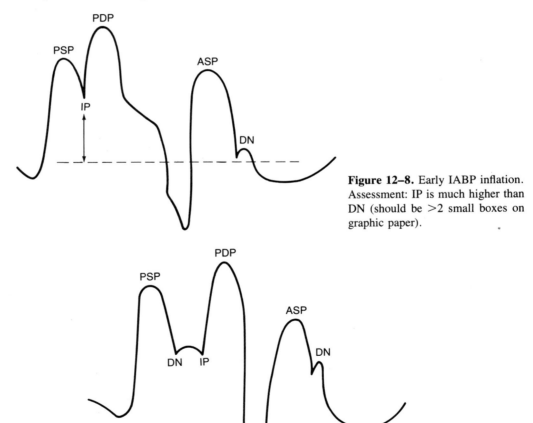

Figure 12–8. Early IABP inflation. Assessment: IP is much higher than DN (should be >2 small boxes on graphic paper).

Figure 12–9. Late IABP inflation. Assessment: DN is visualized at the IP. Absence of V-shaped appearance at the IP.

When the BAEDP is lower than the PAEDP, afterload reduction has been achieved (see A and H on Fig. 12–7). The balloon has deflated just prior to the next systolic beat. The volume of blood ejected into the aorta by the LV has been displaced out of the aorta with balloon inflation, leaving a lower pressure in the aorta upon balloon deflation. A decreased pressure in the aorta means less work has been exerted by the left ventricle and the isovolumetric contraction time has been reduced. This concept is known as systolic unloading (see B and I on Fig. 12–7). The next systolic beat following balloon deflation has been "unloaded" by the afterload reduction induced by balloon deflation.

Deflation Timing Errors

Early. Early deflation occurs far in advance of the next systolic contraction. This situation lowers the aortic end-diastolic pressure, but due to the length of time prior to the next systolic beat, the aortic end-diastolic pressure rises to the normal PAEDP. Because the IAB has deflated early, retrograde blood fills the "space" created by balloon deflation during the remaining diastolic time. No afterload reduction is achieved. It would then follow that no systolic unloading, no shortening of the isovolumetric contraction period, and no reduction in the myocardial oxygen consumption has been achieved either (Fig. 12–10).

Late. Late deflation involves leaving the balloon inflated as the next systolic beat occurs. The result is an increase in the BAEDP above or equal to the PAEDP and, subsequently, an increase in the workload on the left ventricle. A longer period of isovolumetric contraction is required for the generation of enough pressure to overcome not only the aortic valve but also an inflated balloon. The left ventricle is frequently unable to generate the same systolic pressure on late deflation beats as compared with the unaugmented beats. This is visualized by the ASP being lower than the PSP. This occurs, not because of systolic unloading, but because of the impedance to stroke volume ejection (Fig. 12–11).

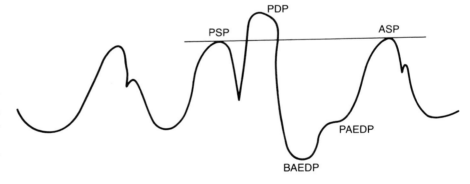

Figure 12–10. Early IABP deflation. Assessment: Absence of V-shaped appearance at BAEDP. PSP is the same as ASP. No systolic unloading.

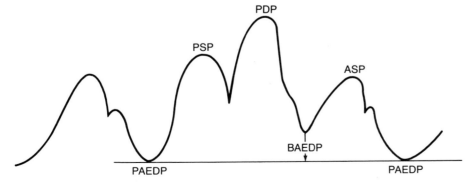

Figure 12–11. Late IABP deflation. Assessment: BAEDP is higher than PAEDP. IVC time is lengthened.

Balloon Waveforms

Balloon waveforms indicate the status of pressure inside the balloon catheter. Balloon waveforms can be used to detect catheter leaks, balloon obstruction, kinking, or overpressurization. Not all IABP consoles provide balloon waveform tracings, but when available and used in correlation with the augmented arterial waveform, they can facilitate troubleshooting of the IABP.

Normal

Landmarks of the normal balloon waveform are shown in Figure 12–12.

The width of the normal balloon waveform is the duration of balloon inflation during the diastolic phase. Therefore, the width of the balloon waveform from baseline to baseline (B to H on Fig. 12–12) should be the same as the distance between the inflation point and the lowest point of the BAEDP on the augmented arterial waveform. The width of balloon inflation will vary depending on the patient's heart rate. The slower the heart rate and longer the diastolic time, the longer the balloon inflation time. Heart rates with a short diastolic phase (tachycardias) will have a narrow balloon pressure waveform (Fig. 12–13).

The balloon plateau pressure should reflect the arterial pressure within the aorta upon IABP inflation. Therefore, the plateau pressure should be within ± 15–25 mm Hg of the PDP on the augmented arterial waveform. The balloon plateau can often be reflected in the augmented arterial waveform (see E and F on Fig. 12–12). Tachycardias will shorten the plateau time in the balloon waveform and also on the arterial waveform to the point where it is indistinguishable.

The height of the balloon waveform represents the driving pressure necessary for balloon inflation. If an increased resistance is transmitted on the balloon catheter, an increased driving pressure will be necessary to inflate the balloon. Hypertensive patients will demonstrate high balloon waveforms. Shorter balloon waveforms indicate that the driving pressure required to fully inflate the balloon was minimal. Hypotensive patients will demonstrate short waveforms.

Many IABP consoles provide the availability of volume control, which allows the operator

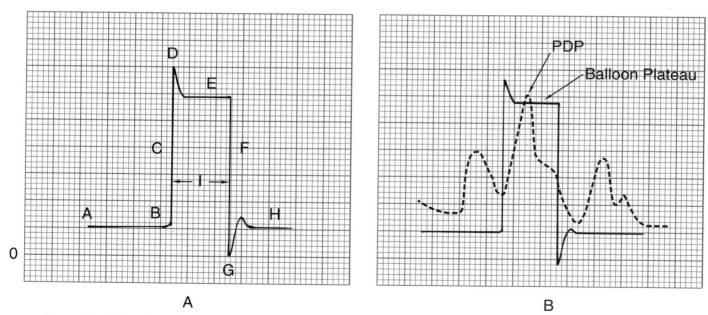

Figure 12–12. *A,* Normal balloon waveform. A = baseline; B = inflation point; C = inflation; D = inflation overshoot (artifact); E = balloon plateau; F = deflation; G = deflation undershoot (artifact); H = return to baseline; I = duration of inflation. *B,* Normal balloon waveform with augmented arterial waveform superimposed.

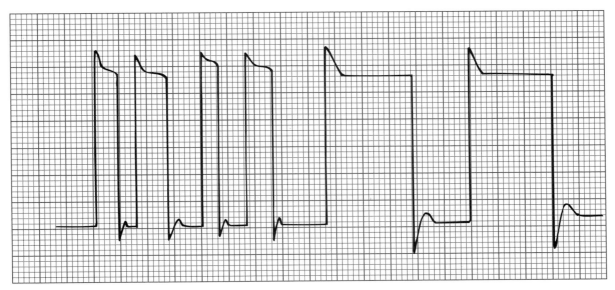

Figure 12–13. The effect of varying heart rate on balloon waveform.

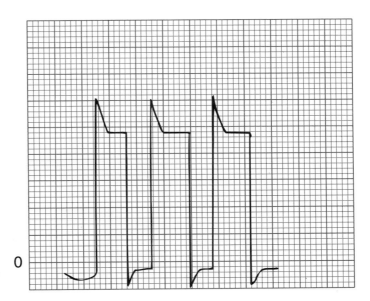

Figure 12–14. A low baseline indicates system leakage.

to determine the percent of gas volume to be delivered to the balloon catheter upon inflation. Some institutions utilize the method of decreasing the volume of gas within the catheter as part of a weaning process from the IABP. When the balloon volume is decreased, a shorter waveform will appear in response to the lower driving pressure required to attain the decreased volume.

Low Baseline

A low or falling baseline on the balloon waveform reflects leakage in the system (Fig. 12–14). Leakage could be in the form of loose connections or balloon rupture. Balloon rupture is usually immediately identified by the presence of blood in the connecting tubing.

High Baseline

A high baseline (above +25 mm Hg) indicates an overpressurized system (Fig. 12–15). IABP consoles have a surveillance system that automatically vents gas pressure accumulated to a dangerous level. If the pressure within the system reaches the level of +25 mm Hg, then the system will automatically shut off and the alarm will sound. Maintenance service of the IABP console may be required.

High Plateau

A high balloon waveform plateau pressure indicates an occlusion of the balloon catheter. The gas shuttled through the catheter upon balloon inflation is obstructed and pressure is reflected back to the IABP console as greatly increased (Fig. 12–16). Conditions that could cause an obstruction are kinked tubing, increased intrathoracic pressure (e.g., coughing, Valsalva), balloon catheter too large for patient's aorta, balloon displacement, and hypertension. Com-

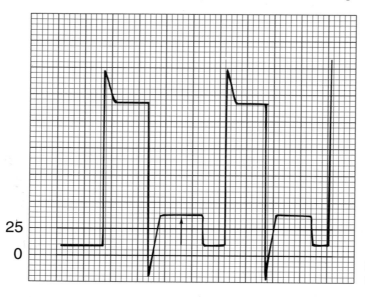

Figure 12–15. A high baseline indicates an overpressurized system.

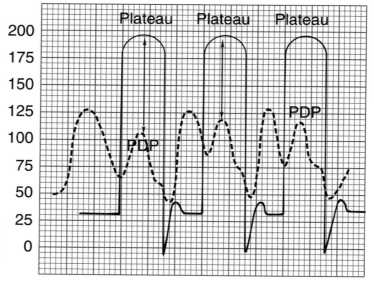

Figure 12–16. A high plateau indicates balloon obstruction. Note the >25 mm Hg difference between balloon plateau and PDP.

paring the patient's augmented arterial waveform with the balloon waveform allows the clinician to identify an obstruction. If the balloon catheter is obstructed and cannot fully inflate, its ability to augment the patient's diastolic pressure is limited. A relatively low PDP will be present on the arterial waveform and a tall, rounded waveform will be present on the balloon pressure waveform. In this situation, the balloon waveform plateau is not within ±15–25 mm Hg of the PDP.

ADVANCED PHYSIOLOGIC CONCEPTS OF COUNTERPULSATION

This section provides the clinician with a broader scientific foundation for understanding counterpulsation physiology.

Factors Involved with Peak Diastolic Pressure (IABP Inflation)

Diastolic Pressure–Time Index

The diastolic pressure–time index (DPTI) is the measurement of time and pressure under the curve of diastole on an arterial waveform. This measurement translates into the amount of blood available for perfusion or, in other words, the availability of oxygen.[119] As illustrated in Figure 12–17, the area under the curve (the diastolic pressure–time index) has greatly increased with balloon inflation. The length of time for diastole did not change, but the pressure

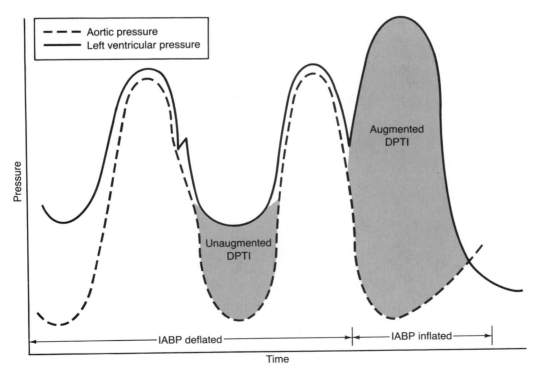

Figure 12–17. Diastolic pressure–time index (DPTI).

during diastole was increased with balloon inflation. The DPTI can be visualized by viewing the area under the PDP curve. The concept of DPTI is summarized in this equation:

$$DPTI = \text{mean diastolic pressure} - \text{duration of diastole}$$

Windkessel Effect

The Windkessel effect involves the stretch of the aortic fibers from the pressure head generated by the ejected stroke volume. This pressure head creates a slight rebound in the aorta, which produces a pulsatile effect in and of itself. IABP inflation enhances the Windkessel effect within the aorta.[120]

Aortic Compliance

Aortic compliance is defined as the elasticity of the aorta. If the aorta is very compliant, the diastolic augmentation upon balloon inflation will be reduced. The energy of IABP inflation and blood displacement may be partially absorbed by the compliant aortic walls. It is very difficult to achieve good diastolic augmentation on children, who have very elastic aortas.[121] Elderly and hypertensive patients tend to have noncompliant aortas, and higher PDPs are easily obtained.

Physical Properties of the IABP Catheter

The higher the volume in an IABP catheter, the higher the augmentation. Also, the more occlusive the catheter is inside the aorta, the higher the augmentation. However, there are limitations due to internal wall damage and red blood cell destruction if the catheter is 100% occlusive within the aorta. Ninety to 95% occlusion is acceptable.

IABP catheter configuration should be a shape that neither traps volume nor causes excessive wall pressure.

The gas used to inflate the balloon needs to be light to ensure fast transit times. Helium is the best choice because of its lower molecular weight.

Factors Involved with Aortic End-Diastolic Pressure (IABP Deflation)

Static and Dynamic Work

As stated earlier, afterload reduction is seen by comparing the BAEDP with the PAEDP. This measurement is also a reflection of static work. Static work refers to the development and maintenance of ventricular pressure prior to the aortic valve opening. The higher the aortic end-diastolic pressure, the greater the static workload. Static work is a reflection of isometric effort, which requires large amounts of myocardial oxygen. If static work and afterload can be measured by comparing the aortic end-diastolic pressures, so can myocardial oxygen consumption. Bolooki[119] states that for every 10–15 mm Hg difference between BAEDP and PAEDP, there is an approximate 5% change in myocardial oxygen consumption.

Dynamic work occurs during the process of ventricular ejection. It reflects the energy required to move the blood out of the heart. This can be measured when assessing systolic unloading by comparing the PSP with the ASP (Fig. 12–18).

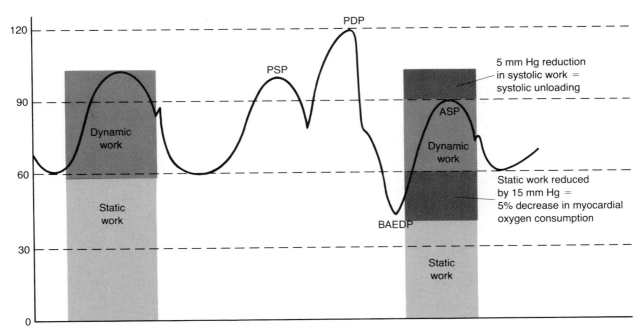

Figure 12–18. Static and dynamic work.

Tension-Time Index

The tension-time index (TTI) refers to the pressure exerted by the left ventricle during systole. This is a reflection of oxygen demand or myocardial oxygen consumption.[122,123] It is measured as the area under the systolic curve on the arterial waveform (from the end-diastolic pressure to the dicrotic notch). If afterload reduction is induced by balloon deflation, systolic unloading or a decreased TTI will follow. TTI and systolic unloading can both be indirectly measured by comparing the PSP and ASP (Fig. 12–19). The equation that summarizes the concept of TTI is:

$$TTI = mean\ systolic\ pressure\ -\ duration\ of\ systole$$

dP/dT Ratio

When afterload reduction is present (as in appropriate IABP deflation), the left ventricle is not required to generate as much pressure to open the aortic valve. If less pressure is required for ejection, then less time is also required. This relationship between changes in pressure and time is referred to as the dP/dT ratio (d = change; P = pressure; T = time).[119] This can be measured and visually observed by looking at the upstroke of rapid ejection on the arterial waveform. If high afterload is present, the period of isovolumetric contraction must be lengthened to allow enough time for the required left ventricular pressure to be generated. The slope of the rapid ejection upstroke will be more horizontal. This reflects the longer time period needed to generate the required pressures to open the aortic valve, thereby causing an increase in MVO$_2$ and a high dP/dT ratio. With afterload reduction present, a more vertical upstroke is observed. Less time is required to generate the pressure needed to open the aortic valve. By

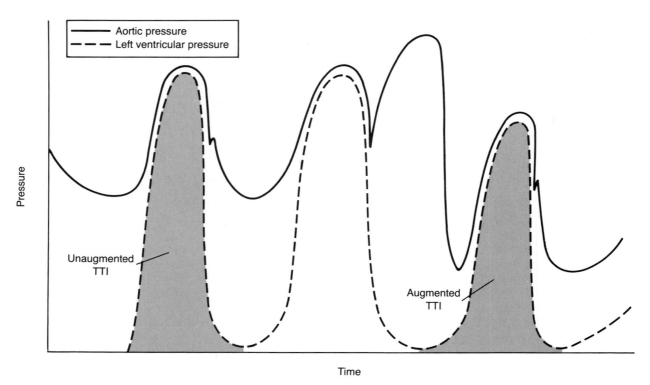

Figure 12–19. Tension-time index (TTI).

comparing the upstrokes of the PSP and the ASP, one can observe the difference in dP/dT ratios as the result of afterload reduction induced by balloon deflation (Fig. 12–20).

Overall Assessment of Cardiac Function

Endocardial Viability Ratio

The endocardial viability ratio (EVR) reflects the balance between oxygen supply and demand by comparing the DPTI with TTI.[124] The DPTI reflects myocardial blood flow with balloon inflation and can be used as an index of oxygen supply. The TTI is related to myocardial oxygen consumption or oxygen demand. The ratio of DPTI to TTI is related to the balance between oxygen supply and demand (Fig. 12–21). An EVR value of 1.0 or higher signifies a normal myocardial supply/demand balance. An EVR of less than 0.7 usually indicates severe myocardial ischemia. It has been suggested that the EVR be used as a prognostic predictor of LV survival and as an early indicator of IABP utilization. Research is still needed to determine the accuracy of the EVR.

SUMMARY

In many institutions, nurses have the primary responsibility for IABP timing and troubleshooting and are frequently the initial assessor of the patient's hemodynamic status. Nurses who are manipulating IABP timing must be aware of how the changes they implement will affect the patient. The physiologic concepts presented in this chapter provide a strong basis for the comprehension of augmented waveform analysis. With this information, the clinician can better

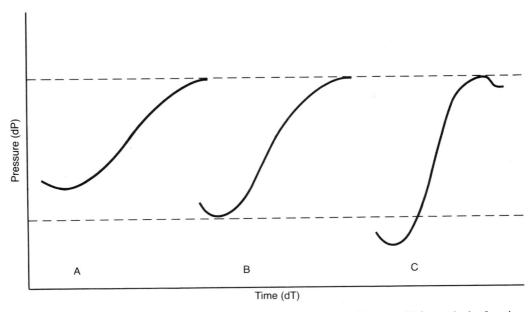

Figure 12–20. dP/dT ratio with arterial pressure waveform upstroke. *A*, Depressed left ventricular function illustrated by a horizontal upstroke. *B*, Normal left ventricular function illustrated by a more vertical upstroke. *C*, Hyperdynamic left ventricular function illustrated by a very sharp upstroke.

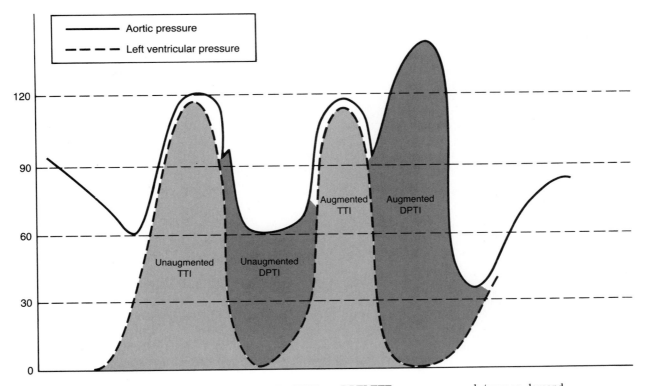

Figure 12–21. Endocardial viability ratio (EVR) = DPTI/TTE = oxygen supply/oxygen demand.

understand and discuss the physiologic and hemodynamic implications of counterpulsation and provide a high level of nursing care to the patient requiring an IABP.

PRACTICE WAVEFORMS

We have provided Practice Waveforms to help the clinician apply the information in this chapter. The four major timing problems are addressed in these waveforms. On the correlating ECG, assist markers are evident. These markers indicate where the IABP is triggering inflation and deflation. The arterial waveform will be the reference for the assessment of IABP timing.

PRACTICE WAVEFORM 12–1. For the following waveform, identify the wean control or assist ratio and describe the balloon's inflation and deflation.

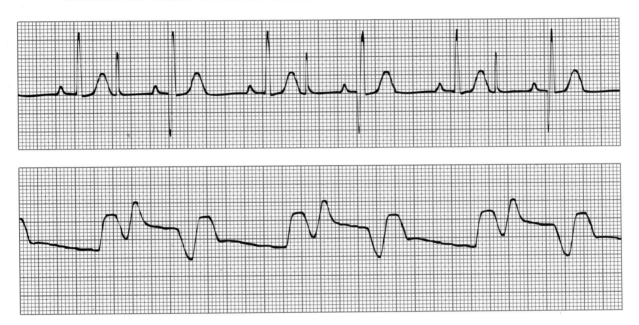

PRACTICE WAVEFORM 12–1. *Analysis:* Wean control: 1:2 or 2:1; the IABP is assisting every other beat.

Inflation: OK.
1. V-shaped appearance at the inflation point (IP).
2. IP within 2 small boxes of preceding beat's dicrotic notch.
3. PDP higher than PSP.
4. Dicrotic notch not visible.

Deflation: OK
1. V-shaped appearance at BAEDP.
2. BAEDP is lower than PAEDP.
3. ASP is lower than PSP.

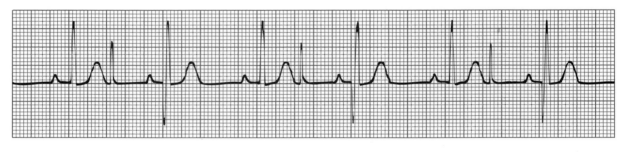

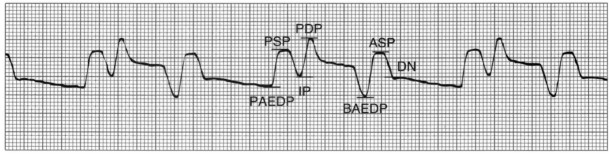

PRACTICE WAVEFORM 12–2. For the following waveform, identify the wean control or assist ratio and describe the balloon's inflation and deflation.

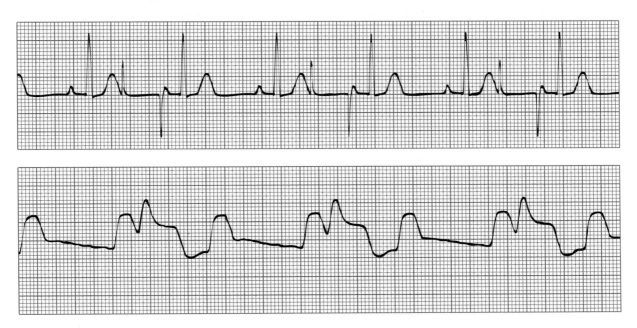

PRACTICE WAVEFORM 12–2. *Analysis:* Wean control: 1:2

Inflation: OK

1. V-shaped appearance.
2. IP within 2 small boxes of dicrotic notch.
3. PDP is higher than PSP.

Deflation: Early

1. U-shaped appearance at BAEDP.
2. Able to visualize PAEDP after BAEDP. Increased aortic pressure after peripheral run-off.
3. No difference in PSP and ASP. No systolic unloading.

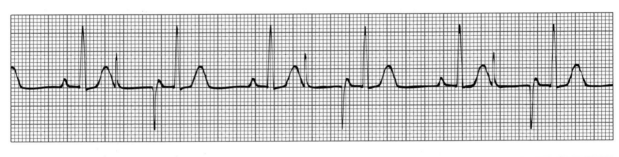

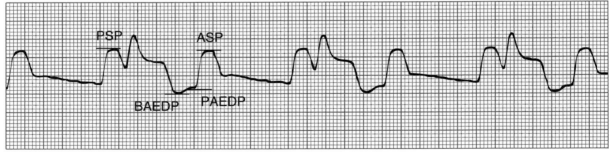

PRACTICE WAVEFORM 12–3. For the following waveform, identify the wean control or assist ratio and describe the balloon's inflation and deflation.

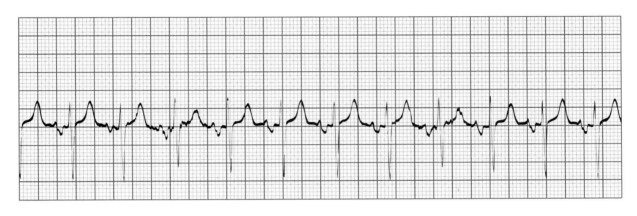

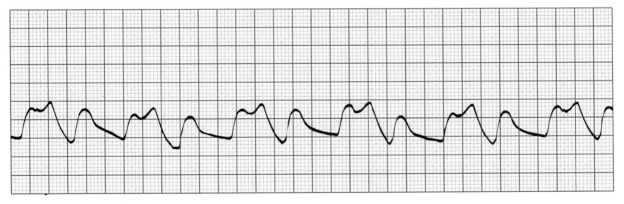

PRACTICE WAVEFORM 12–3. *Analysis:* Wean control: 1:2

Inflation: Early

1. IP is greater than 2 small boxes away from the preceding beat's dicrotic notch. Early inflation is detrimental to the patient and represents balloon inflation prior to aortic valve closure.

Deflation: OK

1. V-shaped appearance to BAEDP.
2. BAEDP lower than PAEDP = afterload reduction.
3. ASP lower than PSP = systolic unloading.

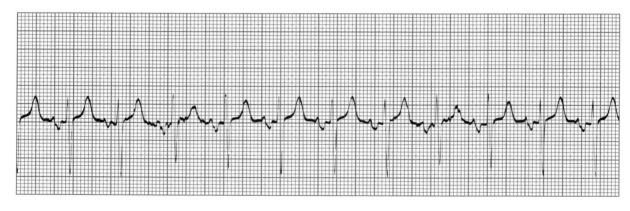

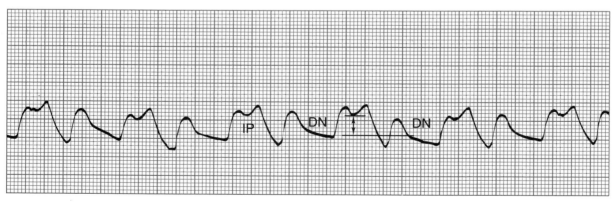

Practice Waveform 12–4. For the following waveform, identify the wean control or assist ratio and describe the balloon's inflation and deflation.

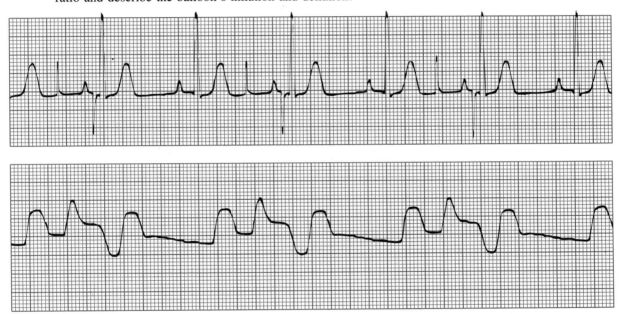

Practice Waveform 12–4. *Analysis:* Wean control: 1:2

Inflation: Late

1. No V-shaped appearance at IP.
2. Dicrotic notch is visible.

Deflation: OK

1. BAEDP is lower than PAEDP.
2. ASP is lower than PSP.
3. More of a U-shaped appearance at the BAEDP, but because afterload reduction and systolic unloading are attained, deflation timing is appropriate.

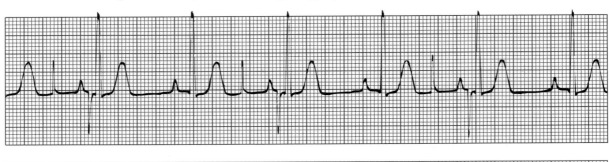

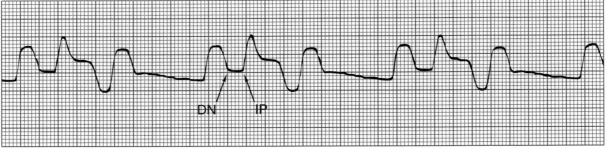

Practice Waveform 12–5. For the following waveform, identify the wean control or assist ratio and describe the balloon's inflation and deflation.

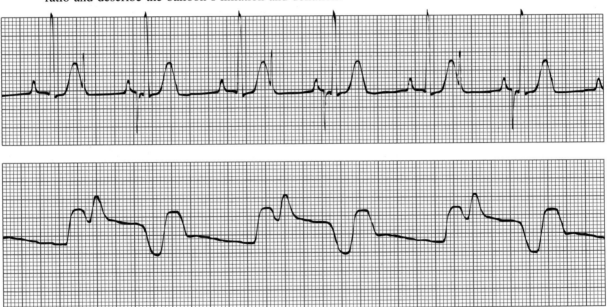

Practice Waveform 12–5. *Analysis:* Wean control: 1:2
Inflation: Early
1. IP is greater than 2 small boxes away from preceding beat's dicrotic notch.
Deflation: OK

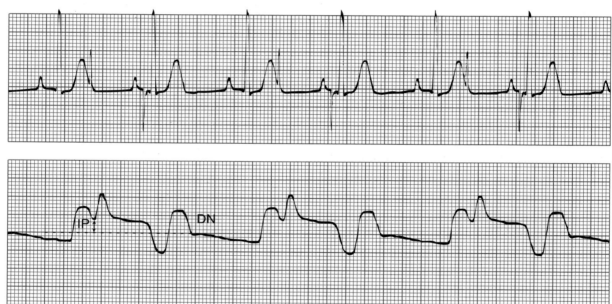

Practice Waveform 12–6. For the following waveform, identify the wean control or assist ratio and describe the balloon's inflation and deflation.

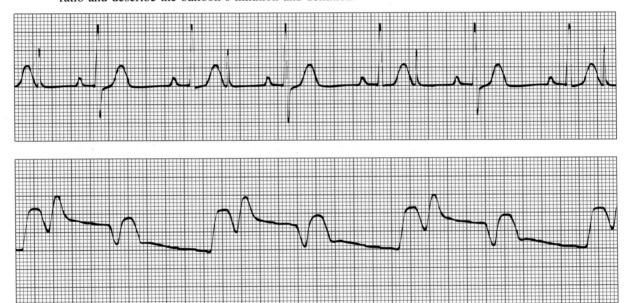

Practice Waveform 12–6. *Analysis:* Wean control: 1:2

Inflation: OK

Deflation: Late

1. BAEDP is higher than PAEDP.
2. ASP is lower than PSP, but not because of systolic unloading. The IAB is still inflated during IVC, limiting the ejection pressure of the next beat. The lower ASP reflects this limited ejection. This is detrimental to the patient.

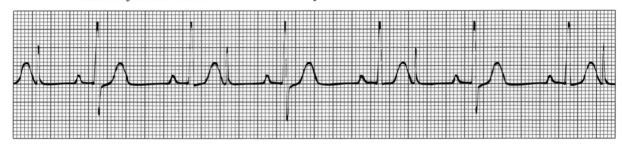

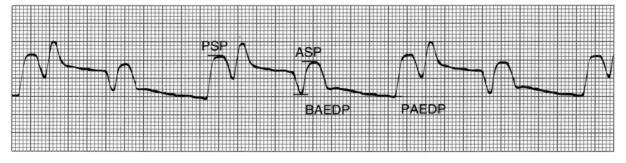

PRACTICE CLINICAL SCENARIOS

Case study scenarios are also included to provide a stronger clinical basis for waveform analysis. The two scenarios discussed involve dysrhythmias that often present difficulty from the standpoint of IABP timing.

Practice Clinical Scenario 12–1. This patient is a 50-year-old white man with the diagnosis of ischemic cardiomyopathy. His past medical history includes coronary artery disease and congestive heart failure with medical regimen of nitrates and calcium channel blocking agent. He presented with angina refractory to medication. A cardiac catheterization revealed 70% right coronary artery, 90% left anterior descending coronary artery, 90% posterior descending artery. Coronary artery bypass grafting was elected. Difficulty was experienced when attempting to wean the patient from the bypass machine. An intra-aortic balloon pump (IABP) was inserted and the patient was transferred to the cardiovascular intensive care unit on the following:

> IABP, wean control at 1:2
> Epinephrine 1.75 μg/min
> Amrinone 13 μg/kg/min
> Norepinephrine 2 μg/min
> Dobutamine 6 μg/min
> Nitroglycerin 100 μg/min

Approximately 6 hours postop, patient experienced two runs of non-sustained ventricular tachycardia (VT) (see waveform). What is your assessment of the IABP timing (wean control or assist ratio, inflation, and deflation) and the rationale for the improper timing with the VT?

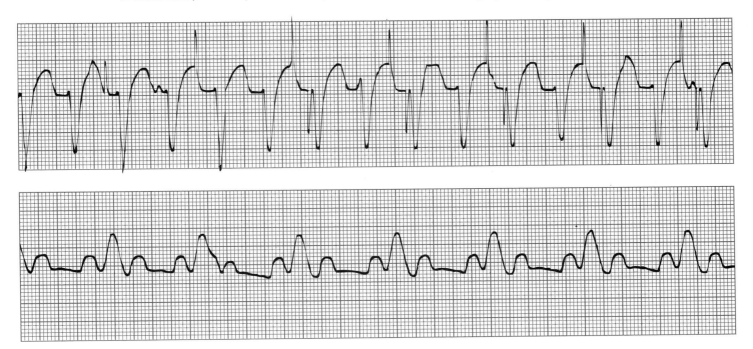

Practice Clinical Scenario 12–1. *Analysis:*

Wean control: 1:2

Inflation: OK

1. V-shaped appearance at IP.
2. IP within 2 small boxes of preceding beat's dicrotic notch.
3. PDP higher than PSP.
4. Dicrotic notch not visible.

Deflation: Late with ventricular tachycardia.

1. BAEDP is higher than PAEDP with VT. The inflate/deflate cycle of the IABP is averaged on a group of approximately 8 beats or more. Sudden changes in heart rate may not be picked up immediately. This accounts for the late deflation. Note at the end of the VT, deflation is starting to occur earlier as the IABP senses this faster rate. Note the last augmented beat's deflation is early. This is secondary to the sudden conversion back into sinus rhythm, which the IABP did not sense immediately.

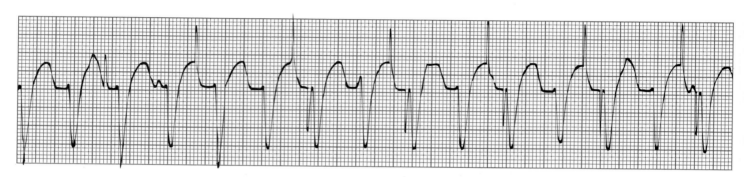

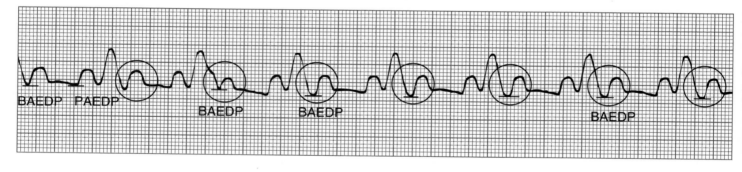

Practice Clinical Scenario 12–2. A 76-year-old woman presented with complaints of squeezing chest pain and shortness of breath. Her past medical history included chronic obstructive pulmonary disease × 20 years, peptic ulcer disease, no prior cardiac history. She displayed pulmonary edema and her ECG revealed sinus tachycardia. Despite therapy with diuretics, nitrates, and oxygen, she became increasingly hypotensive and developed mental confusion. Hemodynamic observations confirmed left ventricular pump failure and cardiogenic shock. Dobutamine was added to the regimen, which temporarily improved stroke volume. The patient soon decompensated further with development of atrial fibrillation. An IABP was inserted and set on a 1:1 wean control. Assess the IABP timing (wean control or assist ratio, inflation, and deflation) and determine the reason for any errors in timing.

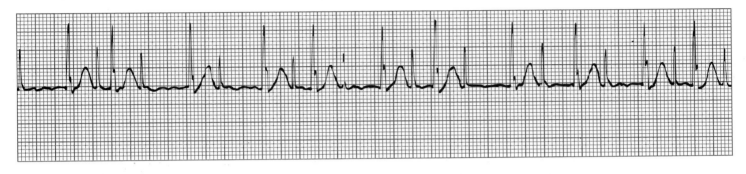

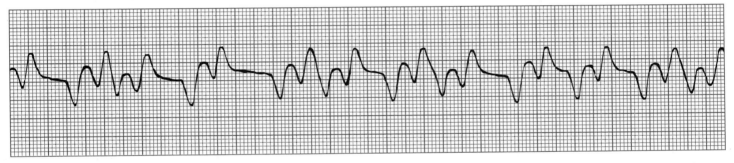

Practice Clinical Scenario 12–2. *Analysis:*

Wean control: 1:1

Inflation: OK

1. V-shaped appearance at IP.
2. IP within 2 small boxes of preceding beat's dicrotic notch.
3. PDP higher than PSP.
4. Dicrotic notch not visible.

Deflation: Late deflation on early R waves. The inflate-deflate cycle of the IABP is averaged on a group of approximately 8 beats or more. Any beats occurring prior to the preset R–R interval that the IABP is expecting will result in late deflation. The recommendation for appropriate timing in this patient is to convert the atrial fibrillation rhythm back into sinus rhythm. IABP provides optimal augmentation with ECG rhythms possessing regular R–R intervals.

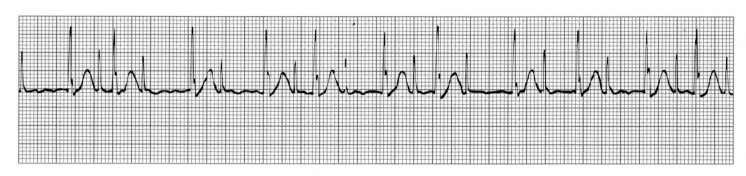

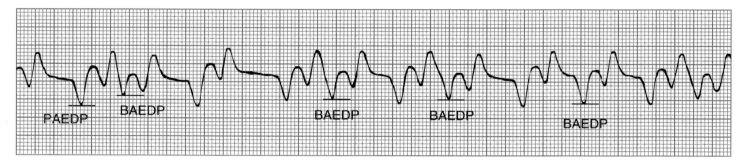

References

1. Maran AG: Variables in pulmonary capillary wedge pressure: Variation with intrathoracic pressure, graphic and digital recorders. Crit Care Med 8:102–105, 1980.

2. Schmitt EA and Brantigan CO: Common artifacts of pulmonary artery and pulmonary artery wedge pressure: Recognition and interpretation. J Clin Monit 2:44–52, 1986.

3. MacKensie J: The interpretation of the pulsation in the jugular vein. Am J Med Sci 134:12–34, 1907.

4. Wiggers CJ: Pressure Pulses in the Cardiovascular System. London: Longmans, Green & Co, 1928.

5. Wiggers CJ and Feil H: The cardiodynamics of mitral insufficiency. Heart 9:149–183, 1922.

6. Wiggers CJ and Katz LN: The contour of ventricular volume curves under different conditions. Am J Physiol 58:439–475, 1922.

7. Dexter L et al: Oxygen content of pulmonary "capillary" blood in unanaesthetized human beings. J Clin Invest 25:913, 1946.

8. Hellems HK et al: Pulmonary capillary pressure in animals estimated by venous and arterial catheterization. Am J Physiol 155:98–105, 1948.

9. Lagerlof H and Werko L: Studies on the circulation of blood in man. VI. The pulmonary "capillary" venous pressure in man. Scand J Clin Lab Invest 1:147–161, 1949.

10. Hellems HU, Haynes FW and Dexter L: Pulmonary "capillary" pressure in man. J Appl Physiol 2:24–29, 1949.

11. Swan HJC et al: Catheterization of the heart in man with use of a flow-directed balloon-tipped catheter. N Engl J Med 283:447–451, 1970.

12. Lappas D et al: Indirect measurement of left atrial pressure in surgical patients — pulmonary-capillary wedge and pulmonary artery diastolic pressures compared with left atrial pressure. Anesthesiology 38:394–397, 1973.

13. Zimmerman HA: Pressure curve analysis. *In* Intravascular Catheterization. Springfield IL: CC Thomas, 1966, pp 294–297.

14. Seely RD: Dynamic effect of inspiration on the simultaneous stroke volumes of the right and left ventricles. Am J Physiol 154:273–280, 1948.

15. Neustadt JE and Shaffer AB: Diagnostic value of the left atrial pressure pulse in mitral valvular disease. Am Heart J 58:675–688, 1959.

16. Constant J: Bedside Cardiology. Boston: Little, Brown & Co, 1985, pp 79–85.

17. Falicov RE and Resnekov L: Relationship of the pulmonary artery end-diastolic pressure to the left ventricular end-diastolic and mean filling pressures in patients with and without left ventricular dysfunction. Circulation 42:65–73, 1970.

18. Haskell RJ and French WJ: Accuracy of left atrial and pulmonary artery wedge pressure in pure mitral regurgitation in predicting left ventricular end-diastolic pressure. Am J Cardiol 61:136–141, 1988.

19. Wilson RR et al: Pulmonary artery diastolic and wedge pressure relationships in critically ill and injured patients. Arch Surg 123:933–936, 1988.

20. Dantzker DR: Diagnosis of secondary pulmonary hypertension: Invasive techniques. Heart Lung 15:423–429, 1986.

21. Goldenheim PD and Kazemi H: Cardiopulmonary

monitoring of critically ill patients (second of two parts). N Engl J Med 311:776–780, 1984.

22. Morris AH and Chapman RH: Wedge pressure confirmation by aspiration of pulmonary capillary blood. Crit Care Med 13:756–759, 1985.

23. Schriner DK: Using hemodynamic waveforms to assess cardiopulmonary pathologies. Crit Care Nurs Clin North Am 1:563–575, 1989.

24. Bloomfield RA et al: Recording of right heart pressures in normal subjects and in patients with chronic pulmonary disease and various types of cardiocirculatory disease. J Clin Invest 25:639–664, 1946.

25. Sapru RP, Taylor SH, and Donald DW: Comparison of the pulmonary wedge pressure with the left ventricular end diastolic pressure in man. Clin Sci 34:125–140, 1968.

26. Braunwald E and Awe WB: Syndrome of severe mitral regurgitation with normal left atrial pressure. Circulation 27:29–35, 1963.

27. Downes TR et al: Frequency of large V waves in the PAWP in ventricular septal defect of acquired (during AMI) or congenital origin. Am J Cardiol 60:415–417, 1987.

28. Picard AD et al: Large V waves without mitral regurgitation. Am J Cardiol 50:1044–1050, 1982.

29. Fuchs RM: Limitation of pulmonary wedge V wave in diagnosing mitral regurgitation. Am J Cardiol 49:849–854, 1982.

30. Vender JS: Invasive cardiac monitoring. Crit Care Clin 4:455–477, 1988.

31. Rushmer RF: Cardiovascular Physiology, 4th ed. Philadelphia: WB Saunders, 1976, pp 180–182.

32. Little RC: Physiology of the Heart and Circulation, 3rd ed. Chicago: Yearbook Medical Publishers, 1985, pp 94–95.

33. Daily EK and Schroeder JS: Hemodynamic Waveforms. St. Louis: CV Mosby, 1990.

34. Milnor WR: Cardiovascular Physiology. New York: Oxford University Press, 1990, p 113.

35. Balcon R, Bennett ED, and Sowton GE: Comparison of pulmonary artery diastolic and left ventricular end diastolic pressures in patients with ischaemic heart disease. Cardiovasc Res 6:172–175, 1972.

36. Ream AK: Mean blood pressure algorithms. J Clin Monit 1:138–144, 1985.

37. Ellis DM: Interpretation of beat to beat blood pressure values in the presence of ventilator changes. J Clin Monitor 1:65–70, 1985.

38. Standards and guidelines for cardiopulmonary resuscitation (CPR) and emergency cardiac care (ECC). JAMA 255:2905–2984, 1986.

39. Rankin JS et al: The effects of airway pressure on cardiac function in intact dogs and man. Circulation 66:108–120, 1982.

40. Pinsky MR: The effects of mechanical ventilation on the cardiovascular system. Crit Care Clin 6:663–678, 1990.

41. Sulzbach LM: Measurement of pulsus paradoxus. Focus Crit Care 16:142–145, 1989.

42. Marini JJ et al: Estimation of transmural cardiac pressures during ventilation with PEEP. J Appl Physiol 53:384–391, 1982.

43. Cengiz M, Crapo RO, and Gardner R: The effect of ventilation on the accuracy of pulmonary artery and wedge pressure measurement. Crit Care Med 11:502–507, 1983.

44. Rice DL et al: Wedge pressure measurement in obstructive pulmonary disease. Chest 66:628–632, 1974.

45. Downs JB: A technique for direct measurement of intrapleural pressure. Crit Care Med 4:207–210, 1976.

46. Ellis EJ, Gauer OH, and Wood EH: An intracardiac manometer: Its evaluation and application. Circulation 3:390–398, 1951.

47. Ahrens T: Airway pressure application in reading hemodynamic waveforms. Crit Care Nurse (in press).

48. Schuster DP and Seeman MD: Temporary muscle paralysis for accurate measurement of pulmonary artery occlusion pressure. Chest 84:593–597, 1983.

49. Riedinger MS, Shellock FG, and Swan HJ: Reading pulmonary artery and pulmonary capillary wedge pressure waveforms with respiratory variations. Heart Lung 10:675–677, 1981.

50. Berryhill RE, Benumof JL, and Rauscher LA: Pulmonary vascular pressure reading at the end of expiration. Anesthesiology 49:365–368, 1978.

51. Wright J and Gong H: "Auto-PEEP": Incidence, magnitude, and contributing factors. Heart Lung 19:352–357, 1990.

52. Pepe PE and Marini JJ: Occult positive end expiratory pressure in mechanically ventilated patients with airflow obstruction: The auto PEEP effect. Am Rev Resp Dis 126:166–170, 1982.

53. Geddes LA: The Direct and Indirect Measurement of Blood Pressure. Chicago: Yearbook Medical Publishers, 1970, pp 46–69.

54. Wiedemann HP, Matthay MA, and Matthay RA: Cardiovascular-pulmonary monitoring in the intensive care unit (Part 1). Chest 85:537–549, 1984.

55. Cromwell L, Weibell FJ, and Pfeiffer EA: Biomedical Instrumentation and Measurements. Englewood Cliffs, NJ: Prentice-Hall, 1980.

56. Boutros A and Albert S: Effect of the dynamic response of transducer tubing system on accuracy of direct pressure measurement in patients. Crit Care Med 11:124–127, 1983.

57. Gardner RM: Direct blood pressure measurement: Dynamic response requirements. Anesthesiology 54:227–236, 1981.

58. Rothe CF and Kim KC: Measuring systolic arterial blood pressure. Crit Care Med 8:683–689, 1980.

59. Gardner R and Hollingsworth K: ECG and pressure monitoring: How to obtain optimal results. In Shoemaker WC et al (eds): Textbook of Critical Care, 2nd ed. Philadelphia: WB Saunders, 1981, p 301.

60. Gardner R and Hollingsworth K: ECG and pressure monitoring. Crit Care Med 14:651–658, 1986.

61. Manketelow RT and Baird RJ: A practical approach to accurate pressure measurements. J Thorac Cardiovasc Surg 58:122–127, 1969.

62. Pedersen A and Husby J: Venous pressure measurement. 1. Choice of zero level. Acta Med Scand 141:185–194, 1951.

63. Russell WJ: Central Venous Pressure. London: Butterworth, 1974, pp 42–51.

64. Shasby DM et al: Swan Ganz catheter location and left atrial pressure determine the accuracy of the wedge pressure when positive end expiratory pressure is used. Chest 80:666–670, 1981.

65. Schermer L: Physiologic and technical variables affecting hemodynamic measurements. Crit Care Nurse 8:33–41, 1988.

66. Groom L, Frisch SR, and Elliot M: Reproducibility and accuracy of pulmonary artery pressure measurement in supine and lateral positions. Heart Lung 19:147–151, 1990.

67. Evaluation: Disposable pressure transducers. Health Devices 14:268–289, 1984.

68. Air embolism during calibration of invasive blood pressure monitoring systems. Health Devices 12:22–25, 1982.

69. Alternatives in calibration. Health Devices 12:22, 1982.

70. Lamantia KR and Barash PG: Arterial pressure monitoring: What are we really measuring? Cleve Clin J Med 55:415–416, 1988.

71. Stern DH et al: Can we trust the direct radial artery pressure immediately following cardiopulmonary bypass? Anesthesiology 62:557–561, 1985.

72. Abrams JH et al: Use of needle valve resistor to improve invasive blood pressure monitoring. Crit Care Med 12:978–982, 1984.

73. Robin ED: The cult of the Swan-Ganz catheter: Overuse and abuse of pulmonary artery flow catheter. Ann Intern Med 103:445–449, 1985.

74. Tachschmidt J and Sharma DP: Impact of hemodynamic monitoring in a medical ICU. Crit Care Med 15:840–843, 1987.

75. Matthay MA and Chatterjee K: Bedside catheterization of the pulmonary artery: Risks compared with benefits. Ann Intern Med 109:826–834, 1988.

76. Eisenberg PR, Jaffe AS, and Schuster DP: Clinical evaluation compared to pulmonary artery catheterization in the hemodynamic assessment of critically ill patients. Crit Care Med 12:549–553, 1984.

77. Daily EK and Schroeder JS: Techniques in Bedside Hemodynamic Monitoring, 3rd ed. St Louis: CV Mosby, 1985, pp 102–103.

78. Sprung CL: The Pulmonary Artery Catheter. Baltimore: University Park Press, 1983, pp 131–132.

79. Halfman-Franey M and Bergstrom D: Clinical management using direct and derived parameters. Crit Care Nurs Clin North Am 1:547–561, 1989.

80. Smith JJ and Kampine JP: Circulatory Physiology. Baltimore: Williams & Wilkins, 1984, p 116.

81. Starling EH: The Linacre Lecture on the Law of the Heart. London: Longmans, Green & Co, 1918.

82. Passmore JM, Byrnes TJ, and Goldstein RA: Hemodynamic support of the critically ill patient. In Dantsker D (ed): Cardiopulmonary Critical Care. Orlando: Grune & Stratton, 1986, pp 354–402.

83. Braunwald E and Ross J: The ventricular end diastolic pressure: Appraisal of its value in the recognition of ventricular failure in man. Am J Med 34:147–150, 1963.

84. Raper R and Sibbald WS: Mislead by the wedge? The Swan-Ganz catheter and left ventricular preload. Chest 89:427–434, 1986.

85. Altschule MD: Invalidity of using so-called Starling's curves in clinical medicine. Perspect Biol Med 26:171–187, 1983.

86. Milnor WR: Hemodynamics, 2nd ed. Baltimore: Williams & Wilkins, 1990, p 144.

87. Ahrens T: Extravascular lung water: Concepts in clinical application. Crit Care Nurs Clin North Am 1:681–688, 1989.

88. Loach J and Thomson NB: Hemodynamic monitoring. Philadelphia: JB Lippincott, 1987, p 9.

89. Passmore MJ and Goldstein RA: Acute recognition and management of congestive heart failure. Crit Care Clin 5:497–532, 1989.

90. Galvao M: Role of angiotensin-converting enzyme inhibitors in congestive heart failure. Heart Lung 19:505–511, 1990.

91. Colucci WS, Wright RF, and Braunwald E: New positive inotropic agents in the treatment of congestive heart failure (mechanisms of action and recent clinical developments). Part II. N Engl J Med 314:349–357, 1986.

92. Stecy P and Gunnar RM: Is intermittent dobutamine infusion useful in the treatment of patients with refractory congestive heart failure? Cardiovasc Clin 17:277–289, 1990.

93. Mueller HS: Management of acute myocardial infarction. In Shoemaker WC et al (eds): Textbook of Critical Care, 2nd ed. Philadelphia: WB Saunders, 1989, p 347.

94. Shoemaker WC et al: Comparison of hemodynamic and oxygen transport effects of dopamine and dobutamine in critically ill surgical patients. Chest 96:120–126, 1989.

95. Kelleher RM: Cardiac drugs: New inotropes. Crit Care Nurs Clin North Am 1:391–398, 1989.

96. Bristow MR et al: Decreased catecholamine sensitivity and β-adrenergic receptor density in failing human hearts. N Engl J Med 307:205–211, 1982.

97. Rice V: Shock management. Part II. Pharmacologic intervention. Crit Care Nurs 5:42–57, 1985.

98. Shoemaker WC: Comparisons of the relative effectiveness of whole blood transfusions and various types of fluid therapy in resuscitation. Crit Care Med 4:71–78, 1976.

99. Tobin MJ: Essentials of Critical Care Medicine. New York: Churchill Livingstone, 1989, p 46.

100. Marini JJ and Wheeler AP: Critical Care Medicine: The Essentials. Baltimore: Williams & Wilkins, 1989, pp 32–33.

101. Falk JL, Rackow EC, and Weil MH: Colloid and crystalloid fluid resuscitation. In Shoemaker WC et

al (eds): Textbook of Critical Care, 2nd ed. Philadelphia: WB Saunders, 1989, pp 1055–1073.

102. Skowronski GA: Hypovolemic shock. *In* Oh TE (ed): Intensive Care Manual. Brisbane: Butterworth, 1990, pp 372–373.

103. Layon AJ and Kirby RR: Fluids and electrolytes in the critically ill. *In* Critical Care. Civetta JM, Taylor RW, and Kirby RR (eds): Philadelphia: JB Lippincott, 1988, pp 461–462.

104. Guyton AC: Circulatory Physiology: Cardiac Output and Its Regulation. Philadelphia: WB Saunders, 1963, pp 355–356.

105. Summers G: The clinical and hemodynamic presentation of the shock patient. Crit Care Nurs Clin North Am 2:161–166, 1990.

106. Burns KM: Vasoactive drug therapy in shock. Crit Care Nurs Clin North Am 2:167–178, 1990.

107. Moulopulas SD, Topoz S, and Kolff NJ: Diastolic balloon pumping (with carbon dioxide) in the aorta: A mechanical assistance to the failing circulation. Am Heart J 63:669, 1962.

108. Kantrowitz A: Clinical experience with cardiac assistance by means of intra-aortic place-shift balloon pumping. Transactions of the American Society of Artifical Internal Organs 14:334, 1968.

109. Angerpointer TA et al: The long term effect of intra-aortic balloon counterpulsation on left ventricular performance. J Cardiovasc Surg 21:399, 1980.

110. Chaterjee S and Rosenweig J: Evaluation of intra-arotic balloon counterpulsation. J Thorac Cardiovasc Surg 61:405, 1971.

111. Akyurekli MD et al: Effectiveness of intra-aortic balloon counterpulsation on systolic unloading. Can J Surg 23:122, 1984.

112. Mueller et al: The effects of intra-aortic balloon counterpulsation in cardiac performance and metabolism in shock associated with acute myocardial infarction. J Clin Invest 50:1885, 1971.

113. Watson JT et al: Temporal changes in collateral coronary blood flow in ischemic myocardium during intra-aortic balloon pumping. Ann Thorac Surg 16:445, 1973.

114. Shaw J, Taylor DR, and Pitt B: Effect of IABP counterpulsation on regional coronary blood flow in experimental myocardial infarction. Am J Cardiol 34:552, 1974.

115. Gill CC et al: Augmentation and redistribution of myocardial blood flow during acute ischemia by intra-aortic pumping. Ann Thorac Surg 16:445, 1973.

116. Saini VK et al: Nutrient myocardial blood flow in experimental myocardial ischemia: Effects of IABP counterpulsation and coronary perfusion. Circulation 52:1086, 1975.

117. Chilian WM and Marcus ML: Phasic coronary blood flow velocity in intramural and epicardial coronary arteries. Circ Res 50:775, 1982.

118. Tyson GS, Davis JW, and Rankin JS: Improved performance of IABP in man. Surgical Forum 37:214, 1986.

119. Bolooki H: Clinical application of IABP. New York: Futura, 1984.

120. Berne RM and Levy MN: Cardiovascular Physiology, 4th ed, ch 5. St Louis: CV Mosby, 1981.

121. Van Breda A: Post-operative care of infants and children who require cardiac surgery. Heart Lung 14:205, 1985.

122. Sarnoff SJ et al: Hemodynamic determinants of oxygen consumption of the heart with special reference to the tension-time index. Am J Physiol 192:141, 1958.

123. Jaron D, Moore TW, and He P: Control of IABP: Theory and guidelines for clinical applications. Ann Biomed Eng 13:155, 1985.

124. Buckberg GD, Fixler DE, and Archie JP: Experimental subendocardial ischemia in dogs with normal coronary arteries. Cir Res 30:67, 1972.

APPENDIX

Abbreviations/Acronyms

A-V	atrioventricular
AMV	assisted mandatory ventilation
APC	atrial premature contraction
ASP	assisted systolic pressure
BAEDP	balloon aortic end-diastolic pressure
BP	blood pressure
bpm	breaths per minute
CI	cardiac index
CO	cardiac output
COPD	chronic obstructive pulmonary disease
CPAP	continuous positive airway pressure
CPR	cardiopulmonary resuscitation
CVP	central venous pressure
DC	damping coefficient
DN	dicrotic notch
DPTI	diastolic pressure–time index
ECG	electrocardiogram, electrocardiograph
EMD	electromechanical dissociation
EVLW	extravascular lung water
EVR	endocardial viability ratio
FR	frequency response
Hz	Hertz
I:E	inspiratory/expiratory [ratio]
IAB	intra-aortic balloon
IABP	intra-aortic balloon pump
IMV	intermittent mandatory ventilation
IP	inflation point
IVC	isovolumetric contraction
LV	left ventricular, left ventricle
LVEDP	left ventricular end-diastolic pressure
MAP	mean arterial pressure
MV_{O_2}	myocardial oxygen consumption
NSR	normal sinus rhythm
P_A	alveolar pressure

PA	pulmonary artery
$Paco_2$	partial arterial pressure of carbon dioxide
PAD	pulmonary arterial diastolic pressure
PAEDP	patient's aortic end-diastolic pressure
PAP	pulmonary artery pressure
Paw	airway pressure
Pco_2	partial pressure of carbon dioxide
PCWP	pulmonary capillary wedge pressure
PDP	peak diastolic pressure
PEEP	positive end-expiratory pressure
Ppl	pleural pressure
PSP	patient's systolic pressure
PSVT	paroxysmal supraventricular [atrial] tachycardia
Ptm	transmural pressure
Pv	venous pressure
PVC	premature ventricular contraction
PVR	pulmonary vascular resistance
RPP	rate pressure product
RR	respiratory rate
RV	right ventricular
RVEDP	right ventricular end-diastolic pressure
SV	stroke volume
Svo_2	mixed venous hemoglobin saturation
SVR	systemic vascular resistance
SVT	supraventricular tachycardia
TTI	tension-time index
VT	ventricular tachycardia

Index

Note: Page numbers in *italics* indicate figures; those followed by (t) refer to tables.